GEROPSYCHOLOGICAL INTERVENTIONS IN LONG-TERM CARE

Lee Hyer, EdD, ABPP is a Professor of Psychiatry at the University of Medicine and Dentistry of New Jersey—Robert Wood Johnson Medical School. He is the director of a geriatric clinic at the University Behavioral Health Care of UMDNJ and directs geropsychology training at UMDNJ. He is the director of a geriatric team that includes geropsychiatry fellows, geropsychology fellows, psychology interns, and graduate students at Rutgers' Graduate School of Applied and Professional Psychology and the Department of Psychology. Clinical work involves nursing homes, assisted living facilities, and outpatient clinics, as well as primary care clinics. Current research includes neuropsychology profiles and memory retraining in dementia, cognitive behavioral therapy in LTC facilities, heart rate variability, and depression and anxiety disorder patterns in older adults. He is the author of over 180 articles and book chapters, and has written two other books. He is a Fellow in American Psychological Association (APA) and Gerontological Society of America (GSA) and has received awards from these organizations, as well as the VA and UMDNJ.

Robert C. Intrieri, PhD, is an Associate Professor in the Department of Psychology at Western Illinois University. He has conducted more than 30 research studies related to aging and the study of emotion, life satisfaction, and perceived stress among differing age groups and has prepared numerous presentations and publications based on this research. He currently holds over 20 peer-reviewed publications, book chapters, and monographs. In the summer of 2003, Intrieri was an invited participant in the American Psychological Association (APA) hometown radio news programs, designed to promote a greater public awareness of the field of psychology, including well-being and wellness issues and current research. He was elected as a Fellow in the Behavioral and Social Sciences (BSS) section of the Gerontological Society of America (GSA), the oldest and largest multidisciplinary scientific organization in the world devoted to the advancement of aging-related research. He was also elected to membership in Sigma Xi, The Scientific Research Society, and Phi Kappa Phi Honor Society. He has been recently elected as president of Division 12, Section 2 (Clinical Geropsychology) of APA.

GEROPSYCHOLOGICAL INTERVENTIONS IN LONG-TERM CARE

Lee Hyer, EdD, ABPP
Robert C. Intrieri, PhD
Editors

SPRINGER PUBLISHING COMPANY
New York

Springer Publishing Company, Inc.
11 West 42nd Street, 15th Floor
New York, NY 10036–8002

Acquisitions Editor: Helvi Gold
Production Editor: Print Matters, Inc.
Composition: Compset, Inc.
Cover design by Mimi Flow

06 07 08 09 10/5 4 3 2 1

Library of Congress Cataloging-in-Publication Data

Geropsychological interventions in long-term care/[edited by] Lee Hyer, Robert C. Intrieri.
p.; cm.
Includes bibliographical references and index.
ISBN 0-8261-3845-4 (hardcover)
1. Geriatric psychiatry. 2. Older people—Long-term care. 3. Older people—Mental health.
I. Hyer, Lee, 1944– II. Intrieri, Robert.
[DNLM: 1. Long-Term Care—psychology—Aged.
2. Dementia—therapy—Aged. 3. Homes for the Aged.
4. Psychotherapy—methods—Aged. WT 31 G3773 2006]
RC451.4.A5G495 2006
618.97'689—dc22

2005049530

Printed in the United States of America by Bang Printing.

We dedicate this book to our wives and grandparents. For Bob, Paige E. Goodwin, whose love, support, and encouraging words allowed him to persist during the entire process. Bob also dedicates this book to his grandparents Josephine Cywinski and Santo Giovanni Intrieri who first taught him about aging.

For Lee, Eileen Hyer, whose unshakable support and caring in life are matchless and who improves with age in body, spirit, and soulfulness. Lee also remembers his grandmother, Margaret Hyndsman, who made aging easy, fun, and important.

Contents

Part IV: Training

Part V: Interventions

Contributors

Erinn E. Beagin, MD
Assistant Professor of Medicine
UMDNJ–Robert Wood Johnson Medical School
New Brunswick, New Jersey

Cameron J. Camp, PhD
Director and Senior Research Scientist
Myers Research Institute
Beachwood, Ohio

Jiska Cohen-Mansfield, PhD
Professor, Department of Health Care Sciences
The George Washington University Medical Center
and Director
Research Institute on Aging
Hebrew Home of Greater Washington
Rockville, Maryland

Amy L. Collins, MA
PhD Candidate
Department of Psychology
Boston College
Chestnut Hill, Massachusetts

Michael Duffy, PhD, ABPP
Professor, Department of Educational Psychology
Texas A&M University
College Station, Texas

Melissa Gartenberg, PsyM
Doctoral Candidate
Rutgers, The State University of New Jersey
Graduate School of Applied and Professional Psychology
Piscataway, New Jersey

Paige E. Goodwin, PhD
Associate Professor, Department of Psychology
Western Illinois University
Macomb, Illinois

Shannon L. Gould, PhD
Postdoctoral Fellow
Long Island Jewish Medical Center
New Hyde Park, New York

John Heath, MDAGSF
Co-Director, Geriatric Medicine Fellowship Program
UMDNJ–Robert Wood Johnson Medical School
New Brunswick, New Jersey

Angela K. Hochhalter, PhD
Postdoctoral Fellow and Project Manager, Division of Gerontology and Geriatric Medicine
University of Alabama at Birmingham
Birmingham, Alabama

Bradley Karlin
PhD Candidate,
Psychology Department
Texas A&M University
College Station, Texas
and Psychology Intern
Department of Psychology
VA Palo Alto Health Care
System
Palo Alto, California

Frederick J. Kier, PhD
Staff Psychologist/Team Leader,
Dementia Special Care Unit
VA Pittsburgh Healthcare
System and Clinical Assistant
Professor of Psychiatry
Department of Psychiatry
University of Pittsburgh
Medical Center
Pittsburgh, Pennsylvania

Debra Liles, BA
Research Coordinator
Houston Center for Quality of
Care and Utilization Studies
Baylor College of Medicine
Department of Surgery
Michael E. DeBakey VA
Medical Center
Houston, Texas

Victor Molinari, PhD, ABPP
Professor, Department of Aging
and Mental Health
Louis de la Parte Florida Mental
Health Institute
University of South Florida
Tampa, Florida

Aleksandra Parpura-Gill, MD, PhD
Project Director
Research Institute on Aging
Rockville, Maryland

David Powers, PhD
Associate Professor
Department of Psychology
Loyola College of Maryland
Baltimore, Maryland

William E. Reichman, MD
Professor of Psychiatry and
Neurology
Robert Wood Johnson Medical
School
Senior Associate Dean for
Clinical Affairs
New Brunswick, New Jersey

Erlene Rosowsky, PsyD
Assistant Clinical Professor of
Psychology
Department of Psychiatry
Department of Psychiatry
Harvard Medical School
Beth Israel Deaconess Medical
Center and Needham
Psychotherapy Associates
Needham, Massachusetts

Shailaja Shah, MD
Clinical Assistant Professor,
UBHC North Building
UMDNJ-UBHC
Piscataway, New Jersey

Joyce Simard, MSW
Geriatric Consultant and
Alzheimer's Specialist
Land O' Lakes, Florida

Michael A. Smyer, PhD
Professor of Psychology and
Dean of the Graduate School
of A&S
Associate Vice-President for
Research
Boston College
Chestnut Hill, Massachusetts

A. Lynn Snow, PhD
Houston Center for Quality
of Care and Utilization Studies
Veterans Affairs Medical Center
Houston, Texas
and Psychiatry and Behavioral
Sciences Departments
Baylor College of Medicine
Houston, Texas

Alan B. Stevens, PhD
Associate Professor of Medicine
and Director of Dementia Care
Research Program
Division of Gerontology and
Geriatric Medicine
University of Alabama at
Birmingham
Birmingham, Alabama

Ladislav Volicer, MD, PhD
Professor, School of Aging Studies
College of Arts and Sciences
University of South Florida
Tampa, Florida

Preface

> You cannot depend on your eyes when your imagination is out of focus.
>
> *Mark Twain*

We are in a remarkable time; 40 years ago, the only anxiety disorders that were considered untreatable were obsessive-compulsive disorder and panic disorder. Things have changed and we had to endure that time, that science, and that conclusion to reach this point. We offer a book that is also captured somewhere in time, one that will certainly change more rapidly than this example, because studies in long-term care (LTC) are now more informative and more evident.

Across the past decade, the typical LTC resident has become frailer, as well as more physically, cognitively, and psychologically vulnerable. Many believe this phenomenon is largely due to a change in the system. Specifically, they highlight the emergence of the Prospective Payment System (PPS) for Medicare hospital expenses. At the time of its inception in 1984, the goal of PPS was to reduce health care costs. Examining its success in achieving this goal, Estes et al. (1993) analyzed the impact of PPS on community-based LTC systems. Their results suggest that PPS leads older adults to return to the community from acute-care settings or to posthospital rehabilitation in LTC facilities "quicker and sicker" than ever before (Estes et al., 1993). Fischer and Eustis (1989) argue that not only does PPS influence the margins of hospital care but it also influences the interactions between acute and LTC facilities. More importantly, Fischer and Eustis (1989) state that PPS has altered the nature of family care. Families are expected to provide care services for increasingly longer periods, often until the family system can no longer sustain the caregiving burden.

The impact of this social policy has been gradual and harmful, especially in relation to the LTC resident's ability to maintain autonomy and dignity within the LTC system. The typical resident suffers from a dizzying array of complicated medical, cognitive, and psychological issues that are agonizingly slow to unravel. For the practice of mental health in

LTC especially, we believe that we are in a borderland between the day-to-day, in-your-face practice in these facilities and empirically supported treatments. Perhaps clinical practice is still too disparate and primitive as a science to be ready to establish best practice guidelines, but we, in this book, argue that we have an improved direction and validated technologies to practice alongside medicine. We offer a book then that examines extant practices, supports or challenges these, and points the way for better care.

We are aware of something else, the complexity of LTC resident him or herself. In the past 5 years, the typical resident in nursing homes has become older and more physically fragile. In fact, there remains much variability in nursing homes. On the one side, 25% of all deaths occur in nursing homes. On the other side, we can assess and treat problems with greater ease and better outcomes. In the middle, we are able to define stability and change among residents and to provide an outlook that allows us to handle these "complex systems," striking a balance between the need for order and the respect for inevitable decline. We are grasping the difference between help and ineluctable loss better, and the creative management of both. In the science fiction novel, *The Lost World,* Michael Crichton commented:

> Complex systems tend to locate themselves at a place we call "the edge of chaos." We imagine the edge of chaos as a place where there is enough innovation to keep a living system vibrant, and enough stability to keep it from collapsing into anarchy. (Crichton, 1996, p. 4)

At present, we have much to go on. Theories of the behavior of residents in LTC now exist and explain the relationship between the aging individual and behavior in these settings. The work of Lawton and Baltes especially has explicated the complexity of this social system and the compensation required of the resident, and provided a guidepost for dialog. These and other theorists address the whole person in a "complete" environment and request us to push the limits of our technology to have a better vision and offer better care. We attempt to accomplish this in the book.

Now more than ever, there is progress and energy in LTC settings. We believe that we have captured this here. We have assembled a group of health care professionals who are dedicated to the care and research of these residents. This group pushes the treatment envelope and opines for the improved use of professional input, time, and effort. Interventions range from the organizational to the personal; psychosocial to the medical; and the theoretical to the practical. This group recognizes that, in our modern information economy, a far higher level of knowledge, education, and skill is required for LTC treatment than in the past. They realize too that this effort demands a much higher level of commitment of human concern and scientific rigor.

To turn a phrase used by Art Linkletter, "long-term care is not for sissies." Working in LTC requires commitment, guile, patience, and knowledge of what works and what does not. To that end, the goal of this book is to provide insight into the psychosocial issues confronting older LTC residents as well as information regarding strategies that are most effective based on the evidence to date. *Who should read this book?* We believe this book provides valuable resource information for physicians and geriatricians who care for older adults in the LTC system and may want to supplement medical treatments with effective psychosocial interventions. Further, we think this book will provide valued and needed information for registered nurses, geriatric nurse specialists, social workers, activity coordinators, as well as physical, occupational, and speech therapists that operate within the LTC setting who are seeking ways to explain behavior and empower the residents that they care for. Finally, psychologists and psychiatrists whose practice focuses on older adults will gain valuable information about the process of working with people in the LTC environment will hopefully further facilitate their effectiveness within the LTC setting. *Who will take care of Mom and Dad when they can no longer take care of themselves?* We hope that it will be someone who understands that maintaining autonomy, respect, and dignity through the end of life is critically important.

We (Lee and Bob) also have our own energies and beliefs. This book was begun under the quixotic skies of hope and change, against the noxious fumes of LTC practice everywhere. No one is at fault. As in health care everywhere, we are strapped to the mast, knowing what can be done and most often helpless to alter practice. As health care providers, we practice in LTC facilities in this country with a rigid, record-based technology that often leaves the resident alone and misunderstood. We know that there is a better way. We believe that this book allows us to look in a clearer way into the cosmos and entrails of LTC facilities, at what we are doing, at bringing awareness to what we are doing, and at explicating our choices and responsibilities. As you peruse the table of contents, and as you complete the book, we hope you agree that you also are more skilled and challenged.

> Most of all we believe in and like what we are doing. We can make a difference. "Blessed is he who has found his work. Let him seek no other blessedness."
>
> *Thomas Carlyle*

REFERENCES

Crichton, M. (1996). *The lost world*. New York: Balantine Books.

Estes, C. L., Swan, J. H., Bergthold, L. A., Binney, E. A., Carrell, D. S., Casper, M. J., et al. (1993). *The long term care crisis: Elders trapped in the no-care zone*. Newbury Park, CA: Sage Publications.

Fischer, L. R., & Eustis, N. N. (1989). Quicker and sicker: How changes in Medicare affect the elderly and their families. *Journal of Geriatric Psychiatry*, 22(2), 163–191.

Introduction

To add spin on a phrase, it takes a village to adequately understand and maximize the quality of life in residents placed in long-term care (LTC) facilities. The natural events of a failing health, general debility, a social milieu that fosters inactivity and lack of control, and an intervention focus on the medical model conspire to prevent adults in LTC to thrive or even adjust marginally. Changing the quality and zeitgeist of care in such a setting requires much effort and some theory. In fact, there are many theories and much speculation on the causative agents involved. Barton, Baltes, and Orzech (1980), for example, proposed specific mechanisms that whereby institutions foster excess disability and a "dependency script." Brandtstadter and Renner (1990) too indicated that a central task of coping for living well is flexible goal adjustment, meaning the view of seeing a positive aspect, or meaning in the failing to achieve one's goals or lower one's level of aspiration.

Applying the one model of care in such settings, Baltes and Baltes (1990) hold that compensation efforts, such as acquiring substitute means to maintain one's level of functioning, indeed do provide a way out, a way to improve quality of life. This is the SOC (selection, optimization, and compensation) model. It takes the global view that every stage of development individuals seek to master life through the application and orchestration of three components—selection, optimization, and compensation. In the action-oriented formulation of SOC (Freund & Baltes, 1998), the focus is on proactive and agentic strategies of life management. It is thereby adaptive to set clear goals, acquire and invest means into the purpose of these goals, and do so persistently even in the face of setbacks and losses.

Perhaps ingenuously, we take the global view that at all stages of development individuals seek to master life through assimilation/accommodation. In LTC this can be seen through the lens of three components—selection, optimization, and compensation. Sometimes this involves an action-oriented formulation of SOC (Baltes & Freund, 2003) where the focus is on agentic, self-regulated strategies of life management; at other times, the focus is elsewhere, on the environment.

In this book, we address the challenge of LTC—how to allow residents to thrive in an environment at the end of life, one with one exit. We have divided the book into five sections; *Overview, Basic Care, "There Is Still a Person in There," Training, and Interventions.*

Overview: We start the book (Chapter 1) with an overview on aging, with a special focus on the lifespan perspective as it assists in an understanding of the "care" in LTC. Behaviors are viewed as the result of the assimilation/accommodation of the whole person and the social environment. We highlight the SOC model in a fluid but closed system, the nursing home. Our concern is the decline progresses, the person usually accommodating by a downward adjustment. How we can undo this is our challenge.

In Chapter 2, a perspective on the care is given by Collins and Smyer. They focus on the ecology in the environment that sets the stage for LTC. Older people are entering nursing homes later, and sicker, than ever before. An understanding of the ecology of LTC allows for a grounding to facilitate optimal aging. The authors initiate the discussion by providing a perspective on the background and modifiable variables that lead to a person to LTC. The authors then examine LTC from an ecological perspective and illuminate the interactions among multiple levels, including the disabled individual and his or her physical and social environment. Their discussion of a hierarchical model of functional assessment implies that level of functioning requires physical, psychological, and social skills. Disabled individuals must manage losses and promote gains based on their individual profiles for risk. Individual characteristics like age, gender, race, marital status, education, and health influence level of risk for disability and the ability to manage disability once it occurs. Finally, the authors discuss Medicaid as an example of a successful program that empowers disabled individuals to choose care based on their changing personal needs.

Basic Care: In the section on medical care, Heath, Gartenberg, and Beagin (Chapter 3) discuss how the family practice physician responds to medical issues in a "nursing home." The import of this chapter is psychosocial care of a human being with multiple medical problems. Importantly, the authors discuss how does the physician overcome the shackles of the medical model in a "nursing" home. Reviews of medical and psychosocial issues related to LTC from a medical perspective set the table for a typology of LTC—actively dying, actively rehabbing, and surviving. The authors finish with typical medical diagnoses and red flag issues, as well as a discussion of the usual models for mental health delivery as inadequate.

In Chapter 4, Shah and Reichman discuss effective psychiatric evaluation and the importance of the contributions of biological, psychological, and social factors to the expression of mental illness. When these are carefully considered, affected residents experience a heightened sense of personal well-being, engagement in the environment, competence, and purpose. The authors provide the reader with a geropsychiatric view that allows for a melding of medical and psychosocial in order to best allow the integrative benefits for residents in LTC. Practical suggestions from medication limits to care interventions are addressed.

In the last chapter of this section (Chapter 5), Duffy and Karlin review the treatment methods for depression in older adults, emphasizing several methods (including exercise), both those that are common to therapy and those that devolve from behaviors. They "push the envelope" to examine a taxonomy of psychological dynamic patterns that exist "within" the depressive symptom profile. Depression at the symptom level then is a "final common pathway" for many distinct dynamic patterns. They discuss depression through the prism of a growth, adaptability, and change model of behavior, the SOC concerns. These authors seek an estimate of the person's available unused psychological and physical capacity to optimize change.

"*There Is Still a Person in There*": In this new section, constructs in LTC related to SOC are considered. These include personality, self-identity, and emotion, as well as the need for ethical deliberation and care in dementia. Molinari, Kier, and Rosowsky (Chapter 6) highlight the importance of personality in LTC. They examine personality and its relationship to the SOC model. Using both research and clinical examples they evaluate how the SOC model meshes with personality factors in the LTC environment, as well as consider the practical implications of the model for enhancing the quality of life of LTC residents.

Next, Parpura-Gill and Cohen-Mansfield (Chapter 7) argue for the pesistence of self in older adults, even in LTC. They discuss the provision of activities in LTC facilities is planned without significant attention to their effects on individuals with dementia. Group activities are then based on "general templates for a range of cognitive abilities, while activities for one-on-one interactions are mostly based on trial and error." In effect, these positions fail to recognize the sense of self. Knowledge of such persons and their roles has practical value for the design of interventions.

Goodwin and Intrieri (Chapter 8) address the important issue of passion in life, emotion. After clearing terminological confusion, they see emotion as referring to the individual's biologically based multidimensional response to a stimulus, leading to changes in physiological functioning, behavior, and subjective experience. Interestingly, this model does not negatively impact on age. The authors find few changes in functioning. In fact, older adults are most capable of intense emotions, despite some decline. Emotion regulation, for example, is suggested as the mechanism through which individuals achieve their emotional goals, specifically, the maximizing of positive affect and/or the minimizing of negative affect. There appears to be an influence of age on emotion regulation, with older adults reporting greater effort to control the experience of emotion in their daily lives. Age differences in mood states then finds older adults enjoy a more positive mood profile with higher levels of positive emotion and lower levels of negative emotion.

In sum, Goodwin and Intrieri suggest that in late life the interaction between the individual and their environment is positive with an adaptive balance between security and autonomy. This can be done modifying the social context to achieve a desired affective state. Importantly, the authors suggest that older adults are adaptive: as personal resources decline, the individual may select a reorganization of emotional goals, emphasizing the construction of a personal environment that limits exposure to negative affective experiences. The nursing home is after all a reservoir of debility and unmet needs.

In the last chapter of this section, Volicer and Simard (Chapter 9) outline the necessity of the SOC model in advanced dementia. The selection of care is based on the knowledge of the burden and benefit of different treatment strategies, and on previous wishes of the individual with dementia or his/her best interest. The ethical mandate to make advanced care plans as early as possible allows for the best care plans to prevent or minimize behavioral symptoms of dementia. This care should be optimized according to the remaining functional abilities of the individual with dementia. The intricate plan of how to prevent an escalation of negative behavior (resistiveness) is discussed. Compensation allows for both habilitation strategies to maintain remaining functions for as long as possible, and executive function interventions to allow for reasonable activity and meaningful activities to occur. The author notes that by paying attention to the SOC model, it is possible to improve dementia care and maintain quality of life throughout the course of the disease.

Training: Staff training is required in LTC facilities and is often offered as an avenue for improving the care and quality of life of nursing home residents. Unfortunately this has not always been the case. The general goal of such interventions is to provide staff with the knowledge and skill to identify and address the unmet needs of residents, particularly residents with dementia.

Gould and Stevens discuss two models that maximize the possibility of staff input, embedded care, and overall satisfaction. Gould and Hyer (Chapter 10) apply an organizational model that specifies steps in the application and process of bottom-up training. They discuss in detail the guiding conception of the individual and organizational competencies of behavior management.

In a similar way, Stevens and Hochhalter (Chapter 11) articulate a general model of staff development called Informed Teams. This model considers the unmet needs of residents and staff. The authors conclude by discussing a project to increase staff member use of care skills that are known to reduce need-driven behaviors, as well as to increase communication about the most effective care strategies for individual residents across shifts and levels of the nursing staff, and to continue this process.

Interventions: In the last section, we have two chapters on care; two methods that, we believe, can make a difference in LTC. First, Snow and colleagues (Chapter 12) discuss the most applied psychotherapy technique in LTC, cognitive-behavioral therapy (CBT). They make a case for its use with persons with dementia for a variety of theory-based and evidence-based reasons. CBT is after all based on the principles of learning and their accommodation to cognitive disability. CBT allows the therapist to flexibily address the range of presenting problems common in dementia, from those that are more common in persons with mild dementia to those that tend to only affect persons with severe dementia.

In the last chapter (Chapter 13), Camp focuses on Montessori-Based Dementia Programming™, a method applied with severely dementing residents. Camp discusses the mechanisms responsible for effects produced by the intervention; in effect, the characteristics of successful activities programming for dementia. The authors discuss the inevitable disconnection between an individual's environment as making demands and the capacity of the person to accommodate these. When environmental press and competence are not in balance, negative affect and maladaptive behavior result. They argue for the Montessori-Based Dementia Programming™ in LTC environments. This program has been implemented at several nursing facilities with success. Interestingly, at the end Camp discusses seven rules for dissemination of innovations within the context of health care delivery systems.

CONCLUSIONS

Increasingly, we can see that the face of LTC is both complex and changing. Nursing homes are now typically filled with residents who are either very impaired or in for a short stay (subacute stays). As such, the health care professional is targeting people who have very different problems. Making glib statements about "residents" is very risky. In fact, it can easily be argued that residents in assisted living facilities also could be considered as targets for the chapters in this book. We are aware then that some chapters will apply to various settings in more or less apt ways, depending on the facility.

We seek to make things better. Psychological well-being is often the goal and it is elusive. This is so because it is hard to define. There is also much heterogeneity at late life, even in LTC. Well-being clearly is a superordinate construct that involves the reaction of a resident to his/her situation. It exists on a continuum. Internal variables that detract from positive well-being include a reduced ability to alter goals, little self-acceptance for who one is and what one has done, inadequate self-protective psychological processes (unable to see perspective or to make favorable comparisons), poor assimilation/accommodation, a lack of emotional regulation, and little capacity for wisdom (Blazer, 2005). Add to this, economic distress, physical diseases, functional impairment, and little social support can make life problematic indeed.

As we shall see, mental health problems are pervasive. They are also added to a sea of physical dilemmas. In fact, if truth is told, mental health is the new kid on the block. Cardiology, for example, has clear mechanisms of pathophysiology and has evolved interventions to address these; psychiatry has the DSM, a symptom-based mechanism for care that is both inappropriate and primitive, especially for LTC needs. A resident who has mild dementia and depression, for example, is one who is both mentally and physically ill. The brain of this resident is different from another resident who has dementia but no depression. Additionally, this depressed resident may have little insight into the state and, for reasons of neurological insult or personological fixity or both, may have "depression without sadness" or depression executive dysfunction (DED) syndrome. This resident may or may not have social support, may or may not like the facility, may or may not be able to negotiate their environment with friendly helpful staff, may or may not. . . . Our mission here is to know as much as we can about such states, appreciate the complexity, and pursue change. To date, we are using a technology that is not sophisticated or in many cases not even helpful.

Swimming against the tide, this book then challenges the reader with the idea of the treatment-refractory resident. All are. We really have "treatment-refractory treatments" and ideas for care. This is truly a challenge. Change almost certainly will not involve cure, but will address the removal of those elements in the care process that interfere with survival-oriented interventions. The reading of *Clinical Applied Gerontological Interventions in Long-Term Care* hopefully will prove worthwhile in better understanding of this condition.

REFERENCES

Baltes, P. B., & Baltes, M. M. (1990). Psychological perspectives on successful aging: The model of selective optimization with compensation. In P. B. Baltes, & M. M. Baltes (Eds.), *Successful aging: Perspective from the behavioral sciences* (pp. 1–34). Cambridge, England: University Press.

Baltes, P. B., & Freund, A. M. (2003). Human strengths as the orchestration of wisdom and selective optimization with compensation. In L. G. Aspinwall, & U. M. Staudinger (Eds.), *A psychology of human strengths* (pp. 23–36). Washington, DC: American Psychological Association.

Barton, E., Baltes, M., & Orzech, M. (1980). Etiology of dependence in older nursing home residents during morning care: The role of staff behavior. *Journal of Personality and Social Psychology,* 38(3), 423–431.

Blazer, D. (2005). Successful aging: A psychological perspective. Paper presented at AAGP, SanDiego, CA.

Brandtstadter, J., & Renner, G. (1990). Tenacious goal pursuit and flexible goal adjustment: Explication and age-related analysis of assimilative and accommodative strategies of coping. *Psychology and Aging*, 4, 58–67.

Freund, A. M., & Baltes, P. B. (1998). Selection, optimization, and compensation as strategies of life management: Correlations with subjective indicators of successful aging. *Psychology and Aging*, 13(4), 531–543.

PART I

Overview

CHAPTER ONE

Perspective on Long-Term Care

Necessary and Unnecessary Practices

Lee A. Hyer and Robert C. Intrieri

The over-65 population of the United States is projected to reach 70 million in 2030. At that time, one in five Americans will be 65 years or older (Older Americans 2004, 2004). Although data indicate rates of chronic disease have not declined, improvements in health care allow for less disability and better quality of life (QOL). The gap between the total life span and healthy life span has narrowed considerably, with the result that people are living longer and enjoying it more.

Despite these facts, the course of aging still tends to be characterized by decline. Heart disease, stroke, and cancer account for 60% of deaths among those 65 and older. Further, over 40% of older people can expect to spend some time in an LTC facility (Hyer & Ragan, 2002). Currently, about 2 million adults are admitted to 17,000 United States nursing homes annually (Rhoades & Krauss, 1999). In a recently published study, Porock et al. (2005) found that 24% of all US deaths occur in nursing homes.

Given the increasing presence of nursing homes in our society, greater attention is being focused on the needs and problems of older people in LTC facilities. Older LTC residents have varied and intense problems and have traditionally received support that under-represented or over-represented those problems. Increasingly, the focus of researchers as well as practitioners is how best to assist older adults so that they may thrive in LTC settings.

There is a stereotypical link between age, aging, disease, and decline. The presence of this stereotype is probably strongest for the LTC environment. But, how accurate is this association? In other words, is aging within an LTC setting truly one of universal decline? At the individual level, aging can be conceptualized as a series of "adjustments." For the most part, age-related diseases are accompanied by meaningful accommodation or the emergence of dysfunction. When stress and loss naturally unfold, a "learned dependence" results where the older person downwardly adjusts and settles for lower life satisfaction. Late in life, psychological and physical resources are increasingly devoted to the regulation and management of decline or loss. How the aging person makes decisions regarding the allocation of increasingly limited psychic and physical resources, as well as how developmental processes assist in this decision-making process, will be a central focus of aging research across the 21st century.

The focal point of this book is the application of clinical interventions in LTC. The "progenitor" of this work is Lawton's Environmental Press Model (Lawton, 1982; Lawton & Nahemow, 1973). From Lawton's perspective, as an individual's environment places demands that cannot be met (environmental press), the individual's (personal capacity) level of competence falters, and problems result. In effect, Lawton believes the well-being of older adults depends on their ability to adapt and modify the social and environmental context to re-establish some degree of equilibrium between their personal competence and environmental demands (Lawton, 1996).

A more recent addition to the field is Baltes' conceptualization of selection, optimization, and compensation (SOC; Baltes & Baltes, 1990). Baltes and colleagues have modified the traditional conceptualization of successful aging, particularly within the nursing home environment. The authors argue that any model which attempts to explain successful aging in LTC must view success as adaptive functioning irrespective of the environmental context (Baltes, Wahl, & Reichert, 1991). The challenge for the LTC resident is to minimize the impact of age-related losses by maximizing potential environmental gains. In an LTC setting, the resident seeks a best-fit interaction between self and environment, one that maximizes strengths while limiting weaknesses. Both Lawton and Baltes believe an adaptive balance between security and autonomy achieves this. In general, the goal of this book is to examine how each resident achieves this balance, as well as identification of the mediators and outcomes of this process. More specifically, this book seeks to encourage practitioners to rethink their beliefs regarding what constitutes successful aging and QOL within the LTC setting so that they may intervene in a more appropriate manner.

QUALITY OF LIFE IN LONG-TERM CARE

Actions in an LTC facility are never solo events that affect one person. They are dynamic and context-specific properties that speak to the concern and philosophy of individual development. In addition to the LTC setting itself, resident characteristics also influence QOL in the LTC environment.

Setting

Over the past few decades, a number of trends have characterized the long-term care environment. First, increased life expectancy has led to an increase in demand for nursing home care. Second, rising health care costs have led to staggering increases in the cost of nursing home care. Third, and perhaps most importantly, regulatory bodies have assumed increasing control over resident QOL. Measures to assess QOL in LTC are now abundant. The Centers for Medicare and Medicaid Services (CMS) contract provides constructs and measures for the evaluation of QOL (Kane, 2001) via quality assurance and regulatory processes as well as internal quality improvement efforts. Indicators of QOL can be found within facility-level structural and process factors that relate to the outcomes of interest, or through the aggregation of resident data, as is done with the minimum data set (MDS). The idea is that nursing homes have some degree of responsibility for QOL and do have the capacity to influence residents' lives for better or worse.

The criticism of attempting to improve QOL through increased regulation stems from the reality that outcomes such as meaningful activity, relationships, etc., are often strongly influenced by social factors outside the control of the home. Further, QOL is also influenced by the nursing home case mix, particularly the physical and mental health, functional and cognitive abilities, as well as sensory abilities, of residents. Although nursing homes can influence factors like pain, functional status, and social interaction, as well as general medical care, they may have difficulty influencing other factors, such as who will be admitted and when.

In the past 15 years, entire industries, as well as federal and state regulatory commissions, have emerged to monitor the application of what is perceived to be quality care (Colenda et al., 1999). To many, this is anything but caring or efficient. Under the direction of CMS, state mandates typically emphasize necessary basic care and prevention of poor care. The result has been the codification of a subtle but powerful stance that is regulation-based, with nursing homes increasingly conforming, antiseptic, and risk averse. "Quality management" often refers to the minimal requirements of state and federal agencies. More cynically, it can be argued the canons of care are profit or maintenance. Most often, the goal of care is to manage residents and appease staff. Penrod, Kane, and Kane (2000) caution that the state can be unforgiving, creating a risk-averse environment in which the desire for perfection is driving out the good, especially when innovations do not correspond to surveyors' criteria. In other words, interventions may be "resident limiting" and "system comforting." Erving Goffman's (1959, 1961) concept of the "total institution" seems to apply. Goffman defines the total institution as one that becomes "a place of residence and work in which a large number of individuals, who are cut off from the wider society for a relatively long time together, lead an enclosed, formally administered round of life."

Research clearly indicates that "usual care" in the nursing home does not seriously address mental health problems (e.g., Binstock & Spector, 1997; Borson, Reichman, Coyne, Rovner, & Sakauye, 2000). Even the thrust of care, once given, is askew. For example, psychological assessment evaluates weaknesses while providing little information regarding an individual's potential for optimal functioning (Camp, Koss, & Judge, 1999). More precisely, the typical psychiatric evaluation seeks to type dementia and evaluate the potential of psychopharmacologic intervention to address problem behaviors. This does not necessarily translate into good care.

Additionally, in a situation that is less than ideal, in LTC the nursing assistant (NA) or licensed practical nurse (LPN) typically provides day-to-day care. LPNs and NAs hold the majority (88%) of full-time positions in hospitals and well over half of all positions in geriatric long-term care (Brannon et al., 1988; Kasteler, Ford, White, & Carruth, 1979). NAs outnumber LPNs 4 to 1 and LPNs outnumber registered nurses (RNs) 3 to 2 (Kasteler et al., 1979). Additionally, turnover among NAs is high, costly to the institution, and has considerable effect on quality of care (Brannon et al., 1988; Kasteler et al., 1979; Waxman, Carner, & Berkenstock, 1984). Turnover rates have been found to be as high as 75% per year (Kasteler et al., 1979). As a group, NAs suffer from low morale, burnout, and stress (Baillon, Scothern, Neville, & Boyle, 1996; Karuza & Feather, 1989). A majority is disenchanted with the understaffing and overwork, along with organizational problems such as poor supervision and communication (Kasteler et al., 1979). In other words, although NAs are heavily involved in difficult patient care, they often feel isolated, ignored, and neglected. Training in this context is often pro forma and perfunctory. In fact, Cohen-Mansfield (2004) labeled most training in LTCs as "placebo," suggesting it is minimally effective and is only offered to satisfy state requirements.

Finally, nursing home administrators are rarely involved in resident care in active and compassionate ways. As system monitors, they look to the bottom line first. In an attempt to change this administrative tendency, motivational systems have targeted the skills of supervisory staff. Performance-based training (Snyder-Halpern & Buczkowski, 1990), competency-based training (del Bueno, Barker, & Christmyer, 1981), mastery learning (Pinkney-Atkinson, 1980), and total quality management (TQM) (Deming, 1986) are popular examples. For example, TQM emphasizes the inter-relatedness of individuals and systems that make up the care setting, as well as customer satisfaction. TQM emphasizes five caring factors: a written statement of philosophy, a structured problem-solving approach including measurement, use of employee teams for the analysis and improvement of processes, assessment of resident satisfaction, and empowerment of employees to identify and respond to quality improvement opportunities. Unfortunately, the system hierarchy within LTC (DONs, RNs, LPN, and NAs) often contradicts these objectives, with all going about their business as if there were no TQM (Burgio & Burgio, 1986; Burgio & Stevens, 1999).

Resident Characteristics

Clearly, characteristics of the LTC setting (e.g., staffing) influence resident well-being and development. As noted previously, characteristics of the resident exercise an independent influence on well-being and QOL within the nursing home. The phenomenology of the LTC facility has changed. In general, LTC residents are both sicker and declining more rapidly than in previous decades. Residents spend less time in the facility, are more ethnically diverse, more likely to be widowed, more likely to suffer from dementia, require more assistance with ADLs, and generally have more choices for care prior to entering the facility. Many have a chronic illness (about 10%), and will iterate through an LTC facility two or more times. The typical resident is more likely to be female (women outnumber men 3:1), more than 50% are cognitively impaired with an additional 19% experiencing a mood or anxiety disorder. The prevalence of mood and anxiety disorders remained relatively stable across approximately 10 years (17% in 1985; 19% in 1997). About 30% of all residents have visual problems despite the use of glasses while a little less than 10% are blind. About 25% of all residents have some difficulty hearing while approximately 5% are completely deaf. The mean number of ADL impairments rose from 3.8 (1985) to 4.4 (1997), although the typical resident's ability to use the phone and secure personal effects (IADLs) remained stable from 1985 to 1997. In sum, older adults' desire to remain in their community for as long as possible has led to a nursing home population that is more disabled than in previous decades (Sahyoun, Pratt, Lentzner, Dey, & Robinson, 2001).

Not surprisingly, resident physical and/or mental impairment has a significant effect on their ability to adjust successfully to life in the facility. Cognitive impairment sufficient to influence physical function affects more than 50% of LTC residents (McConnell, Pieper, Sloane, & Branch, 2002). In a longitudinal analysis, McConnell et al. examined the linear effects of cognitive impairment on admission and the trajectory of dependence in activities of daily living, adjusting for demographic status. Results showed that on average ADL dependence worsened 0.84 points per year. Among long-stay residents, cognitive status had a clinically significant effect on ADL dependence. Using depression as a marker, Hybels, Blazer, and Pieper (2001) applied the Center for Epidemiological Studies–Depression scale (CES-D) and found that subthreshold depression exists at high levels in LTC, especially among women and unmarried residents, and influences physical health, use of psychotropic medications, disability days, and social support.

In a prospective study examining nursing home admissions, Rovner, Steele, Shmuely, and Folstein (1996) noted that after 1 year 50% of residents did not participate in facility activities. In general, this appears to reflect the low social cognitive functioning of LTC residents. Specifically focusing on social cognitive ability, Washburn, Sands, and Walton (2003) assessed 40 residents with and without cognitive decline on 11 social cognition tasks across two occasions. The measure used in this study is unique in that it assesses a collection of cognitive abilities that enable people to make sense of their social world and interact with others. Not only did the measure predict social functioning in the LTC facility, but also residents who scored lower on this measure tended to have more problems. It may be that only with an understanding of the social cognitive abilities associated with cognitive functioning (e.g., affect recognition, social reasoning) a full understanding of social interaction in LTC can be achieved.

Examining the link between illness and social functioning, Binder et al. (2003) used a prospective design to follow residents treated for an acute illness. Of 781 residents, those who survived 30 days of nursing home-acquired lower respiratory tract infection developed new functional declines and were at risk for further decline across 90 days. Doraiswamy, Leon, Cummings, Marin, and Newmann (2002) examined the prevalence of comorbid medical illness in Alzheimer's disease at different severity levels among 679 outpatients. Across patients, 61% had three or more comorbid medical diseases. Medical comorbidity tended to increase with dementia severity and poorer cognitive status.

Problems both physical and mental appear to influence cognitive decline. One interesting study suggests the care equation of the logical lets-get-everyone-active stance may not be generally successful or appropriate. Carstensen, Fisher, and Malloy (1995) assessed social withdrawal and cognitive impairment in nursing homes. Given their belief that social withdrawal in residents reflects cognitive deficits that interfere with the ability to interact with others, they were surprised that social withdrawal was not contingent on intact cognitive functioning. In other words, cognitive deficits do not preclude social activity.

Other studies also indicate resident adjustment in LTC is complex. Residents tend to adjust in ways that reflect their setting, cognitive status, and personality (see Goodwin & Intrieri, 2005). What seems clear is that most residents can make input into their care and do so with some rationality. Feinberg and Whitlatch (2001) found that persons with MMSE scores between 13 and 26 are capable of consistently responding to questions about preferences, choices, and their own involvement in decisions about daily functioning, and can provide accurate demographic information. While it is true that as cognition declines (based upon MMSE scores) choices become more truncated, decisional capacity remains viable until late in the disease process.

The prevalence of disruptive behaviors in LTC is variable and high. Reports of pacing and wandering range from 3 to 59%, rates of noisy and disruptive behavior range from 10 to 30%, while the prevalence of aggressive behavior ranges from 8 to 91% (see Cohen-Mansfield, 2000). Rovner and Katz (1993) indicate that approximately 80–94% of residents have some dementia. Of these, about 40% have psychiatric symptoms that cause behavioral disturbances. Depressive symptoms among residents may be as high as 50% and are strongly associated with increased staff time and resident mortality. Finally, as many as 50% of residents spend more than 50% of their day in bed, especially in homes with low staff ratios (Levy-Storms, Schnelle, & Simmons, 2002).

MODELS OF CARE

Less a theory than a perspective, life-span psychology serves as a framework for a number of promising theses regarding the process of aging. For example, the maturity/specific challenge model of aging (Knight & Satre, 1999) highlights individual differences in the aging process. From this perspective, aging is viewed as a more mature time that brings sociocultural and personal circumstances that require considerable effort and resources to manage. Generally, it is argued that whatever the nature of cognitive deficits, especially regarding memory and fluid intelligence, the performance of older people is sufficient for most tasks including those related to therapy and normal adjustment (Knight & Satre, 1999). Further, older adults appear to utilize emotions in more integrated and complex ways (Carstensen & Turk-Charles, 1994) and can demonstrate intelligence that appears more wise and deliberative (Tornstam, 2000).

Within the context of LTC, theories of aging tend to morph into theories of competence—ecological (Lawton & Nahemow, 1973) and person–environment (Kahana & Kahana, 1982)—underscoring the significance of the match between the person and the environment. In other words, optimal functioning occurs when environmental demands are manageable. From this perspective, models of care within LTC emphasize the practical understanding of how problems emerge and how they can be addressed. In addition, models attempt to identify those factors influencing effective person/environment fit—sound, videos, light, touch, social interaction, to name the more assessed ones.

Medical Model

The most frequently used model in LTC is the medical model, which argues there is a pathogen that can be corrected or alleviated through medical intervention. Becker and Kaufman (1988) suggest the medical model is appealing for LTC because aging is primarily characterized as a physiological event. As such, "medical care" is seen as the appropriate response and is acted upon vigorously and doled out by "nurses" while custodial care is provided by NAs. Given the nature of LTC residents, this is certainly an appropriate response as almost all have multiple medical diagnoses (average number = 4) and are on multiple medications (average number = 6). From the perspective of the medical model, behavior problems are seen to reflect a chemical imbalance and are treated in a prescriptive manner. Highlighting this point, the percentage of residents on psychotropic medication has risen measurably in the last 5 years.

A medical response to psychiatric problems is increasingly the norm in LTC. Use of cholinesterase inhibitors (ChEIs) and selective serotonin reuptake inhibitors is clearly on the rise in LTC (Smyer, Shea, & Streit, 1994). A summary of these medications is given in the accompanying box (Hyer, Carpenter, Bishmann, & Wu, 2005).

- Safe to use, reduce, or stabilize the decline in cognition for 1 year, especially for mild/moderate dementia
- In few studies, ChEIs lead to improvement or delay deterioration in ADLs
- Moderately effective for total problems on behaviors
- Mild effects sustained in severely impaired patients
- Administer early, rather than late

- Equal efficacy but differ somewhat on type of outcome and range and type of dementia
- Efficacy among agents is largely equal as between comparisons cannot be reasonably made as methodology of studies differ.

Caution should be exercised before drawing firm conclusions based on this data. There are large differences in study parameters when placebo groups have been compared with ChEI groups. For example, the percentage of dropouts and adverse reactions is highly variable for both experimental and placebo groups. Often the placebo group exceeds the experimental group with greater than 4 points on standard measures (e.g., ADAS-Cog). It is noteworthy that the level of improvement on standard cognitive, adjustment, and behavioral measures is not translatable to day-to-day gains. An arguable "substantial improvement," a 7-point gain on the ADAS-Cog, occurs in about 20% of donepezil hydrochloride (e.g., Aricept) subjects, and only 3% of subjects when using the CIBIC (the clinical trials gold standard for adjustment over baseline). This occurs only at higher doses for one of the ChEIs (Reminyl [Galantamine]; Reisberg et al., 2003). In sum, findings on the reported data (of ChEIs) are "only suggestive" (Anand, Hartman, Sohn, Danyluk, & Graham, 2003).

Additionally, ChEIs do not appear to be effective for psychiatric symptoms of dementia. In a review of pharmacological treatment of neuropsychiatric symptoms of dementia, Sink, Holden, and Yaffe (2005) conclude that extant medications are not particularly effective for the management of neuropsychiatric symptoms of dementia. Two meta-analyses (Olin & Schneider, 2002; Trinh, Hoblyn, Mohanty, & Yaffe, 2003) and six additional RCTs (Courtney et al., 2004; Erkinjuntti et al., 2002; Holmes et al., 2004; McKeith et al., 2000; Tariot et al., 2001) of various ChEIs for the treatment of neuropsychiatric symptoms have been published. Five of the eight studies report statistically significant benefits for neuropsychiatric symptoms. However, the magnitude of the effect is small and of questionable significance (Sink et al., 2005). These findings also apply to memantine (Reisberg et al., 2003; Tariot et al., 2004), where results indicate nonclinically significant changes.

Problems related to medication are not unique to the cognitive enhancers. Prevalence rates for depression in the nursing home are high, especially in relation to affective symptoms, dysphoria, and mixed depression and anxiety. In outpatients, the SSRIs and SNRIs that address depression and anxiety generally have a 50–60% rate of remission on acute trials with placebo rates at 25–35% (Blazer, 2003). Currently, no RCT studies on depression in LTC residents exist. It should be emphasized that the nature of depression is different in LTC populations characterized by medical comorbidity, multiple medications, failure to thrive, and an inability to act or assert control. In fact, the use of the DSM in LTC as it applies to depression requires rethinking (Hyer, et al., 2005).

There are also issues concerning the use of major tranquilizers. According to the psychiatric model (Tariot, 1999), disturbed behaviors are modal and require a careful diagnosis prior to intervention, most frequently medication to calm the resident and alter brain pathology. Grossberg and Desai (2003) review the use of medicaments with dementia, suggesting they be considered for all psychiatric and cognitive problems. In a meta-analysis of 33 controlled studies of patients with dementia, Olin et al. (1996) identified a response rate of 59% for drug treatment and 41% for placebo. In another meta-analysis of 16 controlled studies, Lanctot, Bowles, Herrmann, Best, and Naranjo (2000) found these rates to be 64 and 38%, respectively. Discussing a consensus panel on treatment guidelines for dementia, Rabins (2000) states meta-analyses indicate neuroleptic medications are better than placebo by 19%. Sunderland (2000) notes that although neuroleptics are more beneficial than placebo, only 20% of patients derived significant benefit.

As noted in Rabins' (2000) summary of the consensus panel on treatment guidelines, current efficacy literature suggests psychotropic medications show only a weak effect. However, this group could not determine whether agents were effective for the treatment of hallucinations or delusions. Nonpharmacological agents, on the other hand, were considered nonefficacious. That said, the panel noted that combining data on a variety of treatments of noncognitive, behavioral, and psychiatric symptoms is important. Therefore, treatments like music therapy, pet therapy, and activity therapy may be modestly effective in specific contexts.

All agree that nonpharmacological interventions are the first line of defense—if only they worked. Mintzer et al. (1997) note that after a thorough review of the medicaments that subserve dementia, nonpharmacologic interventions constitute the basis for care of this disease. The issue is how to have a care plan that is clear, accepted, monitored, and consistently applied. Perhaps psychopharmacology has not fully appreciated the fact that their science is one of complexity, with variance found mostly in the individual and not in the compound. The real world of psychotropic drugs works against a pure deterministic science since not all brains are equal and brains of frail residents are already compromised. Nowhere is this more evident than in LTC.

Psychosocial Models

Perhaps the most appropriate model for the LTC setting is the biopsychosocial model, particularly person–environment interaction models. Kahana and Kahana (1982) warned that we must attend to individual differences or we may unintentionally increase the disparity between person and environment, causing further distress. Carp and Carp (1984) also emphasized that we must acknowledge the role the person plays in the dynamic interplay between individual and context so as not to encourage debility.

As noted above, the seminal understanding of the LTC resident comes from Powell Lawton. Lawton (1999) argued that assessment of residential settings of older adults must fulfill three standard functions: maintaining competence, providing stimulation, as well as offering a sense of security and support. Further, he suggested the goal of LTC should be to keep residents independent and autonomous in a comfortable environment. Therapeutic models should be designed that stabilize and build on the competencies of residents but are challenging enough that the potential for prolonged functioning exists. Parmelee and Lawton (1990) characterized this pivotal issue in terms of a need for balance in LTC, represented by the autonomy-security dialectic. Although both are essential for well-being, it is easier to stress security over autonomy in nursing homes.

More recently, several more general models have been developed to explain the cause of challenging behaviors in LTC settings (Cohen-Mansfield, 2001). The "unmet needs" model proposes that challenging behaviors occur when there is a deficit in the environment. This deficit may lead the resident to become bored, lonely, or deprived of sensory stimulation. As a result, the individual may behave in a challenging way in an attempt to fulfill unmet needs. Cohen-Mansfield (2001) further classified challenging behaviors into four broad categories: physically aggressive behaviors, physically nonaggressive behaviors, verbally aggressive behaviors, and verbally nonaggressive behaviors. Specific to dementia, behavioral symptoms stem from an unmet need or goal of the individual (Algase et al., 1996). Unmet needs have also been linked to several mental health correlates, not limited to depression and aggression. Finally, Talerico, Evans, and Strumpf (2002) suggest aggressive behavior among nursing home residents may be a symptom of inadequately treated depression. In fact, depression in Alzheimer's disease is often undertreated because its detection is difficult in this population.

A second psychosocial model reflects a behavioral or learning perspective in which reinforcement contingencies are seen as the best explanation for behavior (Teri & Gallagher-Thompson, 1991). Teri and colleagues have given us perhaps the one technique that has been evaluated and matches mainstream psychological skills; applied behavioral analysis. This method has merit when it is applied in a validating environment with a motivated staff (Teri et al., 2000). A variant involves the STAR method (Teri et al., 2003), an A-B-C (e.g., antecedent, behavior, & consequence) analysis of a situation and identification of conditions that merit change. As behavior is influenced by a specific antecedent and maintained by a specific consequence, trained staff can apply behavioral principles.

Another model that emphasizes environmental vulnerability/reduced stress threshold as the cause of challenging behaviors is Hall and Buckwalter's (1987) Progressively Lowered Stress Threshold (PLST) model in which people with dementia (as noted previously, rates of dementia among LTC residents is extremely high) become progressively more stressed during the day and more likely to engage in dysfunctional behavior in the evening. According to this model, individuals with cognitive impairment suffer from progressively lower stress thresholds (e.g., a continually decreasing ability to cope with stress). As environmental stress begins to exceed this threshold, individuals become agitated and exhibit challenging behaviors. A reduction in environmental stimulation (e.g., low lighting, quiet, predictable events) is recommended in conjunction with relaxation exercises.

Several authors have advocated for a holistic model. Kitwood (Kitwood, 1995; Kitwood & Benson, 1995) calls for a new culture of dementia care, replacing the medical model with a rehabilitation focus. He proposed a model (D = P + B + H + NI + SP) where D is dementia, P is personality, B is biography and personal history, H is physical health, NI is neurological impairment, and SP is social psychology. He notes, "In a general way the symptomatic presentation of dementia in any individual arises from a complex interaction between all five factors, while the progression of the illness depends primarily on the interplay between NI and SP, and this interplay . . . may properly be characterized as dialectical" (p. 274). This model accounts for a good deal of variance in dementia, complexity of dementia, some with rapid declines, some with slow trajectories, and some with unusual phenotypes of the disorder.

Volicer (Volicer & Hurley, 2003) also argues for an encompassing (holistic) model of dementia in which deviant responses of residents with dementia require assessment and qualification. Primary problems involve functional impairment, delusions, and mood disorders, which in turn lead to secondary problems (inability to initiate activity, ADL dependence, spatial disorientation, and anxiety). Peripheral symptoms, like agitation, vocalization, apathy, food refusal, and repetitive behaviors, develop as a consequence. Interventions should emphasize primary problems first, as these will alleviate secondary and peripheral problems. For example, agitation, a modal response of residents with dementia, should be limited to behaviors that occur outside of caregiving activity and that are not accounted for by other problems. Agitation then is an unpleasant state of excitement unrelated to known physical needs of the person. In contrast, opposition to care occurs when an individual with dementia obstructs caregiving efforts in active care. In effect, they oppose care as provided.

Several writers emphasize the use of continuing abilities. For example, Sifton (2000) suggests that interventions need to focus on how the caregiver can best assist the person with dementia by supporting and reinforcing habitual skills (like humor, emotional memory/emotional awareness, sociability, sensory appreciation, motor function, music responsiveness, and long-term memory). Camp and Stevens (1990) also advocate for the application of these areas, as in errorless learning and spaced retrieval. Others have proposed the introduction of environmental cues to assist in maintaining competence such as memory books (Bourgeois, 1991).

Interventions that emphasize specific and validating responses by the caregiver for the declining resident are plentiful. For example, Feil (1999) posited a method of treatment that maximizes validation. Persons with dementia are attempting to resolve earlier developmental issues in order to die in peace. Zgola (1999) notes the care provider–care recipient relationship is the centerpiece of the caregiving process. From this perspective, a positive environment cannot be cultured without an adequate relationship between the care provider and care recipient. Zgola believes that providing good-quality care to the care recipient is not only positive for the care recipient but also fulfilling for the care provider.

Finally, some consider rehabilitation an option for LTC residents (e.g., Camp, 2000). West, Welch, and Yassuda (2000) summarized the results of several studies on cognitive rehabilitation with older people. Generally, older adults can learn memory strategies (even complex techniques) and this training can lead to lasting memory improvements, although it tends to be task-specific with little or no transfer. In a much-cited meta-analysis of this area, Verhaeghen, Marcoen, and Goossens (1992) endorse training and its effects. This group noted that four factors enhance training: pretraining, group sessions, shorter sessions, and younger participants. They also note modest effect sizes due to training. Hyer and Rebok (2005) argue for a "mild" rehabilitation approach involving the care recipient–care provider dyad. Memory retraining is applied in a problem-solving paradigm where supports are introduced over time. Use of effective communication, validation of emotions, functional assistance, maintenance of social skills, acting to decrease confusion, and a constant effort to understand the person are also beneficial.

INTEGRATING MEDICAL AND PSYCHOSOCIAL CLINICAL INTERVENTIONS

Practicing within an LTC setting does not diminish our obligations as professionals. In relation to any particular resident, the clinical task is to establish and articulate a clear problem list or diagnosis, educate the resident and caregiver regarding prognosis and disease stage, discuss the resident's present state and treatment options, assemble a comprehensive treatment plan (medical, social, financial, legal), establish caregiver support, and confirm the presence of ongoing support across the course of illness. In clinical staff meetings, discussion usually centers on the medical problem, medication effects, presence or absence of cognitive impairment, presence or absence of mental syndrome as well as history and causes, and environment or change in environment.

The idea that any mental health professional can attend to, and oversee, all of the above clinical tasks may strike some as quixotic. Undoubtedly, the multidimensional nature of clinical practice within the LTC setting appears to increase the difficulty of effectively prescribing and monitoring the use of medications. Since OBRA, the established rule of thumb in LTC is that the first intervention should be nonpharmacological. Should psychotropic medications be necessary, they must be justified, monitored regularly, and tapered if possible. Unfortunately, very few health care practitioners really practice this "ideal" care strategy. The reality might be better described as "medicament thinking," in which staff input is biased in the direction of medication. Once a target behavior has been identified, medication is prescribed, and a medication watch ensues. Side effects are considered eventful as the medication is "working." If problems arise, the belief is that the wrong drug was chosen, the dosage was too high or too low, or the trial duration was inadequate. In other words, all attributions of change or lack of change is viewed as a product of the medication. This bias has the unfortunate consequence of shutting down or at least altering dialog about psychosocial intervention.

A second area of concern regarding clinical practice within LTC is the applicability of DSM (a standard in community settings). The DSM is not effective for modal diagnosis and is truly fuzzy in an LTC setting. Volicer and Hurley (2003) note that in LTC, the psychiatric model attempts to overcome shortcomings of the DSM by using a psychobehavioral metaphor that reflects or approximates diagnosis. In effect, a psychological space of clustered behaviors that are considered clinically related is created, similar to a drug-responsive system (Nelson, 1998). According to this perspective, signs and symptoms are identified, classified, and then matched to medications that have the potential to reduce and weaken symptom intensity and frequency. Again, this method of reasoning regarding medication choice is based on poor scientific reasoning and often nondeliberative team discussions.

Mental health professionals are often uninformed about the LTC milieu and associated practice rubrics. When dealing with frail elders, mental health treatment is strikingly different than with younger, reasonably healthy adult patients. The standards of mental health practice in LTC vary not only in the way care is provided and bills are generated, but also in the application of outcomes. One recommendation for improving clinical care within LTC is to provide practitioners with knowledge regarding psychobehavioral models as well as training on their content. The outcome should be a fuller discussion of treatment issues, as well as the use of psychosocial technologies for better care (Hyer & Ragan, 2002).

Strictly speaking, data regarding which interventions are most effective for which persons manifesting which behaviors do not exist. Despite the paucity of efficacy data, failure to provide mental health services is not an option as neuropsychiatric disturbances afflict almost all patients with dementia as well as many without. A "best practice" approach includes a perspective on what to expect and how to predict decline. Extrapolating from current outpatient mental health treatment efficacy data, it is our assumption that nursing home residents will benefit from a combined approach that includes both medication and psychosocial intervention. The key to management is meticulous assessment, conscientious case formulation, interdisciplinary team collaboration, and caring clinical experimentation with clinically informed technologies. At present, medical and nursing care can reasonably address limits in several areas of functioning, including pain, sensory problems, sleep problems, and limits on autonomy.

The following box outlines these concerns.

Practical Considerations for Meds

- Consider use of medication more to stabilize function than to improve cognition/mood.
- Consider meds as an adjunct to psychosocial treatments.
- Consider who is a robust responder, not the mean group effect (it is too modest).
- Do not "medicament think."
- Treatment occurs throughout the entire course of illness and reassessment is ongoing.
- Efficacy relies heavily on team's and caregiver's "clinical global impression."
- Danger: Advanced Management Medication treatment.

Practical Considerations of Psychosocial Therapy

- Integrate care and look for all causes and possible solutions.
- Assemble a team that addresses the person and not the symptom.
- Instruct team on value of meds and psychosocial input.

- Know psychosocial data, models, and behavioral techniques.
- Measure, measure, measure with psychological indices.
- Experiment with best combination of meds and psychosocial treatment.
- Work at multidisciplinary team.
- Consider limits of DSM.
- Know when not to treat.
- Appreciate end of life issues.

TRAINING AND QUALITY OF LIFE

Any discussion of the application of psychobehavioral models in LTC must include attention to the topics of training and QOL. In general, training programs emphasize simple assessment techniques, communication methods, and skills to intervene. Training is typically entrenched within clinical care. A number of scholars argue that training has become reified, taking on a life of its own. The United States Congress passed the Omnibus Budget Reconciliation Act of 1987 (OBRA 87), legislation that discouraged nursing homes from using pharmacological interventions for the management of challenging behaviors. Prior to this legislation, the use of pharmacological interventions, as well as physical restraints, was common. In 1990, the U.S. Health Care Financing Administration (1990) responded to OBRA 87 by recommending staff training and behavior management as first line interventions for challenging behaviors in nursing homes. This recommendation resulted from a growing awareness that a resident's behavior could be influenced by environmental factors (Burgio et al., 2001, 2002).

As noted previously, resident QOL is receiving increased attention. In general, QOL depends on the goodness of fit between a person's unique needs and the facility's ability to meet those needs. In other words, QOL is interactive. Post (2000) argues that caregivers condition the QOL of a dementia victim. If true, enhancing resident QOL cannot be accomplished without attention to the caretaker. Lawton (1991) and Kane et al. (2004) have specified taxonomies, as well as measures, for the construct of QOL. Lawton (1999) outlined six caveats in the measurement of QOL.

1. Documentation indicators of quality: If QOL is limited to what is measurable, then we are impoverished.
2. Incorrect citations have a cost: Surveyors must be trained in new concepts if QOL is to be represented in a broader fashion.

3. The absence of an obvious ultimate validity criterion: Typically, we are rating "hard stuff"—death rates, morbidity rate, etc. Many of the criteria for QOL are process criteria.
4. By whose perspective is QOL to be judged? If the emphases are on the consumer (the resident), there will be problems, as only a few will rate the condition; if only the environment is evaluated, we also miss something.
5. Representing both positive and negative QOL: Most surveys are centered on identifying the negative—deficits, risks. The opposite is the essence of QOL.
6. Does QOL vary by user group? Residents in LTCs are highly variable.

Clearly, QOL is a difficult issue to apply, measure, and optimize. A large body of research suggests that resident QOL is improved by the ability to control, and make autonomous decisions regarding, their environment. However, many residents have basic needs that require a level of assistance that limits autonomy and environmental control. Some research suggests that nursing home staff have an unwitting tendency to provide more help than necessary, leading to even greater declines in autonomy and control (Agich, 1993; Dowd, 1975). Faulk (1988) evaluated QOL using the Life Satisfaction Index with 124 residents in 40 board and care homes. Results demonstrated that once lower level needs were met life satisfaction was enhanced with the meeting of higher level needs. More importantly, if only minimum life satisfaction needs were met, there were no gains in life quality. Improvements in QOL occurred when social integration needs were developed. In summary, it appears that autonomy and control are highly valued by residents and if attained are likely to produce correspondingly high levels of life quality. At the same time, Baldwin (1993) noted that although most LTCs have interventions for the fostering of autonomy, they also have policies that restrict the implementation of these interventions, such as limits on staff time.

Finally, Lawton (1991) and Kane et al. (2004) found that state and federal regulation of nursing homes was associated with better QOL in a number of areas, including social integration, safety, and presence of supportive features. Licensure alone was found to be effective in ensuring that nursing homes provided care at or above state required minimum threshold levels. However, nursing home regulation had no effect on other variables believed to influence resident life quality, like staff training, staff knowledge in any number of areas, availability of licensed nurses, and cleanliness and attractiveness of homes.

The "Holy Grail" of long-term care is to provide a positive residential environment for a declining older adult—in other words, provide a setting that allows for positive QOL. Attempts to identify objective markers of quality care, as well as efforts to appreciate and understand what may be best for a person, are legion. Fortunately, there are increasing efforts to assess QOL beyond that mandated by formal state agencies. QOL as seen from the perspective of the resident (Logsdon, 2000) is being pursued more aggressively. Perhaps the models of intervention advocated in this book, especially SOC, can assist here.

THE POTENTIAL OF SOC FOR CLINICAL INTERVENTION IN LTC

The potential strength of SOC within an LTC setting is its ability to understand the interaction between the individuals and their environment by emphasizing the multiple ways that a context can shape behavior as well as outcomes. Specific to LTC, Baltes, Wahl, and Reichert (1991) argued that nursing homes function as an institutional proxy for SOC. SOC acknowledges that residents may not be physically equipped for extended old age in LTC, but that both the resident and the environment can make adjustments. Baltes and Freund (2003) suggest that a state of "permanent incompleteness" is inevitable as we seek personal change and growth. There are few fixed end states. Baltes and Freund (2003) indicate that the goal of human development is construction of competencies that allow the individual to navigate effectively a changing world. They argue the regulatory processes that are fundamental across the life span are SOC. These processes occur at various levels of analysis or integration ranging from the macrolevel (e.g., society) to the microlevel (e.g., cells). Utilization of these processes can assist in the facilitation of higher levels of functioning, even within LTC.

SOC (Baltes & Baltes, 1980, 1990) represents a holistic view of aging: Aging successfully is reflective of doing the best with what one has. The emphasis is on coping and a positive view of the inevitable consequences of aging (e.g., problems, disease, and loss). The use of SOC to respond adaptively to everyday demands and functional decline in later life is associated with better functioning. Undoubtedly, utilization of SOC requires the use of resources. The more resources an aging individual has, the better is their ability to engage in the use of SOC. Given frailty and ever-increasing morbidity and debility among LTC residents, the challenge is application.

SOC represents a belief in adaptive development. More specifically, SOC provides a framework for understanding processes of developmental regulation across the life span. In an LTC setting, *selection* in everyday life is defined as actively or passively reducing the number of activities, goals, or domains in order to focus on those areas that are most important in one's life. This is a "loss-based selection." *Optimization* is defined as enhancement of the means to refine one's resources in a selected domain. It refers to adaptive processes or strategies where indirect aging losses have occurred and where an actual amelioration or maximization of means can be found. Investing more time and effort in specific tasks or activities that provide meaning as opposed to those that are less salient is most reflective of optimization. Finally, *compensation* involves the use of new and alternative means to reach a goal or to maintain a desired state once a loss has occurred. Compensation emerges when there has been a loss. People may intensify or expand routines once a functional loss has resulted. Again, this occurs best when there are resources available.

Within the LTC setting, selection largely consists of loss-based problems and includes focusing on the most important goals, reconstructing a goal hierarchy, adaptation of standards, in addition to a search for new goals. Optimization involves distinct means-action—attentional focus, seizing the right moment, persistence, acquiring new skills, practice of skills, time allocation, and successfully modeling others. Compensation is the means used to counter a loss—substitute means, use external aids, use therapeutic intervention, acquire new skills and resources, increase effort and energy, increase time allocation, and activate unused skills (Freund & Baltes, 1998). Given the constraints and demands of LTC, implementation of SOC requires creativity.

There is an emerging body of supportive data in relation to SOC. For example, Lang, Rieckmann, and Baltes (2002) found that resource-rich people (e.g., those individuals with positive sensorimotor-cognitive functioning as well as social-personality resources) demonstrated the use of SOC more frequently in their everyday lives and were more likely to survive after 4 years, as compared to resource-poor people. Specifically, resource-rich people were more active in everyday life. It is not surprising that older people with greater resources were more resistant to aging compared to adults with fewer resources. More specific to frail elders in LTC facilities, Brandtstädter and Greve (1994) proposed that older adults use a combination of active, assimilative strategies and passive, accommodative strategies. This dual process model asserts that advancing age results in a shift away from active adjustment of life situations to meet personal preferences (assimilation) and a parallel shift to the accommodation or adjustment of personal preferences to fit situational constraints, making fewer psychological demands on the person's resources. Older adults who replace lost activities with less physically or psychically demanding activities may be viewed as successfully accommodating. If activity levels become unfeasible, accommodative strategies should allow for a change in focus to alternatives.

Using a longitudinal design, Duke, Leventhal, Brownlee, and Leventhal (2002) followed 250 community-dwelling older adults to examine activity loss and replacement due to an important illness episode. In line with the SOC metamodel, reductions in activity were predicted by physical factors. Individual resources like social support and optimism increased the likelihood of taking action to replace lost activities. Conversely, a belief in the need to conserve physical resources reduced the likelihood of replacing activities. Accordingly, older adults who replaced a lost activity experienced higher levels of positive effect 1-year after illness onset in contrast to those who did not replace activities. Physical incapacity was less important for activity replacement than were social factors that influenced the motivation to seek alternatives, like optimism and conservation.

Generally, older people, including those in an LTC setting, manage their own aging process. This self-regulated dependency is an integral part of successful aging (Baltes & Wahl, 1992). SOC proposes that dependency and/or other forms of passive and nonengaged behavior may be considered adaptive within the context of the nursing home. The older person experiencing some form of loss has several choices: (a) give up the activities hampered by functional loss; (b) compensate for them by searching for a means to maintain activities; or (c) become increasingly dependent in the weakened domains to free energy for other more personal areas. In this last strategy, the person recognizes the loss and delegates control to others as a form of proxy control. In effect, only the initial option causes problems.

In other words, SOC makes the intriguing suggestion that lowered performance and behavioral dependency can be adaptive. When effectively coordinated, the three processes (SOC) promote successful aging, even in the presence of losses and reduction of resources. Selection requires age-related losses be identified and compensated for with a wide array of environmental aids which assume a high priority. This often involves a convergence of environmental demands, individual motivations, skills, and biological capacities. Optimization is characterized by the maintenance of high levels of functioning in selected domains through practice and acquisition of new bodies of knowledge and technology. Compensation becomes important when life tasks require a capacity beyond that of current skills. At the risk of repetition, in an LTC facility, even dependency can be self-selected and an outcome of active selection and compensation.

Baltes and Baltes (1990) add one more term here, wisdom. They define human strength as wisdom or knowledge about fundamental pragmatics of life and the implementation of that knowledge through the life management strategies of SOC. The concept of human adaptation is contextually dynamic, because the function of the expression of a person is a function of context (and outcomes). Age, gender, ethnicity, social group, among many others, determine context. Baltes and Freund (2003) point out that the ensemble of multidisciplinary, contextual, and normative factors and perspectives that need consideration when delineating notions of adaptation are legion. This requires a theoretical orientation such as SOC. It is a wisdom-related knowledge that is acquired and translates into developmental-enhancing behavior directed at oneself as well as others. It is then the interplay between SOC and wisdom that determines adjustment.

ADJUSTMENT TO AGING IN LTC

Aging well, especially in LTC settings, requires a series of personal adjustment be made. Fortunately, as humans, we appear to be programmed for growth and change. Over 20 years ago, Block (Block & Block, 1980) noted that one personality dimension, ego-control or ego-resiliency, was moderately consistent across the life span. Research that is more recent indicates that personality, as a trait, is reasonably consistent (Costa & Widiger, 2002) even in the presence of individual differences (Vaillant, 1976). It now seems clear that even into old age, individuals continue to be open to new experiences. We change, but with consistency, and aging allows for unique challenges.

Aging is best characterized as a gradual and natural process, a period of life evaluation and increased freedom, but also a period associated with physical decline and concerns regarding health and loss (Keller, Leventhal, & Larson, 1989). Steverink, Westerhof, Bode, and Dittmann-Kohli (2001) found the aging experience is best represented by physical decline, social loss, and continued growth. Highlighting the importance of individual differences, subjective health, higher income, loneliness, and hope all influence these components. In a sense, aging is an empty variable, a multidimensional construct best accounted for by other factors, particularly those that influence the perception of change.

Philosophically, older people do best when they are self-organizing, proactive, self-reflecting and self-regulating, not just reactive to external events (Bandura, 1999). Usually interactionism involving the person, behavior, and environment is in effect. Perhaps the most parsimonious and realistic view about human actions is that the person is neither driven by traits nor automatically shaped by the environment: They are producers and consumers of their own behavior (Lerner, 1982; Lerner & Busch-Rossnagel, 1981). In addition, this change is not random: It is guided by a person(ality) system that mediates the relationship between types of situations and the cognitive/affective/behavior patterns of the person (Shoda & Mischel, 2000). Thus, there are predictable, characteristic patterns of "variation" in the person's behavior across contexts and age. Organisms self-organize and do so naturally, consistently, and holistically.

The transition to old age is accompanied by increased awareness of what one cannot do in the context of what one can do. This transition influences the type of goals selected in late life. Since the central task of later life is facing decline, one's possibilities adjust accordingly. The choice is probably most often a function of health, identity (personal characteristics), and attachment (social relationships and positive contacts). One example is the concept of possible selves (Markus & Herzog, 1991). Possible selves are defined as highly personal, hoped for and/or feared images that function to encourage the individual towards or away from action (Markus & Herzog, 1991). Using a group of older participants from the Berlin Aging Study (BASE), Smith and Freund (2002) examined the influence of specific hopes and fears regarding health maintenance on the view of possible selves. Their results indicate that possible selves are both stable and discontinuous into old age, suggesting "possible selves" are dynamic throughout the aging process. The importance of this is that as we age, our possible selves adjust to reflect a recreation of "past and anticipated future selves."

In LTC, the operative variables for positive adjustment center on the person and the context. While we have discussed SOC variables, several related constructs also make this point. For example, a sense of control has repeatedly been identified as an important factor in successful aging and emotional well-being. In general, by adulthood, and particularly later adulthood, perception of control has stabilized (Seeman & Lewis, 1995). As a global personality trait, high internal locus of control has been found to be related to greater life satisfaction, more positive self-concept, better ratings of health status, and greater participation in activities among the elderly (Eizenman, Nesselroade, Featherman, & Rowe, 1997; Rodin, Timko, & Harris, 1985). The few studies that have attempted to enhance and examine perceived personal control in residential care settings have found greater levels of choice and internal control are associated with better resident well-being, less reliance on facility services, and greater participation in community activities (Langer & Rodin, 1976; Timko & Moos, 1989).

In the LTC setting, the critical issue concerns enhancing control or at least maintaining the illusion of control. This may involve the use of secondary control strategies, a higher dependence on the environment, as well as accommodation to problems. Schulz and Heckhausen (1996) have suggested successful aging is linked to the development and maintenance of primary control throughout the life course via control-related processes that optimize selection and compensation functions. Primary control is directed outward and targets the external world while secondary control targets the self and attempts to achieve changes within the individual. Although both can involve cognition and action, primary control always involves action. With age, the ratio of gains to losses becomes less favorable and secondary control becomes more important. The person must manage trade-offs across domains and sequential life phases and recognize that resources are a key consideration, as they must be juggled to maintain balance.

However, the reality is that with age, primary control may decrease while secondary control may be more stable and malleable. Elderly individuals who continue to emphasize primary control may experience poorer adjustment to the aging process than those who shift paradigms and gradually increase their reliance on secondary control. When conceptualized in this way, poor adjustment (e.g., general distress, depression, anxiety) may reflect frustration associated with continued attempts to control aspects of one's life that are no longer within the person's control. Put another way, individuals may poorly adjust to changes associated with aging because they continue to place a high priority on controlling their environment, when their ability to control their environment has declined as a function of their life stage. Elderly individuals who accept the declining control that comes with age, and who focus on their ability to control internal states and behaviors, may demonstrate more successful adjustment to aging.

Altering of one's expectation of life in LTC can then be positive. This also applies to a realistically pessimistic perspective, found to be associated with better adaptation to negative life events among older adults, in contrast to typical findings with younger participants (Isaacowitz & Seligman, 2001). Schulz, Bookwala, Knapp, Scheier, and Williamson (1996) followed 238 cancer patients receiving palliative radiation treatment for 8 months. Controlling for site of cancer and level of symptomatology at baseline, the authors examined the independent effects on mortality of pessimism, optimism, and depression. Results indicated that endorsement of a pessimistic life orientation is a more important risk factor for mortality among middle-aged (ages 30–59) than it is among older individuals. For older individuals, endorsing pessimism may simply reflect a coping strategy that has become adaptive in the face of declining ability to control important life outcomes such as health.

CONCLUSIONS

As aging unfolds, the person must adjust to maintain a positive QOL. Evidence suggests this adjustment is not a singular event but continues over the lifetime. Evidence also suggests adjustment can be "for better or worse." The main path to aging adjustment or dysfunction is shaped by imbedded risk factors (behavioral, psychological, and biological factors) and mediated, we believe, by the regulatory processes of SOC. We believe the SOC metamodel is sufficiently cogent and specific to address problems of adjustment in LTC. These involve lifestyle and behavioral actions, as well as appropriate psychosocial attitudes and environmental changes. The burden is on the caregiving to optimize this.

As noted, age itself is best construed as an empty variable. It is not the passage of time alone but various biological and social events that occur with the passage of time that have relevance for change. Unfortunately, the negative consequence of the increased life span is an increased risk for LTC placement. Successful aging within the LTC context requires the individual continuously adjust choices in life via the regulatory mechanisms outlined by the SOC metamodel. Regardless of the model used, however, the many constructs noted above articulate the use of alternative resources and, we believe, a better state of being.

In many ways, this is what occurs in psychotherapy, the psychosocial methodology applied for change. In therapy, internal and external events influence and recreate conditions for positive or negative outcomes. Much of what goes on involves an attempt to shift people's focus to view themselves in their daily lives in different ways. All psychotherapy is an assault on truth. In this way change is a function of having people respond differently to new situations or in response to new contingencies. Optimism-generating, support-assisting, and control-enhancing interventions make a difference in the context of the person. In effect, successful outcomes are represented by altering goals and adjusting to the "new person" they have become. This is what can occur in LTC.

In sum, decline does occur. It has something to do with the disease and something to do with the person with the disease. Finding the "right" intervention and structure is not logically obvious. It is clinical, interactive, and demands a feedback loop of many parties. A resident in bed 18 hr/day, for example, can be gotten up and made to sit in the dayroom. That may be 50% of the battle. The real difficulty comes in the applied behavioral activation in the dayroom. This involves thinking, thoughts about who the person is and what the psychological constructs that can be "SOC-ed." It is here again that our models enter. We may never know the real outcome as defined by satisfaction of the person. Nevertheless, we must persist. The greatest challenge in LTC involves devising strategies for maximizing independent functioning. This should remain a priority for researchers, service care delivery professionals, and policymakers alike in the first decade of the new century (Ory, Yee, Tennstedt, & Schulz, 2000).

ACKNOWLEDGMENT

We thank Dr Paige E. Goodwin for her reading of the manuscript and instrumental editorial suggestions.

REFERENCES

Agich, G. (1993). *Autonomy and long-term care.* New York: Oxford University Press.

Algase, D. L., Beck, C., Kolanowski, A., Whall, A., Berent, S., Richards, K., & Beattie, E. (1996). Need-driven dementia-compromised behavior: An alternative view of disruptive behavior. *American Journal of Alzheimer's Disease, 11*(6), 10–19.

Anand, R., Hartman, R., Sohn, H., Danyluk, J., & Graham, S. M. (2003). Impact of study design and patient population on outcomes from cholinesterase inhibitor trials. *American Journal of Geriatric Psychiatry, 11*(2), 160–168.

Baillon, S., Scothern, G., Neville, P. G., & Boyle, A. (1996). Factors that contribute to stress in care staff in residential homes for the elderly. *International Journal of Geriatric Psychiatry, 1*(3), 219–226.

Baldwin, R. C. (1993). Long term care of elderly people. Dependency increasing in Manchester. *British Medical Journal, 306*(6888), 1338–1339.

Baltes, P. B., & Baltes, M. M. (1980). Plasticity and variability in psychological aging: Methodological and theoretical issues. In G. E. Gurski (Ed.), *Determining the effects of aging on the central nervous system* (pp. 41–66). Berlin: Schering.

Baltes, P. B., & Baltes, M. M. (1990). Psychological perspectives on successful aging: The model of selective optimization with compensation. In P. B. Baltes, & M. M. Baltes (Eds.), *Successful aging: Perspective from the behavioral sciences* (pp. 1–34). Cambridge, England: University Press.

Baltes, P. B., & Freund, A. M. (2003). Human strengths as the orchestration of wisdom and selective optimization with compensation. In L. G. Aspinwall, & U. M. Staudinger, (Eds.), *A psychology of human strengths: Fundamental questions and future directions for a positive psychology* (pp. 23–35). Washington, DC: American Psychological Association.

Baltes, M. M., & Wahl, H. (1992). The behavior system of dependency in the elderly: Interaction with the social environment. In M. G. Ory, R. P. Abeles, & P. D. Lipman (Eds.), *Aging, health, and behavior* (pp. 83–106). Thousand Oaks, CA: Sage Publications.

Baltes, M. M., Wahl, H., & Reichert, M. (1991). Successful aging in long-term care institutions. *Annual Review of Gerontology and Geriatrics, 11*, 311–337.

Bandura, A. (1999). Moral disengagement in the perpetration of inhumanities. *Personality & Social Psychology Review, 3*(3), 193–209.

Becker, G., & Kaufman, S. (1988). Old age, rehabilitation, and research: A review of the issues. *Gerontologist, 28*(4), 459–468.

Binder, E. F., Kruse, R. L., Sherman, A. K., Madsen, R., Zweig, S. C., D'Agostino, R., Mehr, D. R. (2003). Predictors of short-term functional decline in survivors of nursing home-acquired lower respiratory tract infection. *Journals of Gerontology, Series A: Biological Science & Medical Science, 58*(1), M60–M67.

Binstock, R. H., & Spector, W. D. (1997). Five priority areas for research on long-term care. *Health Services Research, 32*(5), 715–730.

Blazer, D. G. (2003). Depression in late life: Review and commentary. *The Journals of Gerontology Series A, Biological Sciences & Medical Sciences, 58*(3), 249–265.

Block, R. W., Block, S. A. (1980). Outreach education: A possible preventer of teenage pregnancy. *Adolescence, 15*(59), 657–660.

Borson, S., Reichman, W. E., Coyne, A. C., Rovner, B., & Sakauye, K. (2000). Effectiveness of nursing home staff as managers of disruptive behavior: Perceptions of nursing directors. *American Journal of Geriatric Psychiatry, 8*(3), 251–253.

Bourgeois, M. S. (1991). Communication treatment for adults with dementia. *Journal of Speech & Hearing Research, 34*(4), 831–844.

Brandtstädter, J., & Greve, W. (1994). Explaining the resilience of the aging self: Reply to Carstensen and Freund. *Developmental Review, 14*(1), 93–102.

Brannon, D., Smyer, M. A., Cohn, M. D., Borchardt, L., Landry, J. A., Jay, G. M., Garfein, A. J., Malonebeach, E., & Walls, C. (1988). A job diagnostic survey of nursing home caregivers: Implications for job redesign. *Gerontologist, 28*(2), 246–252.

Burgio, L. D., Allen-Burge, R., Roth, D. L., Bourgeois, M. S., Dijkstra, K., Gerstle, J., & Bankester, L. (2001). Come talk with me: Improving communication between nursing assistants and nursing home residents during care routines. *Gerontologist, 41*(4), 449–460.

Burgio, L. D., & Burgio, K. L. (1986). Behavioral gerontology: Application of behavioral methods to the problems of older adults. *Journal of Applied Behavior Analysis, 19*(4), 321–328.

Burgio, L. D., & Stevens, A. B. (1999). Behavioral interventions in the nursing home: Motivating staff to apply a therapeutic model of care. In R. Schulz, G. Maddox, & M. P. Lawton (Eds.), *Annual review of gerontology and geriatrics* (Vol. 18). New York: Springer Publishing.

Burgio, L. D., Stevens, A. S., Burgio, K. L., Roth, D. L., Paul, P., & Gerstile, J. (2002). Teaching and maintaining behavior management skills in the nursing home. *Gerontologist, 42*, 487–496.

Camp, C. J. (2000). Clinical research in long term care: What the future holds. In V. Molinari (Ed.), *Professional psychology in long term care: A comprehensive guide* (pp. 401–423). New York: Hatherleigh Press.

Camp, C. J., Koss, E., & Judge, K. S. (1999). Cognitive assessment in late-stage dementia. In P. A. Lichtenberg (Ed.), *Handbook of assessment in clinical gerontology* (pp. 442–467). New York: John Wiley & Sons.

Camp, C. J., & Stevens, A. B. (1990). Spaced-retrieval: A memory intervention for dementia of the Alzheimer's type. *Clinical Gerontologist, 10*(1), 58–61.

Carp, D. R., & Carp, H. J. (1984). Denial and other emotional responses to infertility. *Midwife Health Visit Community Nurse, 20*(8), 286–289.

Carstensen, L. L., Fisher, J. E., & Malloy, P. M. (1995). Cognitive and affective characteristics of socially withdrawn nursing home residents. *Journal of Clinical Geropsychology, 1*(3), 207–218.

Carstensen, L. L., & Turk-Charles, S. (1994). The salience of emotion across the adult life span. *Psychology & Aging, 9*(2), 259–264.

Cohen-Mansfield, J. (2000). Use of patient characteristics to determine non-pharmacologic interventions for behavioral and psychological symptoms of dementia. *International Psychogeriatrics, 12*(Supplement 1), 373–380.

Cohen-Mansfield, J. (2001). Nonpharmacologic interventions for inappropriate behaviors in dementia: A review, summary, and critique. *American Journal of Geriatric Psychiatry, 9*(4), 361–381.

Cohen-Mansfield, J. (2004). Agitation in elderly persons with dementia: Definition, etiology, and treatment. Grand Rounds Lecture Series of the UMDNJ Robert Wood Johnson Medical School in Piscataway, NJ.

Colenda, C. C., Streim, J., Greene, J. A., Meyers, N., Beckwith, E., & Rabins, P. (1999). The impact of OBRA 87 on psychiatric services in nursing homes: Joint testimony of The American Psychiatric Association and The American Association for Geriatric Psychiatry. *American Journal of Geriatric Psychiatry, 7*(1), 12–17.

Costa, P. T., & Widiger, T. A. (2002). *Personality disorders and the five-factor model of personality* (2nd ed.). Washington, DC: American Psychological Association.

Courtney, C., Farrell, D., Gray, R., Hills, R., Lynch, L., Sellwood, E., Edwards, S., Hardyman, W., Raftery, J., Crome, P., Lendon, C., Shaw, H., & Bentham, P. (2004). Long-term donepezil treatment in 565 patients with Alzheimer's disease (AD2000): Randomised double-blind trial. *Lancet, 363*(9427), 2105–2115.

del Bueno, D. J., Barker, F., & Christmyer, C. (1981). Implementing a competency-based orientation program. *Journal of Nursing Administration, 11*(2), 24–29.

Deming, W. E. (1986). *Out of crisis.* Cambridge, MA: MIT Press.

Doraiswamy, P. M., Leon, J., Cummings, J. L., Marin, D., & Newmann, P. J. (2002). Prevalence and impact of medical comorbidity in Alzheimer's disease. *Journals of Gerontology, Series A: Biological Science & Medical Science, 57A*(3), M173–M177.

Dowd, J. J. (1975). Aging as exchange: A preface to theory. *Journal of Gerontology, 30*(5), 584–594.

Duke, J., Leventhal, H., Brownlee, S., & Leventhal, E. A. (2002). Giving up and replacing activities in response to illness. *Journals of Gerontology, Series B: Psychological Sciences & Social Sciences, 57*(4), P367–P376.

Eizenman, D. R., Nesselroade, J. R., Featherman, D. L., & Rowe, J. W. (1997). Intraindividual variability in perceived control in an older sample: The MacArthur successful aging studies. *Psychology & Aging, 12*(3), 489–502.

Erkinjuntti, T., Kurz, A., Gauthier, S., Bullock, R., Lilienfeld, S., & Damaraju, C. V. (2002). Efficacy of galantamine in probable vascular dementia and Alzheimer's disease combined with cerebrovascular disease: A randomised trial. *Lancet, 359*(9314), 1283–1290.

Faulk, L. E. (1988). Quality of life factors in board and care homes for the elderly: A hierarchical model. *Adult Foster Care Journal, 2*(2), 100–117.

Feil, N. (1999). Current concepts and techniques in validation therapy. In M. Duffy (Ed.), *Handbook of counseling and psychotherapy with older adults* (pp. 590–613). New York: John Wiley & Sons.

Feinberg, L. F., & Whitlatch, C. J. (2001). Are persons with cognitive impairment able to sate consistent choices? *Gerontologist, 41*(3), 374–382.

Freund, A. M., & Baltes, P. B. (1998). Selection, optimization, and compensation as strategies of life management: Correlations with subjective indicators of successful aging. *Psychology & Aging, 13*(4), 531–543.

Goffman, E. (1959). The moral career of the mental patient. *Psychiatry: Journal for the Study of Interpersonal Processes, 22*, 123–142.

Goffman, E. (1961). *Asylums; essays on the social situation of mental patients and other inmates.* Chicago: Aldine Publishing.

Goodwin, P. E., & Intrieri, R. C. (2005). The influence of changing emotional goals on the psychological well-being of nursing home residents. In L. A. Hyer, & R. C. Intrieri (Eds.), Geropsychological interventions in long-term care. New York: Springer Publishing.

Grossberg, G. T., & Desai, A. K. (2003). Management of Alzheimer's Disease. *Journals of Gerontology: Series A: Biological Sciences & Medical Sciences, 58*(4), M331–M353.

Hall, G. R., & Buckwalter, K. C. (1987). Progressively lowered stress threshold: A conceptual model for care of adults with Alzheimer's disease. *Archives of Psychiatric Nursing, 1*(6), 399–406.

Holmes, C., Wilkinson, D., Dean, C., Vethanayagam, S., Olivieri, S., Langley, A., Pandita-Gunawardena, N. D., Hogg, F., Clare, C., & Damms, J. (2004). The efficacy of donepezil in the treatment of neuropsychiatric symptoms in Alzheimer disease. *Neurology, 63*(2), 214–219.

Hybels, C. F., Blazer, D. G., & Pieper, C. F. (2001). Toward a threshold for subthreshold depression: An analysis of correlates of depression by severity of symptoms using data from an elderly community sample. *Gerontologist, 41*(3), 357–365.

Hyer, L., Carpenter, B., Bishmann, D., & Wu, H. (2005). Assessment and treatment of depression in long term care. *Clinical Psychology: Science and Practice, 12*(3).

Hyer, L., & Rebok, G. (2005) Memory retraining as add-on to ChEIs.

Hyer, L. A., & Ragan, A. M. (2002). Training in long-term care facilities: Critical issues. *Clinical Gerontologist, 25*(3–4), 197–237.

Isaacowitz, D. M., & Seligman, M. E. P. (2001). Is pessimism a risk factor for depressive mood among community-dwelling older adults? *Behaviour Research & Therapy, 39*(3), 255–272.

Kahana, B., & Kahana, E. (1982). Clinical issues of middle age and later life. *Annals of the American Academy of Political and Social Science, 464*, 140–161.

Kane, R. A. (2001). Long-term care and a good quality of life: Bringing them closer together. *Gerontologist, 41*(3), 293–304.

Kane, R. L., Bershadsky, B., Kane, R. A., Degenholtz, H. H., Liu, J., Giles, K., Kling, K. C. (2004). Using resident reports of quality of life to distinguish among nursing homes. *Gerontologist, 44*(5), 624–632.

Karuza, J., Jr., & Feather, J. (1989). Staff dynamics. In P. R. Katz, & E. Calkins (Eds.), *Principles and practice of nursing home care* (pp. 82–90). New York: Springer.

Kasteler, J. M., Ford, M. H., White, M. A., & Carruth, M. L. (1979). Personnel turnover: A major problem for nursing homes. *Nursing Homes, 28*(1), 20–25.

Keller, M. L., Leventhal, E. A., & Larson, B. (1989). Aging: The lived experience. *International Journal of Aging & Human Development, 29*(1), 67–82.

Kitwood, T. (1995). Exploring the ethics of dementia research: A response to Berghmans and Ter Meulen: A psychosocial perspective. *International Journal of Geriatric Psychiatry, 10*(8), 655–657.

Kitwood, T., & Benson, S. (1995). *The new culture of dementia care.* London: Hawker Publications.

Knight, B. G., & Satre, D. D. (1999). Cognitive behavioral psychotherapy with older adults. *Clinical Psychology: Science & Practice, 6*(2), 188–203.

Lanctot, K. L., Bowles, S. K., Herrmann, N., Best, T. S., & Naranjo, C. A. (2000). Drugs mimicking dementia: Dementia symptoms associated with psychotropic drugs in institutionalised cognitively impaired patients. *CNS Drugs, 14*(5), 381–390.

Lang, F. R., Rieckmann, N., & Baltes, M. M. (2002). Adapting to aging losses: Do resources facilitate strategies of selection, compensation, and optimization in everyday functioning? *Journals of Gerontology, Series B: Psychological Sciences & Social Sciences, 57B*(6), P501–P509.

Langer, E. J., & Rodin, J. (1976). The effects of choice and enhanced personal responsibility for the aged: A field experiment in an institutional setting. *Journal of Personality & Social Psychology, 34*(2), 191–198.

Lawton, M. P. (1982). Competence, environmental press, and the adaptation of older people. In M. P. Lawton, P. G. Windley, & T. O. Byerts (Eds.), *Aging and the environment: Theoretical approaches.* New York: Springer Publishing.

Lawton, M. P. (1991). Planning and designing housing environments for older adults. *Experimental Aging Research, 17*(2), 82–83.

Lawton, M. P. (1996). Quality of life and affect in later life. In C. Magai, & S. H. McFadden (Eds.), *Handbook of emotion, adult development, and aging* (pp. 327–348). San Diego, CA: Academic Press.

Lawton, M. P. (1999). Measuring quality of life in nursing homes: The search continues. Invited address, divisions 34, 5, & 20, Annual Meeting of the American Psychological Association, Boston, MA.

Lawton, M. P., & Nahemow, L. (1973). Ecology and the aging process. In C. Eisdorfer, & M. P. Lawton (Eds.), *The psychology of adult development and aging* (pp. 619–674). Washington, DC: American Psychological Association.

Lerner, R. M. (1982). Children and adolescents as producers of their own development. *Developmental Review, 2*(4), 342.

Lerner, R. M., & Busch-Rossnagel, N. A. E. (Eds.). (1981). *Individuals as producers of their development: A life-span perspective.* New York: Academic Press.

Levy-Storms, L., Schnelle, J. F., & Simmons, S. F. (2002). A comparison of methods to assess nursing home residents' unmet needs. *Gerontologist, 42*(4), 454–461.

Logsdon, R. G. (2000). Enhancing quality of life in long term care. In V. Molinari (Ed.), *Professional psychology in long term care: A comprehensive guide* (pp. 133–159). New York: Hatherleigh Press.

Markus, H. R., & Herzog, A. R. (1991). The role of the self-concept in aging. *Annual Review of Gerontology and Geriatrics, 11*, 110–143.

McConnell, E. S., Pieper, C. F., Sloane, R. J., & Branch, L. G. (2002). Effects of cognitive performance on change in physical function in long-stay nursing home residents. *Journals of Gerontology, Series A: Biological Sciences & Medical Sciences, 57*(12), M778–M784.

McKeith, I., Del Ser, T., Spano, P., Emre, M., Wesnes, K., Anand, R., Cicin-Sain, A., Ferrara, R., & Spiegel, R. (2000). Efficacy of rivastigmine in dementia with Lewy bodies: A randomised, double-blind, placebo-controlled international study. *Lancet, 356*(9247), 2031–2036.

Mintzer, J. E., Colenda, C., Waid, L. R., Lewis, L., Meeks, A., Stuckey, M., Bachman, D. L., Saladin, M., & Sampson, R. R. (1997). Effectiveness of a continuum of care using brief and partial hospitalization for agitated dementia patients. *Psychiatric Services, 48*(11), 1435–1439.

Nelson, J. C. E. (1998). *Geriatric psychopharmacology*. New York: Marcel Dekker.

Older Americans 2004. (2004). Key indicators of well being. Federal Interagency Forum on Aging Related Statistics. Washington, D.C.: U.S. Government Printing Office.

Olin, J., & Schneider, L. (2002). Galantamine for Alzheimer's disease. *Cochrane Database of Systematicr Reviews, CD001747.*

Olin, J. T., Schneider, L. S., Doody, R. S., Clark, C. M., Ferris, S., Morris, J., Reisberg, B., & Schmitt F. A. (1996). Clinical evaluation of global change in Alzheimer's disease: Identifying consensus. *Journal of Geriatric Psychiatry & Neurology, 9*(4), 176–180.

Omnibus Budget Reconciliation Act (OBRA 87). (1987). P.L. 100–203. Subtitle C. The Nursing Home Reform Act. 42 U.S.C. 1395i-3(a)–(h)(Medicare); 1396r (a)–(h) (Medicaid).

Ory, M. G., Yee, J. L., Tennstedt, S. L., Schulz, R. (2000). The extent and impact of dementia care: Unique challenges experienced by family caregivers. In R. Schulz (Ed.), *Handbook on dementia caregiving: Evidence-based interventions for family caregivers* (pp. 1–32). New York: Springer Publishing.

Parmelee, P. A., & Lawton, M. P. (1990). The design of special environments for the aged. In J. E. Birren, & K. W. Schaie (Eds.), *Handbook of the psychology of aging* (3rd ed., pp. 464–488). San Diego, CA: Academic Press.

Penrod, J. D., Kane, R. A., & Kane, R. L. (2000). Effects of posthospital informal care on nursing home discharge. *Research on Aging, 22*(1), 66–82.

Pinkney-Atkinson, V. J. (1980). Mastery learning model for an inservice nurse training program for the care of hypertensive patients. *Journal of Continuing Education in Nursing, 11*(2), 27–31.

Porock, D., Oliver, D. P., Zweig, S., Rantz, M., Mehr, D., Madsen, R., Petroski, G. (2005). Predicting death in the nursing home: Development and validation of the 6-month minimum data set mortality risk index. *Journals of Gerontology, Series A: Biological Sciences & Medical Sciences, 60*(4), 491–498.

Post, S. G. (2000). Key issues in the ethics of dementia care. *Neurologic Clinics, 18*(4), 1011–1022.

Rabins, P. V. (2000). *Neuropsychiatry and Mental Health Services, The American Psychiatric Press Textbook of Neuropsychiatry* (3rd ed.). *American Journal of Psychiatry, 157*(3), 474.

Reisberg, B., Doody, R., Stöffler, A., Schmitt, F., Ferris, S., & Möbius, H. J. (2003). Memantine in moderate-to-severe Alzheimer's disease. *New England Journal of Medicine, 348*(14), 1333–1341.

Rhoades, J. A., & Krauss, N. A. (1999). *Nursing home trends, 1987 and 1996 MEPS Chartbook No. 3.* (AHCPR Pub. No. 99-0032). Rockville, MD: Agency for Health Care Policy and Research.

Rodin, J., Timko, C., & Harris, S. (1985). The construct of control: Biological and psychosocial correlates. *Annual Review of Gerontology & Geriatrics, 5*, 3–55.

Rovner, B. W., & Katz, I. R. (1993). Psychiatric disorders in the nursing home: A selective review of studies related to clinical care. *International Journal of Geriatric Psychiatry, 8*(1), 75–87.

Rovner, B. W., Steele, C. D., Shmuely, Y., & Folstein, M. F. (1996). A randomized trial of dementia care in nursing homes. *Journal of the American Geriatrics Society, 44*(1), 7–13.

Sahyoun, N. R., Pratt, L. A., Lentzner, H., Dey, A., & Robinson, K. N. (2001). The changing profile of nursing home residents: 1985–1997. *Aging Trends, 4*, 1–8.

Schulz, R., Bookwala, J., Knapp, J. E., Scheier, M., & Williamson, G. M. (1996). Pessimism, age, and cancer mortality. *Psychology & Aging, 11*(2), 304–309.

Schulz, R., & Heckhausen, J. (1996). A life span model of successful aging. *American Psychologist, 51*(7), 702–714.

Seeman, M., & Lewis, S. (1995). Powerlessness, health and mortality: A longitudinal study of older men and mature women. *Social Science & Medicine, 41*(4), 517–525.

Shoda, Y., & Mischel, W. (2000). Reconciling contextualism with the core assumptions of personality psychology. *European Journal of Personality, 14*(5, Special Issue), 407–428.

Sifton, C. B. (2000). Searching for Home. *Alzheimer's Care Quarterly, 1*(1), 81–85.

Sink, K. M., Holden, K. F., & Yaffe, K. (2005). Pharmacological treatment of neuropsychiatric symptoms of dementia: A review of the evidence. *JAMA: Journal of the American Medical Association, 293*(5), 596–608.

Smith, J., & Freund, A. M. (2002). The dynamics of possible selves in old age. *Journals of Gerontology, Series B: Psychological Sciences & Social Sciences, 57B*(6), P492–P500.

Smyer, M. A., Shea, D. G., & Streit, A. (1994). The provision and use of mental health services in nursing homes: Results from the National Medical Expenditure Survey. *American Journal of Public Health, 84*(2), 284–287.

Snyder-Halpern, R., & Buczkowski, E. (1990). Performance-based staff development. A baseline for clinical competence. *Journal of Nursing Staff Development: JNSD, 6*(1), 7–11, 24.

Steverink, N., Westerhof, G. J., Bode, C., & Dittmann-Kohli, F. (2001). The personal experience of aging, individual resources, and subjective well-being. *Journals of Gerontology, Series B: Psychological Sciences & Social Sciences, 56B*(6), P364–P373.

Sunderland, T. (2000). Cholinergic contributions to behavioral disturbances in Alzheimer's disease. *International Psychogeriatrics, 12*(Supplement 1), 231.

Talerico, K. A., Evans, L. K., & Strumpf, N. E. (2002). Mental health correlates of aggression in nursing home residents with dementia. *Gerontologist, 42*(2), 169–177.

Tariot, P. N. (1999). The older patient: The ongoing challenge of efficacy and tolerability. *Journal of Clinical Psychiatry, 60*(Supplement 23), 29–33.

Tariot, P. N., Cummings, J. L., Katz, I. R., Mintzer, J., Perdomo, C. A., Schwam, E. M., Whalen, E. (2001). A randomized, double-blind, placebo-controlled study of the efficacy and safety of donepezil in patients with Alzheimer's disease in the nursing home setting. *Journal of the American Geriatrics Society, 49*(12), 1590–1599.

Tariot, P. N., Farlow, M. R., Grossberg, G. T., Graham, S. M., McDonald, S., & Gergel, I. (2004). Memantine treatment in patients with moderate to severe Alzheimer disease already receiving donepezil: A randomized controlled trial. *JAMA: Journal of the American Medical Association, 291*(3), 317–324.

Teri, L., & Gallagher-Thompson, D. (1991). Cognitive-behavioral interventions for treatment of depression in Alzheimer's patients. *Gerontologist, 31*(3), 413–416.

Teri, L., Gibbons, L. E., McCurry, S. M., Logsdon, R. G., Buchner, D. M., Barlow, W. E., Kukull, W. A., LaCroix, A. Z., McCormick, W., & Larson, E. B. (2003). Exercise plus behavioral management in patients with Alzheimer disease: A randomized controlled trial. *JAMA: Journal of the American Medical Association, 290*(15), 2015–2022.

Teri, L., Logsdon, R. G., Peskind, E., Raskind, M., Weiner, M. F., Tractenberg, R. E., Foster, N. L., Schneider, L. S., Sano, M., Whitehouse, P., Tariot, P., Mellow, A. M., Auchus, A. P., Grundman, M., Thomas, R. G., Schafer, K., & Thal, L. J. (2000). Treatment of agitation in AD: A randomized, placebo-controlled clinical trial. *Neurology, 55*(9), 1271–1278.

Timko, C., & Moos, R. H. (1989). Choice, control, and adaptation among elderly residents of sheltered care settings. *Journal of Applied Social Psychology, 19*(8, Pt 1), 636–655.

Tornstam, L. (2000). Transcendence in later life. *Generations, 23*(4), 10–14.

Trinh, N. H., Hoblyn, J., Mohanty, S., & Yaffe, K. (2003). Efficacy of cholinesterase inhibitors in the treatment of neuropsychiatric symptoms and functional impairment in Alzheimer disease: A meta-analysis. *JAMA: Journal of the American Medical Association, 289*(2), 210–216.

U.S. Health Care Financing Administration. (1990). *Report to Congress: Prior and concurrent authorization for home health and skilled nursing facility services.* (HCFA Publication No. 03310) Baltimore, MD: U.S. Dept. of Health and Human Services, Health Care Financing Administration.

Vaillant, G. E. (1976). Natural history of male psychological health: V. The relation of choice of ego mechanisms of defense to adult adjustment. *Archives of General Psychiatry, 33*(5), 535–545.

Verhaeghen, P., Marcoen, A., & Goossens, L. (1992). Improving memory performance in the aged through mnemonic training: A meta-analytic study. *Psychology & Aging, 7*(2), 242–251.

Volicer, L., & Hurley, A. C. (2003). Management of behavioral symptoms in progressive degenerative dementias. *Journals of Gerontology, Series A: Biological Sciences & Medical Sciences, 58A*(9), 837–845.

Washburn, A. M., Sands, L. P., & Walton, P. J. (2003). Assessment of social cognition in frail older adults in its association with social functioning in the nursing home. *Gerontologist, 43*(2), 203–212.

Waxman, H. M., Carner, E. A., & Berkenstock, G. (1984). Job turnover and job satisfaction among nursing home aides. *Gerontologist, 24*(5), 503–509.

West, R. L., Welch, D. C., & Yassuda, M. S. (2000). Innovative approaches to memory training for older adults. In R. D. Hill, L. Backman, & A. S. Neely (Eds.), *Cognitive rehabilitation in old age* (pp. 81–105). Oxford, UK: Oxford University Press.

Zgola, J. M. (1999). *Care that works: A relationship approach to persons with dementia*. Baltimore, MD: Johns Hopkins University Press.

CHAPTER TWO

Evolving Trends in Long-Term Care

The Ecology of Selective Optimization with Compensation

Amy L. Collins and Michael A. Smyer

> Grace Wall . . . has always been independent. But at 83, with a host of health problems that include congestive heart failure, two hip replacements, loss of sight in one eye, and lung cancer, that independence is harder to maintain.
>
> For six years, Mrs. Wall took care of her paralyzed husband before he died in 1991. Now she lives alone in a mobile home. She gets her health care through Medicaid, as well as various personal assistance services, such as help with shopping and housekeeping—things that she has difficulty doing on her own now. (Mahoney, 2003, p.10).

Ms. Wall's situation reflects the dilemma of long-term care in an aging society like the United States. In this chapter, we will provide a framework for thinking about long-term care and will place recent information about changing trends in long-term care within this framework. We focus on the ecology of selective optimization with compensation on an individual, family, community, and policy level.

The recent emphasis on successful aging (Rowe & Kahn, 1998) has renewed attention paid to health promotion and individual risk for long-term care, but it has been criticized for its one dimensional portrayal of disability prevention (Minkler & Fadem, 2002). Its focus on the individual's responsibility to manage health neglects the broader forces that add complexity to an individual's risk profile.

A broader ecological approach calls attention to not only individual aspects, but also the immediate physical environment, including the community and sociopolitical environments in which individuals operate, and the interactions among these levels (Bronfenbrenner, 1979; Bronfenbrenner & Evans, 2000). An ecological approach to disability and long-term care stresses the interaction of person and environment (Lewin, 1935) and the conditions necessary for optimal aging. Although it is true that life style and environmental factors heighten the risk of disability and the need for long-term care in later life, the interdependent nature of individual lives and physical environment cannot be overlooked (Minkler & Fadem, 2002).

In this chapter, we will give an overview of the ecology of disability and long-term care. First, we describe the hierarchical nature of disability and the resulting need for long-term care. Second, we introduce some of the person-level correlates of disability and individual risk for long-term care. Third, we examine the physical environments, including home and community factors that both aid and hinder the ability of disabled elderly to optimize aging. Finally, we discuss some of the larger social structures that enable an aging individual to optimize his or her environment, including government programs like Medicaid and funding for community programs for older adults.

The ecological approach removes the full burden of responsibility of successful aging from the individual while illuminating the tools that individuals and their social structures can use to manage and optimize opportunities for successful aging. This model is consistent with the Baltes and Baltes' (1990) vision of optimal aging as a process of managing losses and promoting gains using selection and optimization with compensation.

The primary source for the disability data reported in this chapter is the American Association for Retired Persons recent report *Beyond 50 2003: A report to the nation on independent living and disability* (American Association for Retired Persons, 2003). The authors conducted or commissioned original data analysis using several nationally representative surveys including surveys conducted by the Agency for Healthcare Research and Quality (AHRQ) (Spector, Fleishman, & Pezzin, 2000), the American Association for Retired Persons Public Policy Institute (American Association for Retired Persons, 2003), the 1984, 1989, 1994, and 1999 National Long-Term Care Surveys (NLTCS) (National Long-term Care Study, 1984–1999), and the 1997 and 1998 Medical Expenditure Survey (MEPS) (Medical Expenditure Survey, 1997, 1998). Although disability and long-term care is relevant to persons of all ages, the data reported in this chapter focuses on age subgroups ranging from 50 years of age and older. Only statistically significant findings are reported.

THE HIERARCHICAL NATURE OF DISABILITY AND LONG-TERM CARE

Disability is difficult to define, and in some cases there are large differences in the way it is measured. An easier point of consensus is functional ability, or what people are capable of doing in their daily lives. The term function encompasses a set of capabilities that are necessary for an individual to survive in the community (Kemp & Mitchell, 1992). This construct is most simply measured as an individual's capacity in terms of activities of daily living (ADLs) (Katz, Ford, Moskowitz, Jackson, & Jaffe, 1963) and instrumental activities of daily living (IADLs) (Lawton & Brody, 1969). ADLs usually include basic personal necessities like eating, dressing, grooming, mobility, toileting, and bathing. IADLs refer to daily activities that allow one to maintain his or her independence, like managing financial affairs, household maintenance, communication, health maintenance, transportation, and personal safety. Patterns of loss in these function categories vary by underlying disorder. For example, people with chronic arthritis will have difficulty with all IADLs and ADLs involving mobility. Individuals with dementia will generally lose IADLs before ADLs, because IADLs require more cognitive skill, whereas individuals suffering from severe depression may lose both ADLs and IADLs simultaneously (Kemp & Mitchell, 1992).

A hierarchical model of disability introduced by Kemp and Mitchell (1992) examines the various determinants of functional ability. A hierarchical model of functional assessment acknowledges that each level of functioning requires certain physical, psychological, and social skills. ADLs and IADLs are assessed as proxy for underlying abilities (see Figure 2.1). The most basic ADLs and IADLs can only be accomplished if the individual is healthy at the most basic levels of functioning, which involves the integrity of the organ system and physical substrates. Physical substrates include endurance, range of motion, strength, and coordination (Kemp & Mitchell, 1992). Similarly, skilled performance in cognitive and motor activities requires competence in previous levels of functioning (Kemp & Mitchell, 1992). For example, driving is a high-level skill that can be accomplished only if an individual has the capacity for lower levels of functioning, like motor strength, endurance, and coordination (see "Elders behind the wheel," 2003).

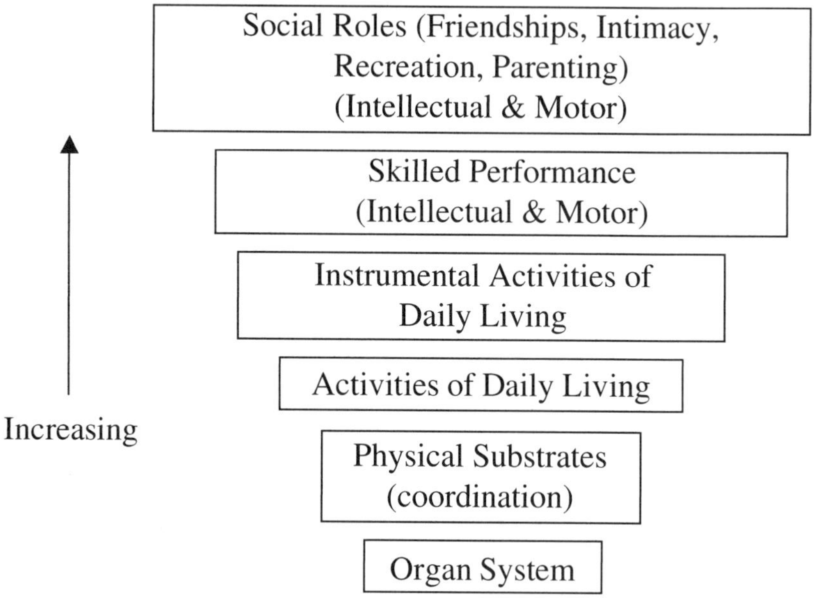

FIGURE 2.1 A hierarchical model of functional abilities.
Source: Adapted from Kemp and Mitchell (1992).

Functional limitations at any of these levels may result in the need for long-term care. Long-term care is an umbrella term that refers to various levels of care offered in informal and formal settings. Nursing homes are only a small proportion of the kinds of services offered to adults who need assistance with daily living. The prevalent political and social climate encourages independent living, which has contributed to a plethora of alternatives to nursing home care, including 600 federally and state funded "Independent Living Centers," private assisted living facilities, and community adult day care programs (American Association for Retired Persons, 2003). Use of formal home care services increases dramatically with age, and persons 65 and older are more likely to use formal home care services at every level of disability (see Figure 2.2).

Trends in nursing home use suggest that individuals over 65 may be living in the community longer and entering nursing homes later and sicker than in previous years (Manton, Corder, & Stallard, 1993). This trend makes it a particularly important goal to understand how to optimize the individual and environmental aspects that contribute to successful "aging in place" (Tillson, 1989). In effect, this becomes an individual, family and community process of selective optimization with compensation.

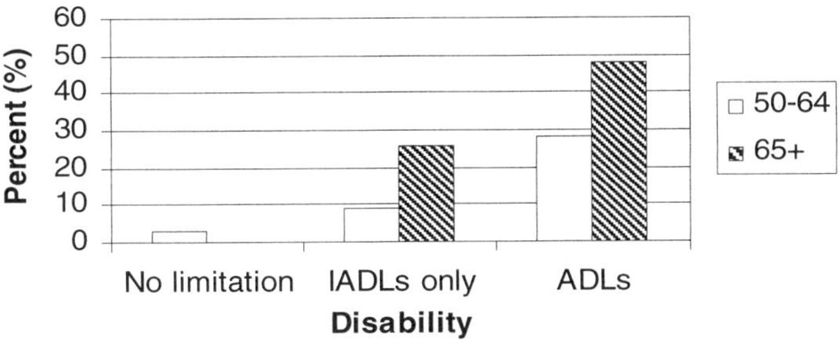

FIGURE 2.2 Persons 50 and older using formal home care services, by age and disability, 1998.

Source: Project HOPE analysis of 1998 Medical Expenditure Survey for AARP Public Policy Institute. From *Beyond 50.03: A Report to the Nation on Independent Living and Disability* (p. 70), by AARP Public Policy Institute, Washington, D.C.: AARP. Reproduced by permission of the publisher.

INDIVIDUAL ASPECTS AND INDIVIDUAL DIFFERENCES

The risk of disability and consequent need for long-term care is dependent on a dynamic interplay of individual characteristics. Individual characteristics are associated with different patterns of risk for loss of function at all levels of the hierarchical model of functioning. In this section, we will briefly review the literature on the association between several individual characteristics like age, gender, race, marital status and education and patterns of disability and service use.

Age

Demographic trends reveal that some older individuals are more vulnerable to functional limitations than others. The loss of independence is a reality for approximately 13% of individuals over 50 who have a limitation in mobility or self-care. Most of these older individuals with disability are aged 65 and older (U.S. Census Bureau Supplementary Survey, 2000). People aged 65 and older are 2.4 times more likely to have some limitations in IADLs, four times more likely to have at least one limitation in ADLs, and 5.4 times more likely to require assistance with more than one ADL (American Association for Retired Persons, 2003).

The NLTCS demonstrates that patterns of disability for different groups have changed since 1989. Increased longevity in the 1990s led to many predictions of higher rates of disability and increased use of long-term care services (Spillman, 2003). Contrary to prediction, increased longevity has not translated into increased levels of disability.

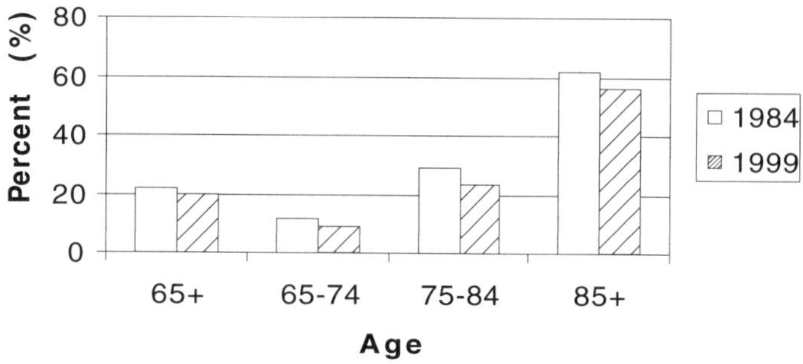

FIGURE 2.3 Percent of persons 65 and older reporting limitations in any IADL or ADL, 1984 and 1999.

Source: Urban Institute analysis of 1984 and 1999 National Long-Term Care Survey for AARP Public Policy Institute. From *Beyond 50.03: A Report to the Nation on Independent Living and Disability* (p. 39), by AARP Public Policy Institute, Washington, D.C.: AARP. Reproduced by permission of the publisher.

The rates of ADL and IADL limitation increased only slightly between 1989 and 1999 and rates of chronic disability declined for individuals 65 and older (American Association for Retired Persons, 2003). Disability rates and long-term care use has declined in recent years, primarily for individuals with higher incomes and higher levels of education (see Figures 2.3 and 2.4) (American Association for Retired Persons, 2003). In addition to age, rates of disability are tempered by other individual characteristics like gender, marital status, race, education, and socioeconomic status.

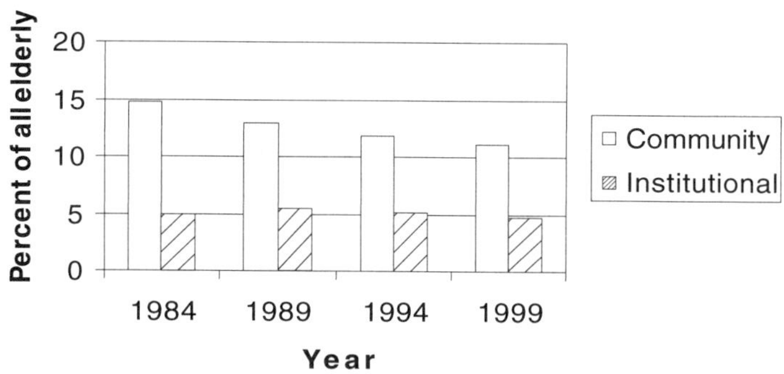

FIGURE 2.4 Long-term care use among adults 65 and older.

Source: Data from the 1984, 1989, 1994, and 1999 National Long-Term Care Survey (Spillman, 2003).

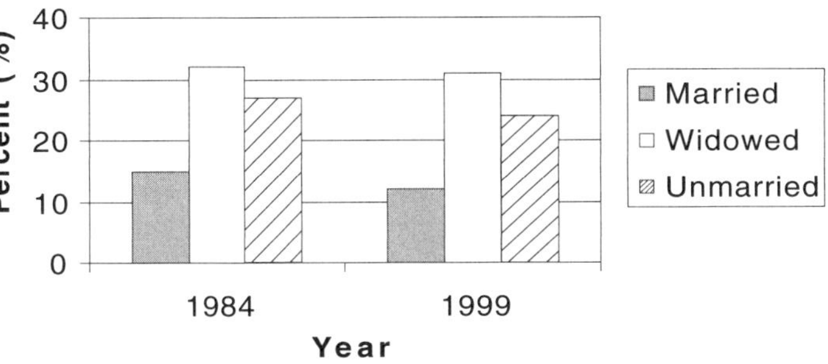

FIGURE 2.5 Percent of persons 65 and older with limitations in any ADL or IADL, by marital status, 1984 and 1999.

Source: Urban Institute analysis of 1984 and 1999 National Long-Term Care Survey for AARP Public Policy Institute. From *Beyond 50.03: A Report to the Nation on Independent Living and Disability* (p. 42), by AARP Public Policy Institute, Washington, D.C.: AARP. Reproduced by permission of the publisher.

Gender

Risk of disability is not evenly spread across men and women. Older women have higher rates of disability than men at all ages and at all levels of disability. In addition, disability rates have declined more for men than for women since 1984. Marital status also relates to disability—married individuals experience lower rates of disability than unmarried individuals (see Figure 2.5). As women tend to live longer then men, they are more likely to be widows and consequently more likely to experience functional limitations. Disability rates declined more modestly for widows and the unmarried than for married individuals since 1989 (American Association for Retired Persons, 2003). In addition, women and those who were widowed or never married are more likely to receive long-term care and be institutionalized (Spector et al., 2000).

Race

The most vulnerable racial group continues to be older Blacks, who tend to be less educated and in lower income brackets than Whites. The decline in reported rates of disability for Blacks between 1984 and 1999 was more modest than the decline for Whites. Blacks are also more likely than Whites to receive long-term care but are less likely to be in institutions (Spector et al., 2000). In contrast, disability rates for Hispanics and Asians may be somewhat lower than for Whites, while disability rates for Native Americans and Alaskans appear to be much higher than for other ethnic groups (American Association for Retired Persons, 2003).

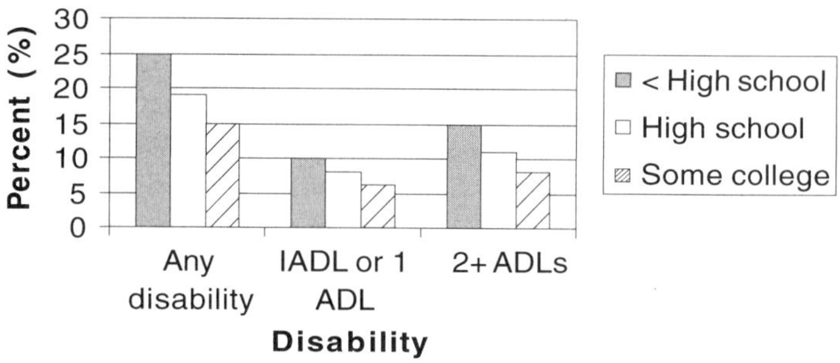

FIGURE 2.6 Disability levels for persons 65 and older, by education level, 1999.

Source: Urban Institute analysis of 1999 National Long-Term Care Survey for AARP Public Policy Institute. From *Beyond 50.03: A Report to the Nation on Independent Living and Disability* (p. 43), by AARP Public Policy Institute, Washington, D.C.: AARP. Reproduced by permission of the publisher.

Education Level

Education levels and socioeconomic status are also strongly related to disability rates in individuals 65 years and older. Education level has a particularly strong association with cognitive disability, work-related injury, access to health care, and smoking and alcohol consumption behaviors. Lower educated individuals show higher rates of any kind of disability (see Figure 2.6). Education is also related to income, which is a strong predictor of disability. Low income is related to higher rates of disability, and individuals in the lowest income bracket are almost three times as likely to experience disability (American Association for Retired Persons, 2003).

Interactions among individual characteristics can also contribute to higher risk of disability. The NLTCS reveals that the effect of education on disability, based on the number of ADLs and IADLs, may be more dramatic for Blacks than for non-Blacks. Disability trends from 1982 to 1999 show that Blacks aged 65–74 showed greater declines in disability for those with up to 12 years of education than non-Blacks (Manton & Gu, 2001). Data from 1999 shows that Blacks 85 and older who have had some college show lower disability than non-Blacks (see Figure 2.7).

The rates of disability for Blacks and non-Blacks by age and education level demonstrates the interaction of multiple determinants of disability. Blacks' risk profile for disability and their need for long-term care are compounded by the fact that Blacks generally have lower incomes and lower education than Whites. However, reducing one of these risk factors, like improving the likelihood that Blacks will achieve secondary

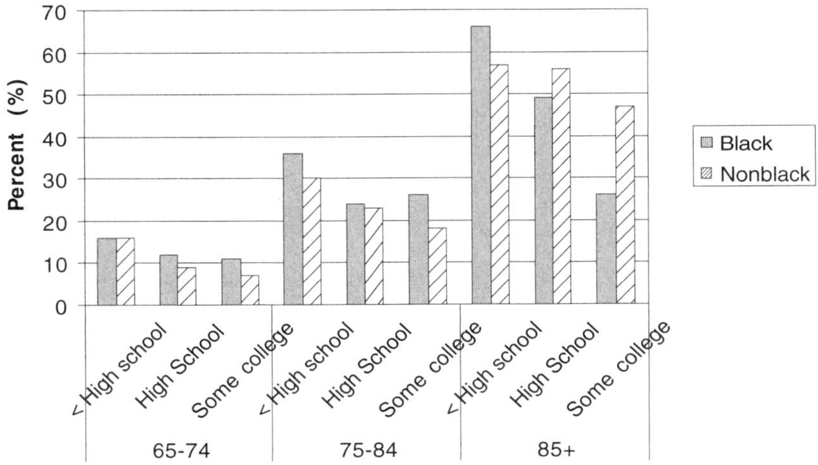

FIGURE 2.7 Blacks and non-Blacks with disabilities by age and education level, 1999.

Source: Data from the National Long-term Care Survey (Manton & Gu 2001, p. 6358).

and higher education, may reduce the risk of disability more substantially for Blacks than for non-Blacks.

Other Risk Factors

Although risk due to demographic group is difficult to prevent at the individual level, adults aged 50 and older can modify risk factors that are related to health behaviors. Eighty-nine percent of adults over 50 have at least one modifiable risk factor, and 19% have three or more modifiable risk factors (Shirey & Summer, 2000). The most common chronic conditions—hypertension, heart disease, diabetes, cancer, and stroke—are associated with modifiable risk factors. These risk factors include obesity, lack of exercise, smoking, high cholesterol, and consuming more than two alcoholic drinks a day (Shirey & Summer, 2000). Older adults with these kinds of risk factors are also more likely to be disabled than those with low risk (see Figure 2.8).

The majority of older adults in America have at least one risk factor. About two thirds of the American population is overweight, about half of the population does not exercise, and over a quarter of adults aged 51–61 smoke cigarettes (Shirey & Summer, 2000). In the year 2000, the nation met only 4 of the 10 Healthy People 2000 targets for the older population (see Table 2.1).

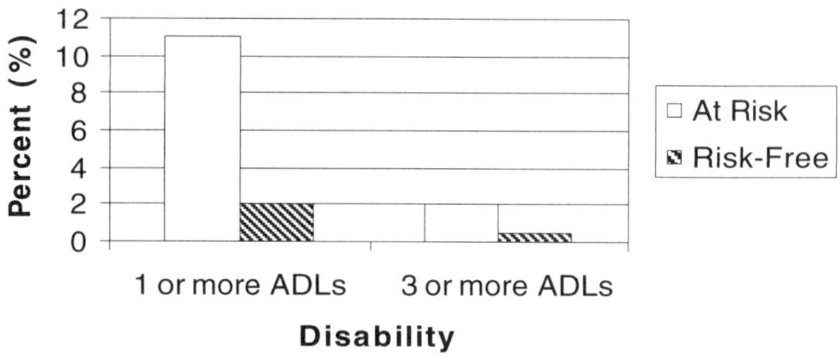

FIGURE 2.8 Proportion of older adults with limitations in ADLs, by risk status.
Source: National Academy on an Aging Society analysis of the 1992 Health and Retirement Study. From *At Risk: Developing Chronic Conditions Later in Life* (p. 3). Copyright© National Academy on an Aging Society. Reproduced by permission of the publisher.

TABLE 2.1 The National Report Card on Healthy Aging

Indicator	Current data for persons age 65 or older (year)	Healthy people 2000 target	Grade
Health behaviors			
1. No physical activity during leisure time in the past month (%)	34.6 (2000)	22	Fail
2. Overweight (%)	37.1 (1999)	20	Fail
3. Eating 5+ fruits/veg. Daily (%)	31.8 (2000)	50	Fail
4. Current smoker (%)	11.1 (1997/98)	15	Pass
Preventive care and cancer screening			
5. Flu vaccine in past year (%)	64 (2000)	60	Pass
6. Ever had pneumonia vaccine (%)	53 (2000)	60	Fail
7. Mammogram within past 2 years (%)	68 (2000)	60	Pass
8. Ever had colorectal screening (%)	48.5 (1999)	40	Pass
Fall-related deaths and injuries (per 100,000)			
9. Hip fractures, 65+	863 (1998)	607	Fail
10. Fall-related deaths, 85+	162.7 (1998)	105	Fail

Source: *The State of Aging and Health in America* (Merck Institute of Aging & Health and the Gerontological Society of America, 2002). Reproduced by permission of the publisher.

Another, less examined risk factor is the stress of work and family life on individuals. Poorer physical and mental health is related to negative "spillover," or intrusions, from work life to family life or vice versa. In contrast, positive spillover between work life and family life results in better physical and mental health (Grzywacz, 2000).

In terms of a long-term care risk profile, there is little one can do about demographic characteristics, but there is much one can do about modifiable risk factors. Still, most people have not planned for their long-term health status or care, despite evidence that early adaptive behaviors can drastically reduce the risk of disability in late life. As researchers and clinicians improve their efforts to educate the public about early life choices and modifiable risk factors, they will aid older adults in their ability to use selection and optimization with compensation to decrease their vulnerability to disability.

Yet, even with this knowledge, individual characteristics such as age, gender, socioeconomic status, race, and education can reduce one's ability to modify risk factors. For example, age, gender, race, and education are all strongly related to socioeconomic status. Low SES in turn is associated with risk factors like poor diet and lack of exercise (Seeman, 2000). Similarly, individual characteristics interact with environmental factors in a way that mounts the odds against individuals with a particular cluster of characteristics. Examples of this will be presented in the next section.

THE ENVIRONMENTAL ECOLOGY OF LONG-TERM CARE

Long-term care is traditionally thought of in terms of medical and institutional services, but the ecology of disability and long-term care actually involves three levels of environmental influences: the individual's immediate environment (home and family), the community, and the social policies that shape the community. The ecological approach to disability and long-term care acknowledges that the physical environment must accommodate disability if optimal aging is to occur (Satariano, 1997).

The face of long-term care has changed considerably because fewer disabled adults are institutionalized and more have access to formal and informal care in their communities. The use of home health care increased 78% from 1992 to 1996 and is expected to continue to increase (Gallagher, 2000). In addition, the increasing use of community services enables disabled individuals to stay longer in their own homes. This section will review the factors in the home, community, and sociopolitical climate that greatly affect an older disabled person's ability to optimize his or her environment.

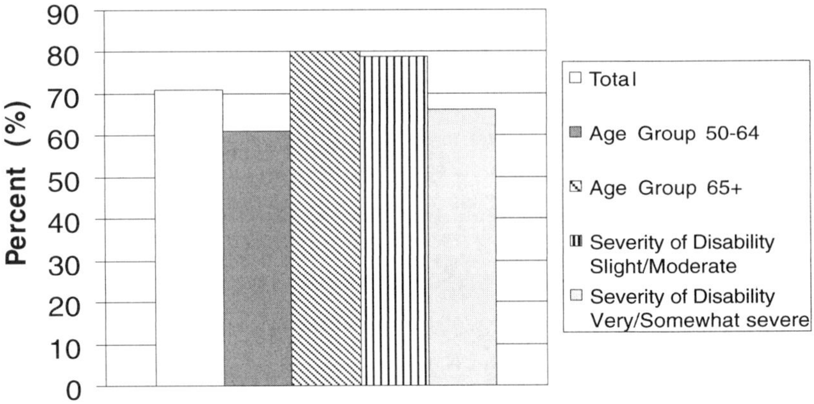

FIGURE 2.9 Persons age 50 and older with disabilities who own their own home.

Source: AARP/Harris Interactive Survey of Persons 50 and Older with Disabilities, September 2002. From *Beyond 50.03: A Report to the Nation on Independent Living and Disability* (p. 143), by AARP Public Policy Institute, Washington, D.C.: AARP. Reproduced by permission of the publisher.

Home

Home can be an isolated and dangerous place for a fragile, elderly person. Yet, disabled persons are twice as likely to live alone (Kaye, 1998). The majority of older persons with disabilities own their home (see Figure 2.9) and an AARP survey found that a large majority of individuals over 50 would like to stay in their current residence as long as possible (AARP Programs/Applied Gerontology Group, 2000) (see Figure 2.10). If they move, persons age 50 and older with disabilities

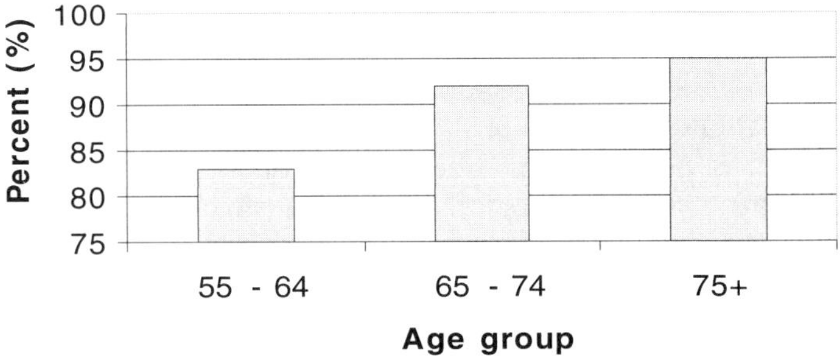

FIGURE 2.10 Percent of older Americans who prefer to stay in their current residences as long as possible.

Source: Data from an AARP survey, *Fixing to Stay: A National Survey on Housing and Home Modification Issues* (AARP Independent Living Program, 2000).

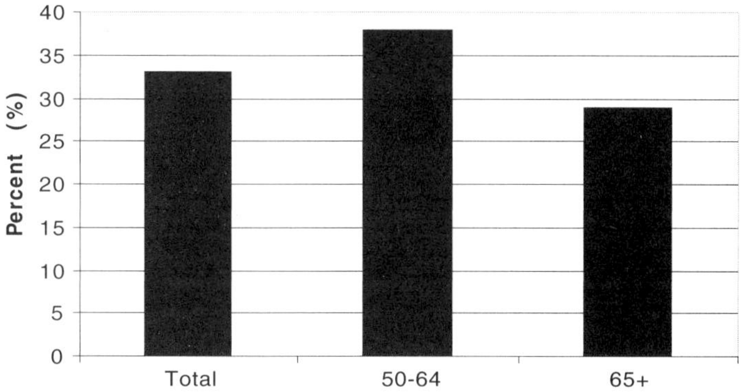

FIGURE 2.11 Proportion of persons 50 and older with disabilities using special equipment or assistive technology to help with daily activities.

Source: AARP/Harris Interactive Survey of Persons 50 and Older with Disabilities, September 2002. Adapted from *Beyond 50.03: A Report to the Nation on Independent Living and Disability* (p. 148), by AARP Public Policy Institute, Washington, D.C.: AARP. Adapted by permission of the publisher.

would like to move to their own home or apartment (AARP Programs/ Applied Gerontology Group, 2000).

Using enabling technologies is one strategy for compensating for a disability. Such technologies may facilitate the process of "aging in place" (Tillson, 1989). A significant number of disabled older adults over the age of 50 use special equipment or assistive technology, and the percent of disabled persons over 65 using assistive technology is

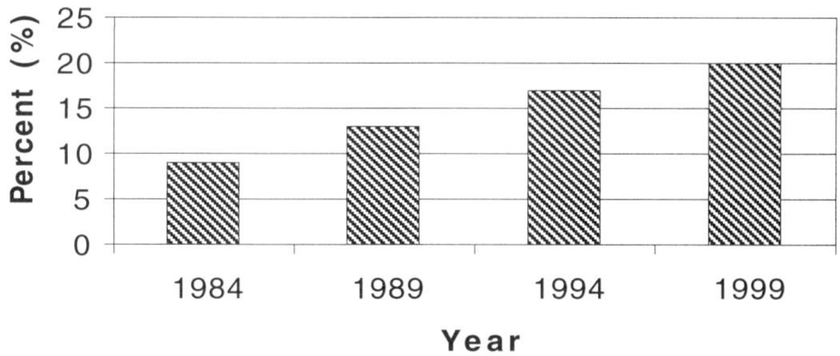

FIGURE 2.12 Percent of persons 65 and older with disabilities using assistive technology only, 1984–1999.

Source: Urban Institute analysis of the National Long-Term Care Survey for AARP Public Policy Institute. From *Beyond 50.03: A Report to the Nation on Independent Living and Disability* (p. 95), by AARP Public Policy Institute, Washington, D.C.: AARP. Reproduced by permission of the publisher.

increasing (see Figures 2.11 and 2.12). Technologies can help older disabled persons achieve independence and simultaneously relieve burden on medical staff and other supportive services. For example, Allen, Foster and Berg (2001) found that older adults' use of canes and crutches saves consumers the cost of formal caregiving services and reduces use of both informal and formal services.

Older persons with more than one ADL limitation use assistive technologies more than persons with lower levels of disability. The most common types of assistance are in the form of walkers, canes, crutches, grab bars, raised toilets, wheelchairs, scooters, railings, ramps, and lifts (American Association for Retired Persons, 2003). Older adults who live alone are more than twice as likely to use assistive technologies than persons who are not living alone. This finding suggests that assistive technologies are substituting for unpaid human help when it is not available (American Association for Retired Persons, 2003).

Architectural features and location of homes can create many barriers for the older person. Older adults are capable of optimizing their environments, however. A study of German older adults found that relocating is not necessarily a stressful event for older adults and that individuals proactively optimize their environments to fit their needs. For example, those who anticipated needing help with basic needs removed barriers to household amenities and moved closer to physicians and their families. In addition, those older adults who were more concerned with higher order needs, like social relations, moved to a location with access to public transportation (Oswald, Schilling, Wahl, & Gang, 2002).

The Oswald et al. (2002) study looked at middle-class older adults. In reality, however, the majority of older adults cannot afford relocation or home improvements. Sixty-nine percent of persons 50 and older with disabilities said they could not afford home improvements. Yet, over a third of individuals 50 and over with disabilities would like to make home improvements such as grab bars in the bathroom, accessible showers, ramps, large hallways and doors, extra handrails or other accessible bathroom features (AARP Programs/Applied Gerontology Group, 2000). Individuals with more chronic disabilities are less satisfied with their homes than those without disabilities, and minorities and those with fewer financial resources are less likely to have home modifications (American Association for Retired Persons, 2003).

Family

When disabled individuals cannot afford assistive technologies or home health care, or when they have multiple disabilities, family members and

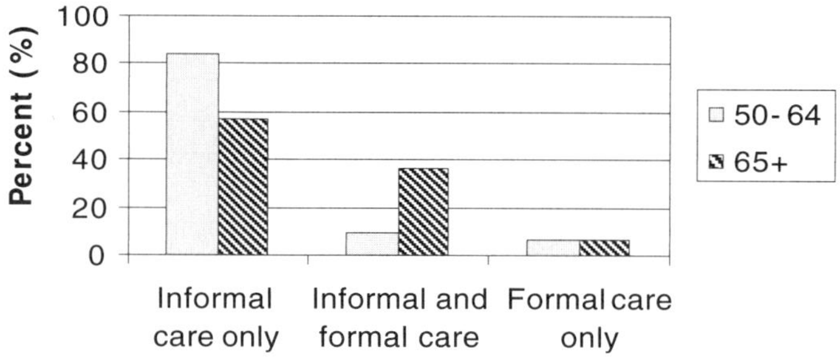

FIGURE 2.13 Percent of persons 50 and older in the community receiving long-term care, by age and type of care, 1994.

Source: 1994 National Health Interview Survey, Disability Supplement, Phase I, National Center for Health Statistics; 1994 National Long-Term Care Survey; AARP Public Policy Institute Analysis of data from W. Spector, J. Fleishman, L. Pezzin et al., *The Characteristics of Long-Term Care Users*, Agency for Health Care Research and Quality Research Report, August 2000. From *Beyond 50.03: A Report to the Nation on Independent Living and Disability* (p. 59), by AARP Public Policy Institute, Washington, D.C.: AARP. Reproduced by permission of the publisher.

friends are often relied on to provide care. Dependence on informal care is greater than on formal care (see Figure 2.13).

Nearly a quarter of American households (22.4 million households) provided caregiving to persons age 50 or over in 1997 (National Alliance for Caregiving, 1997). About 19% of these caregivers lived with the older adult, 46% lived 20 min or less from the care recipient, and 18% lived over 1 hr away (Women's Bureau, US Department of Labor, 1998).

In addition to IADL and ADL assistance, informal caregivers provide socioemotional support, which is an aspect of caregiving that is generally not acknowledged (Walker, Pratt, & Eddy, 1995). Social support is strongly related to health and functioning, and it is often informal caregivers that provide this support (Knickman & Snell, 2002). Men without social support were more likely to die from any cause than peers who had social support, and it is believed that the same relationship holds for women (Eng, Rimm, Fitzmaurice, & Kawachi, 2002).

Informal caregivers are more likely to be a female because of both ideological and practical reasons. Caregiving is thought to be natural and instinctual for the female (Aronson, 1992). Practically speaking, women are paid less in the working world than men, so the financial opportunity costs of providing informal care are lower for them (Walker et al., 1995). Yet, caregiving involves significant financial sacrifices during most caregivers' peak earning years (see Figure 2.14). More than

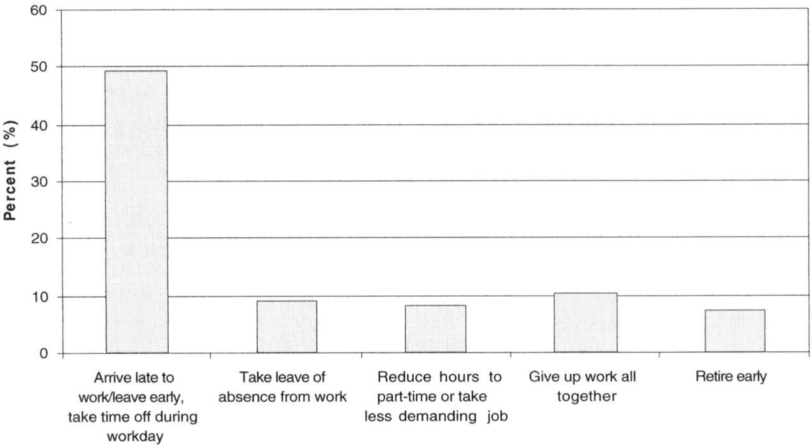

FIGURE 2.14 Changes made by caregivers 50 and older in work life to accommodate caregiving responsibilities, 1997.

Source: National Alliance for Caregiving/AARP Family Caregiving Survey, 1997, previously unpublished data of caregivers 50 and older. From *Beyond 50.03: A Report to the Nation on Independent Living and Disability* (p. 61), by AARP Public Policy Institute, Washington, D.C.: AARP. Reproduced by permission of the publisher.

half of caregivers must change their work schedules in order to accommodate caregiving (American Association for Retired Persons, 2003).

Caregiving can lead to physical or mental health problems for the caregiver. About one in five caregivers reported some physical or mental health problem because of caregiving and sought counseling or professional help (National Alliance for Caregiving, 1997). Caregiving is a significant risk factor for depression (Walker et al., 1995). Caregiving, especially spousal caregiving in late life, can be a chronic stressor that reduces immune response and increases risk for cardiovascular disease and cancer (Kiecolt-Glaser & Glaser, 1999).

Currently, about 23% of persons with disabilities feel they need more help with daily activities than they receive (American Association for Retired Persons, 2003). In addition, the perceived need of help increases with more severe disability (American Association for Retired Persons, 2003). Thus, it is expected that the number of older adults relying on informal caregiving will increase as older adults remain in the community longer.

Community

Another essential aspect to aging well in place is a supportive community. Although there are many factors that contribute to livable communities

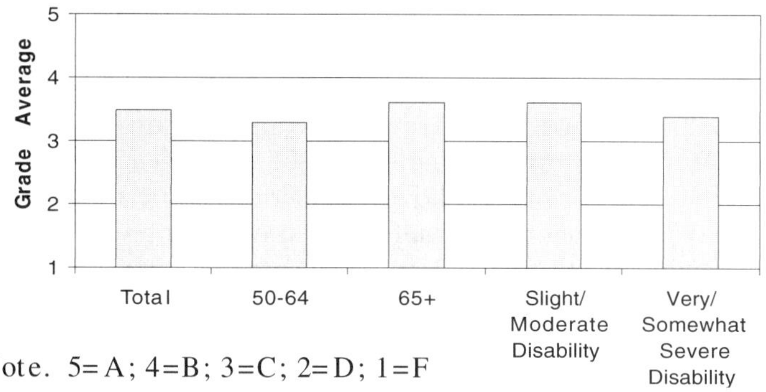

FIGURE 2.15 Report card on communities by persons 50 and older with disabilities.

Source: AARP/Harris Interactive Survey of Persons 50 and Older with Disabilities, September 2002. From *Beyond 50.03: A Report to the Nation on Independent Living and Disability* (p. 141), by AARP Public Policy Institute, Washington, D.C.: AARP. Reproduced by permission of the publisher. Note: 5 = A; 4 = B; 3 = C; 2 = D; 1 = F.

for older disabled persons, we focus on transportation, home security, and community services that enabling communities provide in order to support independence and quality of life for disabled elderly. In essence, these are community-level compensations for the changing abilities of their citizens.

In an interactive survey of persons 50 and older with disabilities, the AARP found that respondents give their communities only satisfactory ratings as a place for people with disabilities to live (see Figure 2.15). Only 52% of residents with disabilities said they are very satisfied with their communities, and Black residents were less likely to say they are very satisfied than White residents.

Of those respondents in communities that received high marks (A or B rating), only slightly more than half of the respondents reported that their communities provide parking for people with disabilities or health conditions like their own. About 50% of the respondents said their communities provide bathrooms accessible to people with disabilities or health conditions like their own, or provide safe and well-run parks, community centers and recreation centers. Only about 35% of the respondents reported that their communities offer accessible, dependable public transportation (American Association for Retired Persons, 2003). In fact, respondents said that transportation was the first thing that they would like improved in their communities (American Association for Retired Persons, 2003).

The dearth of accessible public transportation means that disabled older adults must rely on driving. The majority of individuals age 60 and over (90%) use their own vehicle as a main mode of transportation. The percent of licensed drivers drops substantially at the ages of 70 and 80, to just over 50% (American Association for Retired Persons, 2003). Older adults with disabilities are also less likely to own a vehicle, and about 20% of older disabled individuals 75 and older report that their disability prevents them from driving (American Association for Retired Persons, 2003). When older adults 75 and older stop driving, they are 12 times more likely to not leave their home during a typical week (Ritter, Straight, & Evans, 2002).

Family and friends are often relied on for transportation, especially for those individuals who are 75 and older, have low incomes, have less education, or are female (American Association for Retired Persons, 2003). More than half of individuals with ADL limitations depend on friends and family for transportation (American Association for Retired Persons, 2003). Walking is another option for elders, although 20% of individuals age 50 and older feel that things are too far away to walk to or the sidewalks are in too poor condition for walking (Ritter et al, 2002).

Public safety is another factor that contributes to livable communities. In the years between 1984 and 1999, the proportion of persons 65 and older with ADL or IADL limitations who perceived that crime is a serious problem in their neighborhood rose from 4.5 to 8.2% (American Association for Retired Persons, 2003). Crime is often viewed as a hindrance to walking in the neighborhood and using public transportation (Ritter et al., 2002). Persons 65 and older who live in unsafe neighborhoods are significantly less likely to exercise regularly than persons who live in safer neighborhoods (Weinstein, Feigley, & Pullen, 1999). Thus, even if an older person wanted to modify his or her risk for disability by exercising, an unsafe environment is an unavoidable hindrance.

Finally, community services like senior centers, adult day care, respite care, case management, home delivered meals, and other adult care services are essential to aging well in the community (see Figure 2.16). Not surprisingly, the use of these services increases with age and disability. Among persons 50 years and older, 81% of community service users are 65 and older. Low-income individuals, individuals who live alone, females, and Blacks are more likely to use community services (American Association for Retired Persons, 2003)

Public Policy Contexts

Individual patterns of service use and service preference affect and are affected by public policy options. In this section, we will focus on one

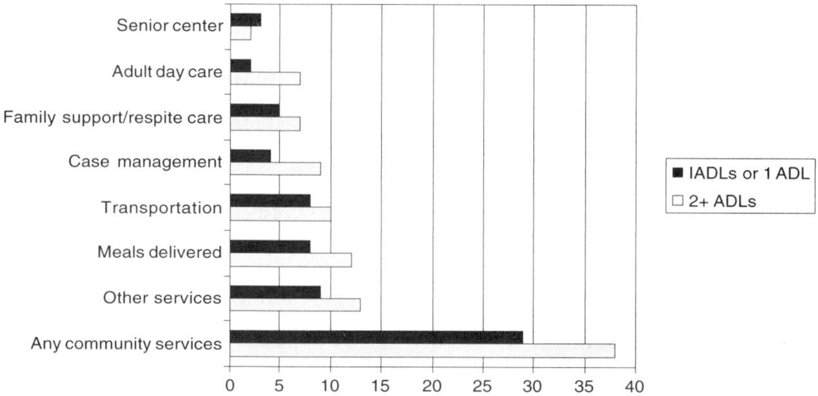

FIGURE 2.16 Use of community services by persons 50 and older, by level of disability, 1998.

Source: Project HOPE analysis of 1998 Medical Expenditure Panel Survey for AARP Public Policy Institute. From *Beyond 50.03: A Report to the Nation on Independent Living and Disability* (p. 72), by AARP Public Policy Institute, Washington, D.C.: AARP. Reproduced by permission of the publisher.

public policy program, Medicaid, to illustrate current efforts to optimize the ecology of long-term care. Medicaid is the major public financing program for low-income individuals' health and long-term care services in the United States (Kaiser Commission on Medicaid and the uninsured, 2001). In fiscal year 2002, total Medicaid spending was $222.9 billion, 11.4% more than in the previous fiscal year (National Association of State Budget Officers, 2003). Medicaid is funded through a combination of state and federal funds.

Both the size and the rate of growth of the Medicaid budget pose significant challenges to state governments. For example, since 1990 Medicaid expenditures have been the second largest state program. In fiscal year 2002, Medicaid accounted for 20.8% of state expenditures, just behind elementary and secondary education (21.6%) as major elements in state budgets (see Figure 2.17).

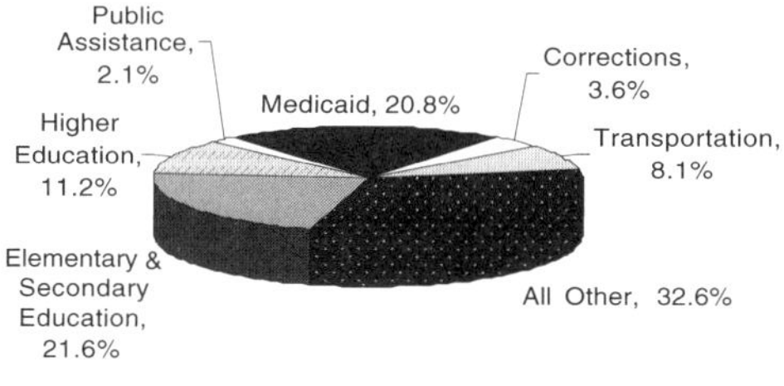

FIGURE 2.17 Composition of state budgets, fiscal year 2002.

Source: From *State budget expenditures, 2002* (p. 4) by National Association of Budget Officers (2003). Reproduced by permission of the publisher.

During fiscal year 2002, 25 states experienced Medicaid shortfalls. This is one indicator of the budgetary challenge posed by the Medicaid program (National Association of State Budget Officers, 2003). Another challenge is the alignment of service recipients and service costs: one quarter of Medicaid beneficiaries are elderly and disabled citizens and three quarters are children and nondisabled adults. The costs are just the opposite: approximately three quarters of Medicaid service costs are for the elderly and disabled, one quarter for children and nondisabled adults (National Association of State Budget Officers, 2003).

In response to these challenges, states are pursuing several strategies simultaneously: attracting additional revenue sources to pay for services; changing eligibility rules to limit access to services; increasing the cost-effectiveness of service management; and altering the range of services covered by the Medicaid program (National Association of State Budget Officers, 2003; Wiener, 1996; Wiener & Stevenson, 1998). At the same time, the federal government has proposed streamlining its contributions to states, through a "block grant" mechanism, giving states greater control and flexibility over the use of federal funds. The block grant proposal was greeted with skepticism in scholarly and popular media (e.g., Weil, 2003; Cohn, 2003)—viewed as an attempt to limit eventually the federal commitment to services for poor and disabled.

One strategy, however, has garnered substantial support from consumer groups, state legislators, and federal policy makers: a "consumer driven" health care purchasing process, accomplished by experimentation at the state level (Waldholz, 2003). The Cash and Counseling Demonstration and Evaluation (CCDE) is an ongoing project jointly funded by the Robert Wood Johnson Foundation (RWJF) and the Office of the Assistant Secretary for Planning and Evaluation (ASPE) in the U.S. Department of Health and Human Services (Dale, Brown, Phillips, Schore, & Carlson, 2003; Mahoney, 2003). CCDE operates under a research and demonstration waiver granted to states by the Centers for Medicare and Medicaid Services (CMS). The CCDE allows states to change the process of service reimbursement and service organization, with a goal of enhancing service impact and cost effectiveness.[1] In some ways, the CCDE is a state-level policy attempt at selective optimization with compensation for elderly and disabled recipients of personal care services through Medicaid.

The CCDE focuses on an important question: do cash allowances maximize consumer choice and promote program efficiencies? (Mahoney,

[1]http://www.hcbs.org/state_by_state.htm

2003). To answer this important question, three states—Arkansas, Florida, and New Jersey—undertook experiments in 1998 to assess the impact of allowing consumer-directed approaches compared to traditional agency-directed approaches for hiring PCS. As Dale and her colleagues summarized it:

> . . . The Cash and Counseling model of consumer-directed supported services give eligible beneficiaries who choose to participate a flexible monthly allowance to purchase disability-related goods and services (including hiring relatives as workers). The program also provides counseling and fiscal assistance and allows consumers to designate representatives (such as family members) to make decisions on their behalf. These features make the model adaptable to consumers of all ages and with all types of impairments. (Dale et al., 2003, p. 567)

CCDE takes a different form for each person. But a case description gives a sense of how the program might work for each individual recipient. Remember Grace Wall, whose experiences started this chapter?

> Grace Wall . . . has always been independent. But at 83, with a host of health problems that include congestive heart failure, two hip replacements, loss of sight in one eye, and lung cancer, that independence is harder to maintain.
>
> For six years, Mrs. Wall took care of her paralyzed husband before he died in 1991. Now she lives alone in a mobile home. She gets her health care through Medicaid, as well as various personal assistance services, such as help with shopping and housekeeping—things that she has difficulty doing on her own now.
>
> Mrs. Wall used to get those services through a Medicaid contractor. But in September 2000, she enrolled in Consumer Directed Care (CDC), Florida's Cash & Counseling program. Mrs. Wall says that CDC has changed her life.
>
> "I just feel better," she says. "This gets what I need to get done without much fuss."
>
> Now Mrs. Wall can hire people she knows and trusts to help her. A good portion of her $437 monthly budget goes toward buying medications and health care supplies. She also uses the money for transportation and to maintain her home.
>
> At first, Mrs. Wall admits that she was daunted by the paperwork. But her CDC consultant has helped her through that and Mrs. Wall says the rewards have been well worth the effort.
>
> Mrs. Wall says that CDC has enabled her to do things she wouldn't otherwise have been able to do and made difficult tasks simpler for her. She also feels more secure with help that is close at hand and accountable to her. Agency workers, she notes, were not always

> there for her when she needed them. "Now I can rely on my worker, and I couldn't before. I can get help when I need it." (Mahoney, 2003, pp. 10–11)

The most detailed assessments of CCDE have focused on the impact in one state, Arkansas in its IndependentChoices program. 2,008 beneficiaries in Arkansas were randomly assigned to the CCDE or to standard treatment (Dale et al., 2003). Initial assessment of CCDE has been positive. Consumer satisfaction with the program is high. In Arkansas, for example, 96% of clients say they would recommend the program to others, 82% say the program has improved their lives, and 65% say the program has improved their lives a great deal (Mahoney, 2003). IndependentChoices greatly increased the likelihood that beneficiaries received paid assistance and received assistance in the evening hours (Dale et al., 2003). Economically, the initial Medicaid expenditures under IndependentChoices were higher, but projections are that the state of Arkansas will save money on total long-term care expenditures in the long run (Dale et al., 2003).

Through CCDE the federal government and several states have tried to change the policy context of the ecology of long-term care. By providing greater consumer-directed choice, the CCDE program hopes to enhance individual, community, state, and federal functioning. CCDE represents a policy-level attempt to selectively optimize individual functioning while compensating for changing personal care needs of long-term care beneficiaries.

CONCLUSIONS

Examining long-term care from an ecological perspective illuminates the interactions among multiple levels, including the disabled individual and his or her physical and social environment. Apparent within these levels is the selection and optimization with compensation required to enable disabled individuals to optimize their functioning. Disabled individuals must manage losses and promote gains based on their individual profiles for risk. Individual characteristics like age, gender, race, marital status, education, and health influence level of risk for disability and the ability to manage disability once it occurs. Communities are pressed to adapt their programs and services to the needs of older disabled adults. Few communities presently receive high ratings for meeting the needs of their disabled citizens. This discrepancy in turn affects its disabled citizens' abilities to function well independently. Finally, state and federal programs directly impact the potential for individuals and their communities to optimize the functioning of older disabled adults. IndependentChoices in Arkansas is an example of a successful program that empowers disabled individuals to choose care based on their changing, personal needs.

We began this chapter by describing an important trend in long-term care over the past decade: the dramatic increase in disabled elderly living in the community and corresponding decrease in the number of institutionalized elderly. Older people are entering nursing homes later, and sicker, than ever before. A more thorough understanding of the ecology of long-term care makes clear that to facilitate optimal aging, this shift from dependence to independent living requires the education and efficacy of aging individuals, their families, their communities, and society.

REFERENCES

AARP Independent Living Program. (2000). *Fixing to stay: A National Survey on housing and home modification issues*. Washington, DC: AARP.

Allen, S., Foster, A., & Berg, K. (2001). Receiving help at home: The interplay of human and technological assistance. *Journal of Gerontology, 56B*(6), S374–S382.

American Association for Retired Persons. (2003). *Beyond 50 2003: A report to the nation on independent living and disability.* Washington, D.C.: AARP Public Policy Institute.

Aronson, J. (1992). Women's sense of responsibility for the care of old people: "But who else is going to do it?" *Gender and Society, 6*, 8–29.

Baltes, P. B., & Baltes, M. M. (1990). Psychological perspectives on successful aging: The model of selective optimization with compensation. In P. B. Baltes, & M. M. Baltes (Eds.), *Successful aging: Perspective from the behavioral sciences* (pp. 1–34). Cambridge, England: University Press.

Bronfenbrenner, U. (1979). *The ecology of human development: Experiments by nature and design.* Cambridge, MA: Harvard University Press.

Bronfenbrenner, U., & Evans, G. W. (2000). Developmental science in the 21st century: Emerging questions, theoretical models, research designs and empirical findings. *Social development, 9*, 115–125.

Cohn, J. (2003, March 6). How Medicaid Was Set Adrift, *The New York Times*, Late Edition-Final , p. 31, C2.

Dale, S., Brown, R., Phillips, B., Schore, J., & Carlson, B. L. (2003). The effects of cash and counseling on personal care services and Medicaid costs in Arkansas. *Health Affairs* (Web exclusive), *W3*, *566–575*.

Elders Behind the Wheel. (2003). Elders Behind the Wheel (2003, July 27). The New York Times, Late Edition–Final, p. 12, C1.

Eng, P. M., Rimm, E. B., Fitzmaurice, G., & Kawachi, I. (2002). Social ties in relation to subsequent total and cause-specific mortality and coronary heart disease incidence in men. *American Journal of Epidemiology, 155*, 700–709.

Gallagher, R. (2000). How long-term care is changing. *American Journal of Nursing, 100*, 65–67.

Grzywacz, J. (2000). Work-family spillover and health during midlife: Is managing conflict everything? *American Journal of Health Promotion, 14*(4), 236–243.

Kaiser Commission on Medicaid and the uninsured. (2001). *The role of Medicaid in State budgets.* Policy brief available @ www.kff.org

Katz, S., Ford, A. B., Moskowitz, A. W., Jackson, B. A., Jaffe, M. W. (1963). Studies of illness in the aged. The index of ADL: A standardized measure of biological and psychosocial function. *Journal of the American Medical Association, 185*, 914–919.

Kaye, H. S. (1998). Is the status of people with disabilities improving? *Disability Statistics Abstract, 21*, 1–4.

Kemp, B., & Mitchell, J. (1992). Functional assessment in geriatric health. In J. Birren, R. B. Sloane, & G. Cohen (Eds.), *Handbook of mental health and aging*. New York: Academic Press, Inc.

Kiecolt-Glaser, J. K., & Glaser, R. (1999). Chronic stress and mortality among older adults. *JAMA: Journal of the American Medical Association, 282*(23), 2259–2260.

Knickman, J. R., & Snell, E. K. (2002). The 2030 problem: Caring for aging baby boomers. *HSR: Health Services Research, 37*(4), 849–884.

Lawton, M. P., & Brody, E. M. (1969). Assessment of older people: Self-maintaining and instrumental activities of daily living. *Gerontologist, 9*, 179–186.

Lewin, K. (1935). *A dynamic theory of personality: Selected papers of Kurt Lewin.* New York: McGraw Hill.

Mahoney, K. J. (2003). *Cash and counseling demonstration and evaluation.* Statement before the U.S. Senate Special Committee on Aging. Washington, D.C.

Manton, K., Corder, L., & Aragon, C. (2000). Chronic disability trends in the elderly United States population: 1982–1994. *Proceedings of the National Academy of Sciences, 94*, 2593–2598.

Manton, K., Corder, L., & Stallard, E. (1993). Estimates of change in chronic disability and institutional incidence and prevalence rates in the U.S. elderly population from the 1982, 1984, and 1989 National Long Term Care Surveys. *Journal of Gerontology, 48*, S153–S166.

Manton, K., & Gu, X. (2001). Changes in the prevalence of chronic disability in the United States black and nonblack population above age 65 from 1982 to 1999. *Proceedings of the National Academy of Sciences, 98*, 6354–6359.

Medical Expenditure Panel Survey, (1997–1998). Public use data set. Rockville, MD: Agency for Healthcare Research and Quality [Producer and Distributor], http://www.meps.ahrq.gov/

Merck Institute of Aging & Health and the Gerontological Society of America. (2002). *The State of Aging and Health in America*, p. 20.

Minkler, M., & Fadem, P. (2002). "Successful aging:" A disability perspective. *Journal of Disability Policy Studies, 12*(4), 229–236.

National Academy on an Aging Society. (2000). *Challenges for the 21st century: Chronic and disabling conditions,* (4), 6.

National Association of State Budget Officers. (2003). *State budget expenditures, 2002.* Washington, D.C. www.nasbo.org

National Long Term Care Study. (1984–1999). [Public use data set]. Duke University Center for Demographic Studies with funding from the National Institute on Aging [Producer and Distributor].

National Alliance for Caregiving and AARP. (1997). *Family caregiving in the U.S.: Findings from a national survey.* Bethesda, MD: National Alliance for Caregiving.

Oswald, F., Schilling, O., Wahl, H., & Gang, K. (2002). Trouble in paradise? Reasons to relocate and objective environmental changes among well-off older adults. *Journal of Environmental Psychology, 22*, 273–288.

Ritter, A., Straight, A., & Evans, E. (2002). *Understanding senior transportation: Report and analysis of a survey of consumers age 50+.* Washington, DC: AARP Public Policy Institute.

Rowe, J., & Kahn, R. (1998). *Successful aging.* New York: Random House.

Satariano, W. (1997). The disabilities of aging: Looking to the physical environment. *American Journal of Public Health, 87*, 331–332.

Seeman, T. E. (2000). Health promoting effects of friends and family on health outcomes in older adults. *American Journal of Health Promotion, 14*, 362–370.

Shirey, L., & Summer, L. (2000). At risk: Developing chronic conditions later in life. In Challenges for the twenty-first century: Chronic and disabling conditions, no. 4 (pp. 1–6). Washington, DC: National Academy on an Aging Society.

Spector, W., Fleishman, J., & Pezzin, L. (2000). *The Characteristics of Long-Term Care Users.* Agency for Healthcare Research and Quality, AHRQ Pub. No. 00–0049.

Spillman, B. (2003). *Changes in Elderly Disability Rates and the Implications for Health Care Utilization and Cost.* U.S. Department of Health and Human Services report.

Tillson, D. (Ed.). (1989). *Aging in place.* Glenview, IL: Scott Foresman.

U.S. Census Bureau Supplementary Survey. (2000). Public use data set. Washington, DC: American Community Survey Office of the U.S. Census Bureau [Producer and Distributor].

Waldholz, M. (2003). A consumer approach to Medicaid. *The WallStreet Journal* Online http://online.wsj.com/public/us

Walker, A., Pratt, C., & Eddy, L. (1995). Informal caregiving to aging family members: A critical review. *Family Relations, 44*(4), 402–411.

Weil, A. (2003). Putting Medicaid at risk. *Hastings Center Report, 33*(3), 49.

Weinstein, A., Feigley, P., & Pullen, P. (1999). Neighborhood safety and the prevalence of physical inactivity—selected states, 1996. *Morbidity and Mortality Weekly Report, 48*, 143–146.

Wiener, J. M. (1996). Can Medicaid long-term care expenditures for the elderly be reduced? *Gerontologist, 36*, 800–811.

Wiener, J. M., & Stevenson, D. G. (1998). State policy on long-term care for the elderly. *Health Affairs, 17*(3), 81–100.

Women's Bureau, U.S. Department of Labor. (1998). *Work and elder care: Facts for caregivers and their employers*. U.S. Department of Labor, Washington, DC.

PART II

Basic Care

CHAPTER THREE

Blending Mental Health Services into the Geriatric Medical Care of Long-Term Care Facility Residents

John Heath, Melissa Gartenberg, and Erinn E. Beagin

The decision to relocate to a long-term care facility, such as a nursing home or assisted living residence, is a major transition point in an older adult's life. Institutionalization is a very tangible response to an imbalance between an individual's functional ability and the resources available for their care. This imbalance can result from limitations of their environment, caregivers, and resources available in their home settings and is often compounded by demands related to an accumulation of both medical and mental health issues.

Long-term care settings provide a unique platform upon which to explore the interaction and blending of mental health issues of aging with geriatric medicine. Consider the term "nursing home": in addition to striving to meet "home" criteria for being a home as a familiar, stable place where an individual lives, it is also a setting where increasingly complex medical treatments occurs. Many life events, whether they are physically or psychologically motivated, play out in such settings, in front of a cadre of nurses, doctors, aids, activity coordinators, nutritionists, and social workers. Each staff member has an opportunity to assess and interact with more dimensions of an individual than they would outside of the institutional setting. The lines between the psychological and the medical treatments are blurred.

Mental and medical pathologies often share a common expression and function. For example, an explicit diagnosis of dementia, or an indication that a dementing process is in place is often the reason for long-term care placement. Other medical events, including those that include the onset or progression of difficult to care for physical changes like those seen in Parkinson's disease, also have definite medical etiologies, but fall into the domain of mental health, given their neuropsychological properties and high incidence of comorbid depression (Dening & Bains, 2004).

HEALTH CARE ISSUES IN LONG-TERM CARE: THE BIG PICTURE

Medical Diagnoses

Various medical conditions are seen in nursing home residents and many residents have multiple medical problems. All Medicare or Medicaid certified nursing homes are required to complete a comprehensive assessment of each resident's functional capabilities, diagnoses, and interim complications called the Minimum Data Set (MDS). This assessment must be completed routinely on admission, quarterly, and yearly. It is important to note that the nature of the assessment causes some diagnoses to be over or under-reported. For example, the chart may have stroke listed as a problem, but may omit hemiplegia. Despite these shortcomings, the MDS is the best source of information available regarding nursing home residents' current medical problems. Table 3.1 presents the top 20 disease diagnoses reported in the MDS Active Resident Information Report (Centers for Medicare and Medicaid Services, 2004).

Admissions diagnoses change as a resident progresses in the long-term care facility. In a comparison of the 1985 and 1997 surveys, it was noted that almost all residents had more than one condition present at admission and more than half had three or more admitting diagnoses (Sahyoun, Pratt, Lentzner, Dey, & Robinson, 2001). The prevalence of mental and cognitive disorders including depressive disorders, anxiety disorders, and organic brain damage is striking (Jones, 2002).

An inability to function independently is a theme that underlies the many different diseases found in long-term care settings (Williams, 1998). Observed difficulties or self-perceived difficulties are the definition of a functional decline (Arseven, Chang, Arseven, & Emanuel, 2005). While assessing patients, it is important to determine the overall impact of their conditions as it relates to their ability to interact with

TABLE 3.1 Most Frequent Nursing Home Disease Admission Diagnoses

Hypertension	60.70%
Depression	44.00%
Conditions/diseases of mood or behavior	39.20%
Dementia	37.30%
Arthritis	31.40%
Diabetes mellitus	27.60%
Allergies	26.80%
Anemia	23.70%
Congestive heart failure	22.20%
Cerebrovascular accident (stroke)	21.90%
Other cardiovascular	19.70%
Alzheimer's disease	17.70%
Hypothyroidism	17.60%
Emphysema/COPD	16.40%
Anxiety disorder	14.60%
Cardiac dysrhythmia	13.40%
Arteriosclerotic heart disease	12.30%
Peripheral vascular disease	11.70%

Note: Center for Medicare and Medicaid Services. (2002). *Revised Long-Term Care Resident Assessment Instrument User's Manual for the Minimum Data Set (MDS), Version 2.* Atlanta, GA: Center for Medicare and Medicaid Services.

the environment. One patient may have suffered a cerebral vascular accident, have underlying hypertension, diabetes, and coronary artery disease, and be able to continue to work as an executive in a large corporation. Another patient with the same diagnosis may need maximum assistance, including placement in a long-term care facility. The difference between these two patients with the same medical conditions is their functional status.

Functional assessment is typically classified into basic and instrumental domains. The ordinary activities of basic functional daily living tasks can be categorized as self-care activities, activities involving moving around independently, and maintenance of bladder and bowel function. A person who can carry out all of these functions independently does not need the assistance of anyone else. Inability to perform any of these activities necessitates external assistance. Clearly, many patients are between these two ends of the spectrum. The amount of assistance necessary is a function of their level of dependence. For example, a person who only needs help bathing often requires assistance for 1–2 hr per day. A person who needs help feeding themselves is unable to move independently and is incontinent of bowel and bladder requires almost constant attendance.

The instrumental activities of daily living (IADL) evaluate individuals' ability to manage their living environment. These needs generally require more planning and higher levels of execution. Examples include ability to shop for and prepare food, clean the house and do the laundry, get to places beyond walking distance, use the telephone, manage money, and take medications. Again, a limitation in any of the above necessitates help from an outside source. Often limitations in these areas do not require daily assistance and are less expensive for the person to employ outside help. Many communities have meals-on-wheels, bus services to local shopping centers, and volunteers to help with light housekeeping, all for a nominal fee. Family members are often able to help manage the check book and arrange medications in pill boxes for their loved ones. As more IADLs are impaired, independence is often decreased and limitations of activities of daily living are also seen.

Commonly used instruments to assess one's functional status are the Katz Index of Activities of Daily Living (Katz, Ford, Moskowitz, Jackson, & Jaffe, 1963) and the IADL developed by Lawton and Brody (1969). These scales serve as instruments that can easily be performed in a short amount of time, with consistent results. Information is structured in a way that can be easily communicated to all members of the patient's care team. The scales are also useful in documenting changes over time and need for services and reimbursement. In using these scales, the sum is not equal to whole. The total score neither serves any use in the development of a plan nor does it give an impression of the degree of disability. It is each independent variable and the needs associated with it that are useful in guiding specific therapeutic plans (Williams, 1998).

Functional status can also be used to monitor treatment responses and provide prognostic information for a care plan (Arseven et al., 2005). As an example, a patient admitted to a long-term care facility after a stroke may not be able to toilet independently at admission. Goals set forth by the treatment teams, such as ability to transfer and walk 20 feet, translate into increased independence, exemplified by a restoration of independent toileting abilities in a home environment. Such outcomes are tracked as part of quality monitoring of the care provided by long-term care settings (Agency for Healthcare Research and Quality, 2004).

The goals of a patient in subacute rehabilitation and the patient who is a long-term resident are different in respect to their functional status. Common to both is the maintenance of the maximum amount of independence. In subacute rehabilitation, specific functional disabilities are identified and goals are set to regain independence in those areas. Alternatively, for many long-term care residents, independence in certain areas is not obtainable, and therefore these areas are identified as functions necessitating assistance or total help. The therapeutic goal is to provide assistance to compensate for the identified functional disability or disabilities, thus ensuring continued independent living to the maximum extent possible (Williams, 1998).

Psychiatric Diagnoses

Psychiatric diagnoses are quite prevalent in long-term care settings. As many as 80% of nursing home residents will have dementia or another diagnosable psychiatric disorder (Rovner et al., 1990). Furthermore, anywhere between 6 and 24% have a major depressive disorder diagnosis, 30 and 50% have minor depression or dysthymia, and as many as 35 and 45% manifest depressive symptoms. MDS reports 14.6% of long-term care patients have been diagnosed with anxiety disorder, though this rate may be deceptively low, given limitations in reporting anxiety symptoms within the MDS (Centers for Medicare and Medicaid Services, 2004). Despite the high rate of psychiatric disorders, most residents are not under the care of a mental health clinician. Typically, these services are provided by independent psychiatric consultants who see specific residents on an as needed, on call basis (Bartels, Moak, & Dums, 2002).

Psychiatric concerns are addressed in different ways by the team of professionals who care for the individual. Behavioral interventions may be made by recreation staff; social workers may provide therapeutic or supportive services to the resident and the family; and physicians participate in decisions about behavioral and psychosocial interventions as well as provide pharmacologic treatment (Depla et al., 2003). The Centers for Medicare and Medicaid Services (Boyle et al., 2004) report a 97% increase in antidepressant medications for all residents from 12.6 to 24.9%. Datto et al., (2002) suggest that current 35–60% of nursing home residents receive antidepressant medication.

Psychosocial Factors

New residents arrive at long-term care facilities with a long, complex life behind them. As such, they are likely to come with poorly defined premorbid issues. There could be mental health problems that may or may not have been diagnosed, acknowledged, and treated prior to the onset of change that brought them to the facility. Other psychosocial concerns that may not be obvious from reading a medical chart can also greatly impact a resident's physical and mental well-being. It is important to consider confounding issues related to the resident's transition to the long-term care facility, family dynamics that might be compounded by physical distance, discontinuity of medical care by a primary care physician and themes related to the resident's cultural background. An exploration of these factors highlights the importance of seeing each resident as a whole person.

The transition to the long-term care facility can often be a traumatic one, signifying loss of autonomy, physical and cognitive decline, failure of children to fulfill obligations of filial piety, a loss of familiar physical surroundings, and much more. Groger (1995) found that when the psychological preparation for relocation occurs before the actual move to the institution, transitional issues are mitigated. Furthermore, better outcomes are associated with a greater degree of empowerment on the part of the future resident regarding decisions to relocate. The way in which a resident is prepared to enter a long-term care facility can greatly influence the ease in which subsequent medical treatment decisions are determined.

Many patients arrive at a long-term care facility with an unclear prognostic status; for example, they experienced a medical event (i.e., stroke), are ready to be released from the hospital, but have not gotten better "enough" to return to noninstitutional living. This can result in denial of the reality of need for longer term institutional placement and conflict among family members with regard to decisions about their relative's treatment.

Moving a family member to a long-term care facility can challenge the strengths of the healthiest family system and can magnify deficits among those who are functioning more poorly to begin with. Conventional wisdom that a caregiver will be relieved of a great burden when a family member is moved to a nursing home has been challenged (see Schulz et al., 2004). For example, a daughter who no longer has to bathe, dress, and feed her mother, now has to negotiate for her parent's care at the facility, worry that she is being well cared for, and deal with her own guilt over "putting mother away."

Many times relocation to a long-term care facility requires moving to another part of the country. The phenomena of returning "snowbirds" in LTC facilities in the Northern US climates is increasingly recognized: individuals who had previously established a full life in retirement in Sunbelt states later return to colder climates for younger relatives to provide care. Though the resident has gained the closer care of his relative, he has lost the friends and care providers with whom he is most familiar. Different issues arise when family members live far from the long-term care facility. Family planning meetings are often seen as a primary way of assuring optimal care for a particular resident. Logistically, this is much harder to do when key decision makers live out of town. Though technology makes virtual meetings easier, conflict is more likely to ensue between relatives and care providers in the absence of face to face contact.

Another area impacting the transition process to a long-term care facility is the discontinuity in health care providers systems between acute care hospital and a long-term care setting (McGilton, 2002) The acute health care provider team that an older patient in a hospital has come to know—the physicians from various specialties, the nursing, professionals, and rehabilitative therapists—are all changed upon long-term care facility admission. Mold, Fryer, and Roberts (2004) present several benefits of continuity of care including: improved patient, physician, and staff satisfaction, increased trust of physician, better identification of medical problems, better coordination of care, more preventative services, decreased cost of care, and greater likelihood of patient disclosure of emotional problems. These benefits are particularly relevant for older adults who are likely to have several comorbid diseases, increased frailty, and require careful management of multiple medications.

It is also important to consider the cultural congruency of the decision to place a family member in long-term care. Historically, older adults with dementia from ethnic minorities were less likely to be placed in nursing homes. Data still reveal that White people are more likely than Black or Hispanic people to be placed in nursing homes (Kersting, 2001). This is sometimes explained by the "African–American Subculture Theory" suggesting that stronger ties to family and community within African–American communities would lead to an increased likelihood of frail elderly being cared for by family and community services (Belgrave, Wykle, & Choi, 1993 as cited in Kersting, 2001). Kersting (2001) also quotes Angel and Angel (1992) finding that elderly Blacks and Latinos "are more likely to live with family and less likely to live alone than Whites regardless of health levels" suggesting that family attitudes tend toward the young caring for their elderly within the family or community before considering institutional placement.

Other issues of ethnicity, beyond whether it is acceptable within a culture to place a family member in long-term care, exist once placement is made. A relative might be concerned that family members from an ethnic minority group would not be able to get the foods to which they are accustomed, participate in familiar prayer services, or have a peer group with whom to share a common language. This trend might be changing as a critical mass of minority individuals live in nursing homes. Other problems related to a history of previously cloaked or controlled prejudicial beliefs often come up with demented patients sharing a room with someone from a different ethnicity. A resident with dementia, who may not consider himself prejudiced, may have regressed to an earlier post-traumatic state reacting to a staff member of a different race in a violently prejudiced way. An example frequently given is that of an adverse reaction to a Southeast Asian staff member by a resident having served with the military in the South Pacific.

TYPOLOGY OF LONG-TERM CARE FACILITY RESIDENTS

A useful typology to consider the interaction between the mental and medical health needs of long-term care facility residents is based on the "trajectory" of the anticipated course of care within the facility. In this context, most residents can be considered to be actively rehabilitating, actively dying, or surviving. Table 3.2 presents a summation of the features of three broad categories of LTC residents. Following the discussion of each category, a clinical scenario is presented to illustrate the geriatric medical and mental health interface within the case history.

Actively Rehabilitating

The first category reflects the role that long-term care facilities play within the broader health care system in providing a site for rehabilitation following an acute illness. Acute care hospitals are the site where many such "rehab" patients start their recovery after an acute medical or surgical

TABLE 3.2 Typology of Long-Term Care Residents

Nature of resident	Typical medical diagnoses	Characteristic mental health issues	Common red flag presentations
Actively rehabilitating	Acute stroke; joint fracture/ replacement; major surgery; limb amputation; deconditioning after prolonged medical hospitalization	Self-care challenges; conflicts over body image; pain management	Slowed progress in rehabilitation; accelerating somatic complaints; anorexia
Actively dying	Metastatic cancers; end-stages of progressive chronic diseases	Pain; depression; anxiety; psychiatric features of brain lesions	Isolation and withdrawal; hallucinations; delirium
Surviving	Dementias; heart disease; Stroke; advanced Parkinsonism; emphysema	Learned helplessness; adjustment reactions; restlessness	Dementia-related behaviors; weight loss; resistance to care; excessive call bell use

experience. Indeed, in the context of elective surgical procedures such as joint replacement of an arthritic hip or knee that has been contemplated for some time by a patient and their physician, prehospital phase rehabilitation may have occurred before the actual surgical procedure.

More often, however, an acute traumatic event such as a hip fracture, heart attack, acute pneumonia, motor vehicle accident, or other serious and unexpected event is addressed initially in the acute care hospital. The acute recovery phase after such events then typically involve the discharge planning efforts on the collaborative part of both the hospital-based providers and the patient and/or their family. Depending upon the functional status of the patient and the resources available to them at home, further rehabilitation may be recommended to take place in a variety of different settings. Individuals who are ready to return home might receive treatment on an outpatient basis. Other, typically younger, individuals with both the required tolerance and motivation for aggressive and intensive rehabilitation efforts may spend time in a specially designated rehabilitation hospitals. Finally, others will go to what is termed subacute rehabilitation provided within long-term care facilities.

It is in this later category that many older adults, whose functional impairments resulting from their acute medical or surgical events preclude a return to a home, first face the prospect of "going to a nursing home." This often poses a conflict between frequent preconceived notions of nursing homes as being a destination rarely considered desirable versus the site where further progress in the recovery phase from their acute illness will occur. Many of the mental health issues confronted by these rehabilitating residents of long-term care facilities may arise from such conflicts between the preconceived negative images of nursing homes and the need to continue the recovery process while moving out of the acute care setting.

The role of physicians, central to much of the direct acute care issues provided in the hospitals, is very much diminished in long-term care settings. Physician involvement in the treatment of long-term care rehabilitation residents is still important in the monitoring of chronic conditions that may influence the trajectory of the rehabilitation process; however, having helped establish the game plan and priorities, physician care is largely supplanted by the nursing and rehabilitative therapists who are delivering the actual services, such as wound care, medications and the physical, occupational, speech and swallowing training, and other interventions that may be prescribed as part of the rehabilitation process. Many of these interventions are intended to require greater participation by the individual resident to demonstrate recovery of function and health. This can pose challenges to the self-care skills and desires of the resident, especially those whose initial passivity were fostered in the hospital setting but are now being pushed by the rehabilitation process to take on increasing responsibility for their own care and recovery.

Other common mental health issues that arise among the rehabilitating population in long-term care facility involve the conflict over an altered self-image facing their own physical changes and/or recognition of the vulnerability of their health and future welfare, given the recent acute health events. In the former category, perhaps the most obvious example is the adjustments required by individuals who have suffered a limb amputation, either on a traumatic basis or as part of a progressive vascular impairment condition like peripheral vascular disease or advanced diabetes. The challenges of bodily integrity perspectives must occur concurrent with the often demanding and physically exhausting efforts to regain mobility to varying degrees, whether mechanically aided and assisted with a wheelchair or prosthetic devices such as artificial limbs.

A more common manifestation however is the role that pain and physical discomfort play for the actively rehabilitating resident. Pain is viewed through many different lenses including cultural, past health experiences, and religious perspectives. The interaction between the views of the resident undergoing active rehabilitation and their therapists as it relates to pain management can play a large role in the degree of successful outcomes. A "no pain–no gain" attitude once prevalent in the rehabilitation setting has largely been replaced by an attempt to individualize the tolerance of all forms of physical discomfort with the needs for joint mobility, required skin wound care, or other specific rehabilitation measures that are often part of the daily routine within long-term care rehabilitation units (Feldt, 2004).

In this latter context, one of the common "red flag" indicators among rehabilitating populations that trigger the involvement of mental health professionals into their care is the perceived change in the rate of achieved rehabilitative progress. For example, an individual admitted into long-term care facility after a stroke, whose functional impairments in mobility and swallowing are being addressed by both physical therapy and speech pathology, will have periodic rehabilitation goals established by the therapists involved in their care. Such individualized therapeutic goals are often expressed in very concrete tasks such as the ability to ambulate 20 feet using a rolling walker or verbal spoken word fluency or a set number of percentages to be achieved by a certain date. Such specific goals are used within the long-term care facility's interdisciplinary care team to document the progress of the rehabilitation over time as well as to provide justification for the continuation of financial payment from sources such as Medicare or commercial insurances paying for the rehabilitation effort. The "failure" of a resident to meet specified rehabilitation goals is immediately identified by many members of the institution's health professional and administrative team as a cause for concern. Although in some instances, the mismatch between the resident's performance on the rehabilitative goals may reflect an unrealistic goal, most often the initial focus is to try to identify and correct any barriers that may prevent or impede the successful rehabilitation of the resident. Pain issues and less-than-optimal motivation for participation are often prime triggers for the enlisting of mental health care providers.

Clinical Case: Actively Rehabilitating

MB is an 85-year-old female who was admitted to subacute rehabilitation after a 4-day acute hospital stay for a large, acute cerebral stroke. On admission to the facility, MB had severe dysphasia, was nonverbal, did not seem to recognize her family, and was unable to dress herself, ambulate, or help with transfers. She was incontinent and had a dense right-sided motor weakness of both arm and leg. Feeding was accomplished by a nasal-gastric tube. MB is a widow with no children. Before admission to the hospital, MB lived in an apartment and was independent in activities of daily living. She required the assistance of a live-in companion and a niece for shopping and food preparation as well as management of medications and finances. The niece describes MB as a very proud woman who cherished her independence. When long-term goals were discussed with the niece, she indicated a desire to have MB return to her own apartment, with long-term care in a skilled nursing facility considered a last resort.

During the first few days, MB did not try to help herself, despite indications that she was physically able to do so. When utensils were placed in her left hand she made no attempt to feed herself, though she would be seen coughing into her left hand. She would not move when asked to stretch her left foot, but was able to move it when she was in an awkward position. The care team met early in MB's stay to discuss her lack of progress. Even though it was unclear whether she would understand, it was decided to include MB in a discussion of her treatment goals, reflecting her desire to maintain her independence with an eye toward returning MB to her own home.

The day after the meeting, MB began to try to feed herself with the speech therapists help. It was determined that her swallowing function was improving, and MB was provided with foods her niece suggested she preferred. Within 1 week, MB was able to swallow thickened liquids and pureed food. It was determined that she would be able to maintain hydration and nutritional status through her own improved swallowing skills and her feeding tube was removed.

Over the course of the next month MB continued to progress, showing signs of recognizing her niece by smiling when she would walk on the floor to visit and interacted more positively with the nursing staff. She also gained some mobility of her right arm and leg. Her aphasia remained, though she began to speak when she read a sign or label, but did not seem to understand what she was reading. She learned to feed herself with her left hand, assist with transfers, propel herself in a wheelchair using her left leg and help with dressing and toileting. MB's prior home aide companion was brought into the treatment plan and taught by the facility staff about her care needs, spending 8 hr a day at the facility. MB eventually was successfully discharged to her own apartment with her companion.

Actively Dying

In contrast to those long-term care facility residents undergoing active rehabilitative efforts, there exists a smaller proportion of facility residents who have been identified as being in the end stages of their health condition. Although, obviously, many older residents within long-term care are nearing the end of their natural life, the health care perspective for this particular group of residents is classified here as "actively dying;" those formally recognized as no longer "living with" their conditions but rather now "dying from" their ailments. This construct is obviously a fluid distinction, in that medical science's ability to make accurate prognostic judgments about a given patient's immediate future course is quite limited beyond the final few hours and days of life. Despite this, the MDS data collection tool used in nursing homes does identify those residents with a limited prognosis of 6 months or less. The most commonly cited diagnoses among these residents include those with solid cancers of various cellular types which have been identified as having metastasized or widely spread throughout the body so that interventions focused on curing through either surgical treatments cutting out the lesion or the use of radiation, chemical chemotherapies, or immunological/genetic interventions can no longer be considered effective (Buchanan, Choi, Wang, & Ju, 2004). In addition to cancer diagnoses, however, recent efforts have also sought to better define the end stage of noncancer chronic conditions such as advanced AIDS, ischemic heart diseases, or progressive neurological conditions.

Many long-term care facilities will seek a contractual relationship with a hospice organization to assist the facility in the care of dying residents who may choose to have their insurance switched into a hospice organization. In 2000, about 60% of the newly admitted long-term care facility residents whose MDS indicated a limited prognosis were formally under a hospice organization's care (Miller, Mor, & Teno, 2003). Hospice organizations require a physician determination of an estimated prognosis of less than 6 months of life be made, though in practice most individuals who are admitted into a hospice care entities die much sooner. Many long-term care facility residents who are actively dying, however, will not be formally under the care of a hospice organization during their terminal long-term care facility stay and the mental health issues mentioned here are not applicable just to those clients.

Mental health issues that arise among such residents whose care is explicitly centered on terminal care is first and foremost one of relief of pain and discomfort, along with its associated depression and despondency (Miller et al., 2003). The dying process is highly individualized and will often incorporate the attitudes and approaches of those surrounding the dying individual, including the professional care giving staff of the facility as well as the family, caregivers, and friends.

Challenging issues that also arise within the mental health care of such individuals can stem from organic brain lesions associated with the terminal illness. Structural brain lesions can produce unique and often quite disabling behavioral manifestations. Features such as personality changes can result from frontal brain lobe lesions. Hallucinatory or delusional perceptions can also be associated with delirium episodes related to metabolic endocrinologic effects of some cancers. Although the occurrence of these rather dramatic events are evident to all discussed typologies, other more subtle red flag triggers in this population of long-term residents include the isolation and withdrawal from the institutional life.

Clinical Case: Actively Dying

CK is a 79-year-old African–American female who was admitted to the long-term care facility for hospice care after a short hospitalization. CK had a long history of dementia and had previously been taken care of by her daughter in her daughter's home. CK also had a history of hypertension and hypercholesterolemia. Her dementia had progressed so that she was no longer ambulatory, unable to help in transfers, was nonverbal, and completely dependent for all needs. Her daughter worked outside the home 8 hr a day, during which time an aide came to stay with the patient. At baseline, the patient spent all day in bed, ate, and drank only if food was brought to her mouth, and responded only to painful stimuli. CK's daughter reported that approximately 1 week prior to admission she began to not open her mouth during feeding. She also noted that the patient had had a small sacral decubitus pressure skin ulcer, which had recently become painful. Additional pressure sores on both hips as well as both heels and lateral ankles were also diagnosed during the hospital stay just prior to long-term care facility admission. The geriatric team and CK's daughter discussed the grave prognosis of such end stage markers of advanced dementia and it was elected to pursue LTC facility admission for hospice services.

CK was admitted to the long-term care facility and immediately started on a long-acting narcotic agent for pain control delivered by a transdermal patch, along with a short-acting buccal morphine preparation for breakthrough pain. Her family brought in some items of significance to her, including an afghan and pictures of her family. Food and drink were offered to CK frequently, but she was not forced to eat or drink. Effective pain control was evidenced by CK no longer yelling out in pain during routine care, and her gradual willingness to eat and drink. When she began to take oral medications, she was started on a low dose of a selective serotonin reuptake inhibitor (SSRI) to address what was felt to be underlying depression and anxiety. CK's face was noted to be more relaxed, no longer with a furrowed brow. If she indicated at all that she was in pain, medications were adjusted accordingly. She also began to turn her head toward the door when she would hear her daughter's voice. CK died approximately 5 weeks after her admission.

"Surviving"

The largest proportion of long-term care facility residents compromise those which here are being classified here as surviving. This term is intended primarily to reflect the fact that such residents are not undergoing rehabilitative efforts actively, due to the static nature of their impairments or the chronicity of the conditions; however, their prognosis has not been formally determined to be immediately limited. The most typical of these residents are those with various stages of dementias such as Alzheimer's disease. Such slowly progressive dementias often have caused an extent of functional impairment that requires institutional care but has not yet led to immediate threats to continued survival. Such dementing illnesses may either be explicitly identified as the primary diagnosis for the individual or be listed among a variety of chronic conditions that have accumulated to an extent that institutional placement was required. Often the coexistence of dementia with depression further complicates the therapeutic prioritization, as both highly prevalent and interactive conditions are often not formally recognized among the "more medical" admitting diagnoses (Burrows, Satlin, Salzman, Nobel, & Lipsitz, 1995).

The institutional approach to the mental health needs of such surviving residents may include concerns of learned helplessness. One manifestation of this is illustrated by the use of wheelchairs for mobility within many nursing home settings. Many communal activities within long-term care facilities occur within the time constraints of staff and institutional protocols that often do not easily adapt to the extra time required for the most independent ambulation techniques. Therefore, though the extent of mobility functional impairment is highly variable, often ranging from those who could make use of canes, walker, or other standing mobility assistance and self-propel themselves standing to those who could also self-propel but use a wheelchair, many surviving long-term care facility residents find themselves being pushed about in wheelchair to meals, activities, toileting or bathing requirements, and other settings. The extent of such enforced helplessness may vary greatly across facilities with differing perspectives staffing and institutional intent.

Clinical Case: Surviving

CL is a 75-year-old male who was admitted to a skilled nursing facility as a long-term care patient. He previously lived at home with his daughter and son-in-law before the worsening of his chronic breathing problems and the placement of a urinary bladder catheter exceeded the ability of his family to care for him. CL often felt short of breath and during acute exacerbations of his emphysema would call for his daughter, seeking reassurance. He also began to worry in anticipation of his next "attack," constantly seeking assurance that his daughter there "just in case." He required six routine nebulizer bronchodilator breathing treatments daily, as well as frequent "rescue" treatments for episodic periods of perceived breathlessness. At least one treatment was necessary during the night. CL also suffered from acute anxiety in the late afternoon and evening, frequently referred to as "sundowning." During these periods CL would become very anxious and occasionally verbally abusive. CL was resistant to taking medications, stating adamantly that medications made his breathing worse. Other concurrent diagnoses included mild dementia and moderate sensory impairment of both hearing and vision.

CL's daughter was becoming increasingly distressed by her father's situation and felt that her marriage and health were suffering. CL refused the help of aides hired by his daughter. CL's daughter eventually told him that she was not able to take care of him at home any longer.

CL's experience increased upon arrival at the long-term care facility. He pressed the call button approximately once every 15 min, requesting a drink of water or a tissue or a cough drop. He refused to come out of his room and insisted on having his meals in bed, stating that if he got out of bed he would have a "breathing attack." When his daughter visited, he would talk incessantly about his medical problems. His daughter attended the first team meeting and expressed concern that her father seemed even more anxious. CL was brought in the meeting and was able to hear his daughter share these concerns. CL related that he was afraid that no one would respond to his "breaking attacks" and that he would die. It was brought to his attention that his call bell was always answered promptly and that he had yet to suffer an attack. A plan was made with the team, CL, and his daughter to initiate an acetylcholinesterase inhibitor focused on his dementia diagnosis as well as try an antidepressant from among the SSRI class. His daughter was encouraged to ask her father to only talk about his medical problems for a set amount of time during her visits and insist on talking about other topics. The nursing staff committed to CL that they would deliver his routine treatments on time, as well as follow-up with him after any physical activity to see if he required additional treatments. CL has since been seen often in the dining room and at activities. His daughter reports that he only discusses his medical problems approximately five times a week and for less than 15 min each time. CL's attacks have decreased in frequency and he no longer becomes agitated in the evenings.

MODELS FOR PROACTIVE GERIATRIC MEDICAL MENTAL HEALTH DELIVERY

A collaborative effort by the American Geriatric Society and American Association of Geriatric Psychiatry (2003) focused on the perceived inadequacies of delivering mental health services in long-term care facilities. Two major publications resulted from this effort: the first was a detailed listing of specific recommendations for the care of long-term care facility residents with both depression and behavioral symptoms caused by dementing illnesses; the second provides policy recommendations that could support the delivery of the quality-driven recommendations. In the former document, the importance of depression was clearly recognized as being at such a prevalence level, estimated at 22% of the nursing home residents, this screening was recommended as part of the initial 2-week admission process and then repeated on a semiannual basis thereafter. The expert panel recognized that this was in part the intent of existing regulatory instruments utilized as part of the federal financing and administrative structure within nursing homes, namely, the MDS. The clinical utility of this essentially administratively driven data collection instrument in accurately detecting depression was held suspect and a more clinically focused screening was suggested. Once recognized, the interaction of mental health providers with the facility-based staff of nurses and other disciplines were encouraged to develop combined approaches of nonpharmacologic and antidepressant medication interventions. The role of the geriatric physician in coordinating and supporting these interventions is stressed, as is the need to consider enlisting formal psychiatric physician involvement if the depressed resident's clinical improvement is not apparent within the initial 6 weeks of treatment.

The recommendations for dementia-related behavioral symptom management are based on an even greater prevalence of mental health needs, in that an estimated 40% of those residents of nursing homes with diagnosed dementia will have significant behavioral and/or psychiatric symptoms. Although depression can have a myriad of presentations and features among the various concurrent illnesses, functional impairment profiles, and premorbid personality issues seen in long-term care facility residents, there exist even greater heterogeneity among the dementia-linked behavioral disturbances. Alzheimer's disease, Lewy body dementia, vascular dementias, frontal-temporal lobe dementias, chronic alcohol abuse-induced dementia states, metabolic dementias syndromes arising from vitamin deficiencies, infectious-induced encephalopathy dementias, cognitive impairments resulting from chronic exposures to occupational toxins, and traumatic brain injury states—all represent disease states that, either in isolation or combination, give rise to dementia syndromes seen among long-term care residents (Camp, Cohen-Mansfield, & Capezuti, 2002).

This considerable heterogeneity among the types of dementia processes seen in long-term care is matched by the range of inappropriate behaviors observed among residents with such dementia. One useful construct in considering the behavior concerns of dementia includes a hierarchical grouping based on severity and disruption. Aggressive behaviors such as hitting, biting, and cursing are considered to be of highest priority and in the past have served as justification for some of the infamous and inappropriate interventions by nursing homes of the past to control behavior, such as the widespread use of physical restraints and indiscriminate dosing of powerful antipsychotic agents in a blanket attempt to "tranquilize away" such behaviors. Physical nonaggressive behaviors such as wandering, restlessness, and inappropriate fondling constitute a second, less obtrusive grouping of dementia behaviors that also are somewhat disruptive within an institutional setting. The final grouping includes verbal agitation, whether consisting of actual language or simply frequent sound expressions.

The response to such dementia-related behaviors, like that of depression described earlier, is deemed optimal when involving both a mix of disciplines from the start, as well as blending of interventions. Nonpharmacologic measures are often considered of primary importance in such responses, involving a mental health care provider in helping the long-term facility staff identify any unmet needs on the part of the resident who is "acting out," is an important first step. Interventions that have been shown, to varying degrees of effectiveness, to provide some relief include enhancing social support and physical contact in a preventive effort before the escalation of the targeted behavior, providing diverting engaging activities that seek to substitute and acceptable outlet for the inappropriate behavior, and assuring that the behavior is not in itself an expression of discomfort, pain, or another medically relevant symptom that, because of the dementia, is being expressed aberrantly (Ellet, 2005). The various disciplines that constitute the interdisciplinary teams used within LTC settings are often encouraged to contribute outcome markers for judging the effectiveness of such interventions, often looking at the combined results from pharmacologic agents along with such behavioral strategies (Cafiero & Hajjar, 2005).

CONCLUSIONS

Annually with the U.S., almost 2 million adults are admitted to one of the 16,800 nursing homes in the United States (Rhoades & Krauss, 1999). The recent growth of assisting living facilities—now estimated at over 36,000 facilities serving about 1 million residents (Stefanacci, 2005)—complements these nursing homes within the spectrum of long-term care facilities. The challenge of integrating mental health into the care of the aging within these varied long-term care settings is a reflection of the nomenclature. Nursing homes are not "hospitals" from the perspective of the residents, many of whom will spend their final phase of life in such settings (Bergman-Evans, 2004); but the level of supportive services provided in them, as well as within the assisted living setting as well far exceeds what is provide in homes, given the range of diagnostic conditions and their resulting functional and mental health limitations imposed on the elderly resident. The presented typology of existing models of integrating mental health services into the care of residents and the proactive models focused on high impact issues of depression and dementia will facilitate the optimal integrated care provision of both medical and mental health providers for the care of future long-term care residents.

REFERENCES

Agency for Healthcare Research and Quality. (2004). National Healthcare Quality Report. AHRQ Publication #05-0013. US Department Health and Human Services December 2004.

American Geriatric Society, American Association for Geriatric Psychiatry. (2003). Consensus statement on improving the quality of mental health care in U.S. nursing homes: Management of depression and behavioral symptoms associated with dementia. *Journal of the American Geriatric Society, 51*(9) 1287–1298.

Angel, J. L., & Angel, R. J. (1992). Age at migration, social connections, and well-being among elderly Hispanics. *Journal of Aging & Health, 4*(4), 480–499.

Arseven A., Chang, C. H., Arseven, O. K., & Emanuel L. L. (2005). Assessment instruments. *Clinics in Geriatric Medicine, 21*(1), 121–146.

Bartels, S. J., Moak, G. S., & Dums, A. R. (2002). A model of mental health services in nursing homes: A review of the literature. *Psychiatric Services, 53*(11), 1390–1396.

Bergman-Evans, B. (2004). Nursing homes, not nursing hospitals. *Journal of Gerontological Nursing, 30*(6), 3.

Belgrave, L. L., Wykle, M. L., & Choi, J. M. (1993). Health, double jeopardy, and culture: the use of institutionalization by African-Americans. *Gerontologist, 33*(3), 379–385.

Boyle, V. L., Roychoudhury, C., Beniak, R., Cohn, L., Bayer, A., & Katz, I. (2004). Recognition and management of depression in skilled-nursing and long-term care settings: evolving targets for quality improvement. *American Journal of Geriatric Psychiatry, 12*(3), 288–295.

Buchanan, R. J., Choi, M., Wang, S., Ju, H. (2004). End-of-life care in nursing homes: Residents in hospice compared to other end-stage residents. *Journal of Palliative Medicine, 7*(2), 221–232.

Burrows, A. B., Satlin, A., Salzman, C., Nobel, K., & Lipsitz, L. A. (1995). Depression in a long-term care facility: Clinical features and discordance between nursing assessment and patient interviews. *Journal of the American Geriatrics Society, 43*(10), 1118–1122.

Camp, C., Cohen-Mansfield, J., & Capezuti, E. A. (2002). Mental health services in nursing homes: Use of nonpharmacologic interventions among nursing home residents with dementia. *Psychiatric Services, 52*(11), 1397–1404.

Cafiero, A., & Hajjar, E. (2005). Beyond dispensing: The role for the clinical pharmacist in assisted living facilities. *Assisted Living Consult, 1*(1), 30–33.

Centers for Medicare and Medicaid Services. (2002). *Revised long term care resident assessment instrument. User's manual for the minimum data set (MDS), Version 2*. Atlanta, GA: Center for Medicare and Medicaid Services.

Centers for Medicare and Medicaid Services. (2004). *MDS Active Resident Information Report: Fourth Quarter 2004*. Retrieved March 8, 2005 from http://www3.cms.hhs.gov/states/mdsreports/res2.asp.

Datto, C. J., Oslin, D. W., Streim, J. E., Scheinthal, S. M., DiFilippo, S., & Katz, I. R. (2002). Pharmacologic treatment of depression in nursing home residents: A mental health services perspective. *Journal of Geriatric Psychiatry & Neurology, 15*(3), 141–146.

Dening, T., & Bains, J. (2004). Mental health services for residents of care homes. *Age and Aging, 33*, 1–2.

Depla, M., Polsm, J., de Lange, J., Smits, C., deGraad, R., & Heeren, T. (2003). Integrating mental health care into residential homes for the elderly: An analysis of six Dutch programs for older people with severe and persistent mental illness. *Journal of American Geriatric Society, 51*(9), 1275–1279.

Ellet, A. (2005). Caring for those with dementia in assisted living. *Assisted Living Consult, 1*(1), 8–13.

Feldt, K. S. (2004). The complexity of managing pain for frail elders. *Journal of the American Geriatrics Society, 52*(5), 840–841.

Groger, L. (1995). A nursing home can be a home. *Journal of Aging Studies, 9*(2), 137–153.

Jones, A. (2002). The National Nursing Home Survey: 1999 Summary. *National Center for Health Statistics. Vital Health Stat 13*(152). Retrieved March 8, 2005 from http://www.cdc.gov/nchs/data/series/sr_13/sr13_152.pdf.

Katz, S., Ford, A. B., Moskowitz, R. W., Jackson, B. A., Jafffee, M. W. (1963). Studies of illness in the aged. The index of ADL: A standardized measure of biological and psychosocial function. *Journal of the American Medical Association, 185*, 914–919.

Kersting, R. C. (2001). Impact of social support, diversity, and poverty on nursing home utilization in a national representative sample of older Americans. *Social Work in Health Care, 33*(2), 67–87.

Lawton, M. P., & Brody, E. (1969). Assessment of older people: Self-maintaining and instrumental activities of daily living. *Gerontologist*, 9, 179–186.

McGilton, K. S. (2002). Enhancing relationships between care providers and residents in long-term care: Designing a model of care. *Journal of Gerontological Nursing, 28*(12), 13–21.

Miller, S. C., Mor, V., Teno, J. (2003). Hospice enrollment and pain assessment and management in nursing homes. *Journal of Pain & Symptom Management, 26*(3), 791–799.

Mold, J. W., Fryer, G. E., & Roberts, A. M. (2004). Why do older patients change primary care physicians? *Journal of the American Board of Family Practice, 17*(6), 453–460.

Rhoades, J. A., Krauss, N. A. (1999). *Nursing home trends, 1987 and 1996 MEPS Chartbook No. 3.* (AHCPR Pub. No. 99-0032). Rockville, MD: Agency for Health Care Policy and Research, Public Health Service, US Department of Health and Human Services.

Rovner, B. W., German, P. S., Broadhead, J., Morriss, R. K., Brant, L. J., Blaustein, J., Folstein, M. F. (1990). The prevalence and management of dementia and other psychiatric disorders in nursing homes. *International Psychogeriatrics, 2*(1), 13–24.

Sahyoun, N. R., Pratt, L. A., Lentzner, H., Dey, A., Robinson, K. N. (2001). The changing profile of nursing home residents: 1985–1997. *Aging Trends, 4*, 1–8.

Schulz, R., Belle, S., Czaja, S. J., McGinnis, K. A., Stevens, A., Zhang, S. (2004). Long-term care placement of dementia patients and caregiver health and well-being. *Journal of the American Medical Association, 292*(8), 961–967.

Stefanacci, R. G. (2005). Assisted living consult: What's in a name? *Assisted Living Consult, 1*(1), 6–7.

Williams, T. F. (1998). Comprehensive geriatric assessment. In E. H. Duthie, Jr., & P. R. Katz (Eds.), *Practice of geriatrics* (3rd ed., pp. 15–22). Philadelphia: WB Saunders Co.

CHAPTER FOUR

Psychiatric Intervention in Long-Term Care

Shailaja Shah and William E. Reichman

Effective psychiatric evaluation and treatment relies on an appreciation of the important contributions of biological, psychological, and social factors to the expression of mental illness. The biopsychosocial approach (Engel, 1980), so broadly embraced in contemporary psychiatric intervention, represents a vital component of care in the long-term residential setting. In the nursing home, mental disorders such as depression, anxiety, psychosis, verbal and physical agitation, aggression, and seemingly purposeless motor behaviors such as pacing, are often the consequence of patient attributes such as dementia, physical discomfort, and sensory deprivation interacting with the environmental and social influences of the surrounding milieu. When the biological, psychological and social determinants of mental disorder are effectively addressed in the long-term care setting, affected residents are more functionally adept and are more able to experience a heightened sense of personal well-being, engagement in the environment, competence, and purpose.

This chapter will briefly review the prevalence and phenomenology of mental disorder in the long-term care setting, some of the biological, psychological, and social factors that are contributory and emerging approaches to diagnosis and treatment.

In a review of the literature, Bartels, Maok, and Dums (2002) identified three possible models for mental health care delivery: psychiatrist-centered models that emphasize the role of the psychiatrist as the primary and often sole provider of direct consultation and clinical services; multidisciplinary team models that include a variety of mental health clinicians with different roles and responsibilities (typically a psychiatrist, most commonly in combination with nurses, social workers, and/or psychologists); and nurse-centered models that revolve around a geropsychiatric nurse specialist who coordinates the services of extrinsic mental health professionals while providing training to develop the mental health skills of intrinsic nursing staff. Unfortunately, there are no data on the prevalence of these or other models of delivery, and no data on which models are most efficacious or cost-effective. The intent of this chapter is to provide the reader with a view that allows for a better understanding of the integrative benefits of geropsychiatry in the application of the psychosocial treatments in LTC.

THE SCOPE OF THE PROBLEM

The contemporary nursing home in the United States resembles a long-term, geropsychiatric hospital with rates of diagnosable mental illness in the resident population ranging from 65 to 91% (Rovner, Kafonek, Filipp, Lucas, & Folstein, 1986). Nearly two thirds of nursing home residents have dementia of which 30–40% demonstrate associated behavioral and psychiatric symptoms (Tariot, Podgorski, Blazina, & Leibovici, 1993). Dementia's cognitive and psychiatric features account for nearly 50% of admissions to nursing homes. Some commonly observed dementia-associated disturbed behaviors that appear to occur in more than 20% of nursing home residents include depression, restlessness, active aggression, passive aggression, verbal aggression, and wandering (Burrows, Satlin, Salzman, Nobel, & Lipsitz, 1995; Rovner et al., 1986). Kim and Rovner (1996) reported that approximately 30–50% of nursing home residents are clinically depressed, with 15% meeting the criteria for a current major depressive episode by the application of structured diagnostic criteria, and the remainder experiencing significant, but subsyndromal depressive symptoms (minor depression).

Psychiatric disorders translate into other day-to-day problems in LTC settings. Dementia with its associated psychiatric and behavioral symptoms and depression has significant consequences for the affected individual and the long-term care milieu. Affected residents have comparatively worse health outcomes, a greater likelihood of physical injury, increased hospitalization rates, and greater use of emergency services (American Geriatrics Society and American Association for Geriatric Psychiatry, 2003). Dementia and depression also interfere with the staff's ability to provide care to the resident, contributing to lowered staff morale and increased staff turnover (Snowden, Sato, & Roy-Byrne, 2003).

Despite a wealth of studies demonstrating the significant prevalence of mental disorders in nursing homes, access to comprehensive mental health assessment and care remains elusive for many facilities and their resident populations. Reichman et al. (1998) surveyed nearly 2000 nursing homes in six states to examine the availability and perceived adequacy of psychiatric consultation in nursing homes, as reported by Directors of Nursing. They found that within the 900 facilities that responded to the survey, 38% of residents were reportedly in need of formal psychiatric evaluation and treatment. Psychiatric services were noted to be adequately available in only half of the responding nursing homes. Two thirds of the facilities reported that their residents received "adequate" psychiatric diagnosis and medication treatment, while nonpharmacologic interventions for mental illness were reported as adequate by less than one third of the facilities. Effective staff education, assistance with facility–family conflicts, and help with staff stress were reportedly inadequately provided in two-thirds of the facilities. The greatest unmet need for psychiatric services existed in smaller sized and rurally placed nursing homes. Analyzing the same survey data, Borson et al. (2000) reported on nursing home staff expertise in managing mental health problems among the residents under their care. These investigators noted that the Directors of Nursing in 900 skilled nursing facilities reported that 49% of nurses had "a good deal of expertise" in "managing disruptive behavior" as compared to 56% of social workers, 32% of medical directors, 32% of aides, and 22% of attending physicians. No data were available on the presumed expertise of psychologists or pharmacists.

Other investigators have drawn attention to the gap that exists between the need for formal mental health interventions in nursing homes and the lack of available manpower. Colenda et al. (1999) reported that only 1.7% of general psychiatrists provide services in nursing homes. Only 3% of practicing psychologists see older patients as their primary work (Qualls, Segal, Norman, Niederehe, & Gallagher-Thompson, 2002) and less than 3% of master's degree candidates in social work specialize in aging (Browne, Braun, Mokuau, & McLaughlin, 2002). In a study of mental health service delivery, Burns et al. (1993) reported that over a 1-month period, only 4.5% of mentally ill nursing home residents received mental health services. Other investigators reported that only 19% of mentally ill residents, excluding persons with dementia, received treatment at least once during their total length of stay (Smyer et al, 1994). Shea, Clark, and Smyer (1995) noted that 5 years after the enactment of OBRA'87, only 29% of the residents with a mental illness, other than dementia, received treatment by mental health professionals during the year.

OPTIMIZING MENTAL HEALTH IN LONG-TERM CARE

A number of authors then have drawn attention toward the prevalence of mental disorders in the long-term care setting and the barriers to care that have existed for decades (Emerson, Fogel, Robinson, & Weiss, 1996). A consistent theme in the literature is that environment plays an important role in provoking and exacerbating problem behaviors. Nursing homes, where the active identification and attention to resident needs are the primary focus of providing care, tend to perform well in terms of the overall quality of care. Unfortunately, some nursing homes rely too heavily on psychotropic medication interventions to manage behavior problems. Other nursing homes utilize a multimodal treatment strategy, including observation, monitoring, addressing environmental factors, and implementing behavior management techniques. In order to utilize both behavioral and pharmacologic interventions, one needs to adequately diagnose the underlying problem taking into consideration the interaction between biological, psychological, and social factors. Nursing homes need adequate staffing to identify and intervene with behavioral problems. They need to encourage and provide staff training in nonpharmacologic interventions for behavior symptoms. However, as behavior management is not listed as a separate billable entity under Medicare and Medicaid, this serves as a disincentive to the provision of this crucial intervention (Emerson et al., 1996).

Regulatory and other stakeholder efforts continue to strive to improve the recognition and treatment of mental health problems in the nursing home environment. With the recognition that the identification and treatment of mental disorders in the long-term care setting must be done in partnership across professional disciplines (medicine, psychiatry, psychology, social work, nursing, pharmacy, and administration), a number of professional associations have begun to issue collaborative position papers. Under the leadership of the American Geriatrics Society and the American Association for Geriatric Psychiatry, an expert panel has published a consensus statement on "Quality Mental Health Care in Nursing Homes" (American Geriatrics Association and American Association for Geriatric Psychiatry, 2003). The panel established a number of overarching principles to guide the improvement of policy and practice in caring for the mental health needs of nursing home residents. These principles reinforce the need for the nursing home milieu to be structured and operated in such a way as to promote the mental health of the resident population. These principles assert that:

- Persons living in nursing homes should be allowed to maintain an autonomous and pleasant lifestyle. They should also be treated with respect and dignity.
- High-quality mental health care relies on the presence of high-quality medical care.
- State and Federal regulatory efforts must focus on treatment as well as on assessment.
- Appropriately qualified mental health specialty providers must be adequately reimbursed to assess and treat residents with mental health problems.
- An atmosphere that encourages residents to develop trusting relationships, feel supported, and feel that they are productive must be cultivated by staff at all levels and supported by the leadership of the nursing home. Residents need to retain as much autonomy as possible. They need to be allowed to make choices as to when they wake up, when they take care of daily chores, or whether they want to be alone or to participate in the day's group activities.
- Nursing homes must maintain adequate and permanent staffing in order to personalize and strengthen staff–resident relationships.
- A nursing home environment that is less institutional and more homelike with the presence of pets, plants, and children promotes a higher quality of life and aids the management of resident depression and behavioral symptoms.

ASSESSMENT OF THE RESIDENT: GENERAL PRINCIPLES

Psychiatric assessment of the nursing home resident involves a search for all biological, psychological, social and environmental factors that may underlie the expression of mental illness. Assessment involves a comprehensive review of medical records, interview of all potential informants (nurses, aides, administration, family members), and physical and mental status examination of the resident. The assessment is focused on ruling out underlying medical etiologies (e.g., urinary tract infection) and looking for any evidence of environmental stressors or precipitating factors that could have triggered the psychiatric symptoms. Important evaluation components include a pain assessment, exploration of sensory deficits, investigation of drug interactions and side effects, and a determination of whether the psychiatric or behavioral symptoms represent an unmet physical need (e.g., hunger, need to void).

It is also important to evaluate other patient-centered factors that may be contributory to the mental symptoms that are under scrutiny. The cognitive portion of the mental status examination should explore the patient's capacity to express thoughts and feelings verbally and to comprehend spoken language. Impairment in language ability (aphasia) can contribute to inadequate communication between the resident and other residents and between the resident and the nursing home staff. Such labored communication can contribute to staff frustration and resident expressions of disturbed behavior such as resisting assistance, overt hostility, or anxiety. In addition to language, the domains of memory, attention, concentration, executive functioning (planning and organization), and visuospatial ability should also be formally assessed. Impairments in these cognitive areas, as are seen in dementia, can undermine the resident's ability to successfully participate in care and to cope with the demands and potential deprivations of the nursing home milieu. The mental status examination must also focus on assessment of the resident's mood and sense of well-being, autonomy, mastery and control. Aside from what the resident is able or not able to verbalize, close scrutiny of the resident's affect, physical appearance and psychomotor behavior is of paramount importance (e.g., sadness, apathy, anxiety, anger, fear, signs of physical discomfort, restlessness, slowness). The interview also assesses whether there is voiced or behavioral evidence of psychosis, such as paranoid delusions or hallucinations.

The importance of a thorough evaluation of potential environmental or social influences on the resident's observed display of mental illness cannot be overstated. It is essential to determine whether the disturbed behavior or expression of depressive symptoms occurs in certain settings within the facility, at a particular time of day, during specific activities, or when the resident is in the company of certain staff members, family members, other visitors, or other residents of the facility. It is very important to determine whether there are adequate opportunities for the resident to experience privacy, make decisions, and access those social and recreational activities that promote and support pleasure, gratification, autonomy, independence, mastery, and a sense of self-worth and importance.

ASSESSMENT OF DEPRESSION

As depression so frequently complicates the care of nursing home residents, but often goes unrecognized (NIH, 1992), consensus guidelines for the screening of these symptoms have been recently developed by an expert panel convened by the American Geriatrics Society and the American Association for Geriatric Psychiatry (American Geriatrics

Association and American Association for Geriatric Psychiatry, 2003). These guidelines state that depression screening should be done 2–4 weeks after admission and at least every 6 months, thereafter. In addition, the new onset of depressive symptoms should prompt an assessment of psychological, situational, and medical factors.

Depression screening instruments must be utilized for the identification of depressed residents and assessment of treatment effectiveness. The Minimum Data Set (MDS) is inadequate by itself as a screening tool. However, self-reporting scales such as the Geriatric Depression Scale (GDS) (Yesavage, 1998) or Beck Depression Inventory (Beck et al., 1961) are indicated in patients with mild-to-moderate dementia. Observer-rated scales, such as the Cornell Scale for Depression in Dementia (Alexopoulous, Abrams, Young, & Shamoian, 1998b), are indicated in patients with moderate-to-severe dementia. Importantly, the resident who tends to be quiet and withdrawn, and may not be especially help-seeking or demanding, may be depressed and prone to be overlooked. Symptoms of lethargy and social withdrawal have been noted in the nursing home to be predictive as possible indicators of depression (Fenton et al., 2004). Residents with new-onset depression or worsening of depressive symptoms should receive an evaluation focusing on those current symptoms constituting a mood disorder, any past history of depression and treatment, current response to treatment, suicidal ideation, changes in cognitive function, and any contributory changes in the resident's social or family situation. In addition, the possibility of new stressors or situational factors, such as a change in staff, identification of unmet needs, availability of meaningful social, and recreational activities, and other positive well-being reinforcing activities are to be evaluated.

As mentioned above, a thorough medical examination should be included in the assessment of new-onset depression or worsening of depression. This exam must focus on pain assessment, nutritional status, worsening of chronic medical conditions, recent onset of a new medical condition, and the administration of medications that can possibly alter mood or cognition. Unless recent results are available, one must consider laboratory and diagnostic testing as determined by the findings of the history and physical examination. Testing may include a complete blood count, thyroid function, electrolytes including serum calcium and magnesium, Vitamin B12 level, and urinalysis (for evidence of a urinary tract infection). The guidelines also note that the presence of suicidal thoughts or psychosis or failure to respond to 6 or more weeks of treatment should initiate a referral to a mental health professional.

The Clinical Practice Guidelines (CPG) Project initiated by the American Medical Directors Association (AMDA) (American Medical Directors Association, 1996) has provided a recommended approach to assessment and treatment of depression in long-term care settings. The AMDA guidelines state that an interdisciplinary assessment is crucial to identifying signs and symptoms of depression. Further, they recommend the use of scales like GDS, Cornell Scale for Depression in Dementia, or the Center for Epidemiologic Studies of Depression Scale (CES-D) (Radloff, 1977). In addition, the significance of obtaining data from other sources, such as rehabilitation and recreation personnel, is stated. When conducting an assessment, it is important to provide a private and confidential setting and be sensitive when asking the resident questions that are of a personal nature. Importantly, the guidelines recommend consideration of consultation from a geriatric psychiatrist when there is uncertainty regarding the diagnosis of depression, or when severe, urgent, or emergent situations arise. These situations include presence of suicidal ideation, homicidal ideation, refusal to eat or drink because of depression, or the presence of psychotic symptoms. The decision regarding the need for a thorough medical evaluation of depressive symptoms must be made on an individualized basis. If the evaluation would not change the management of a terminally ailing resident or end-stage of a resident's condition, then it may not be indicated. However, medication use must always be ruled out as a contributing etiologic factor. Specifically, levodopa-carbidopa, clonidine, beta-adrenergic blockers, benzodiazepines, and barbiturates are among the medications that are known to cause depression as a side effect.

Case vignette

Mr A was an 82-year-old male with a significant past medical history that included chronic obstructive pulmonary disease requiring continuous oxygen supplementation, hypertension, and diabetes. He had been living in the nursing home setting for several years. Nursing staff noticed the new onset of social withdrawal, deteriorating hygiene, irritability, and weight loss of 7 lbs over the preceding 4 weeks. Mr A had uncharacteristically refused to leave his bed and get dressed or bathed in the morning. Upon questioning by the staff, he denied feeling especially ill and asked to be "just left alone." A mental health consultation was requested. On evaluation by a consulting psychiatrist, it was noted that potential precipitants to Mr A's change in condition included the recent death of his roommate at the same time that Mr A had been briefly hospitalized for pneumonia. Review of this resident's most recent blood work was nonrevealing except for some mild macrocytic anemia; his serum vitamin B12 level was borderline low and his serum homocysteine was elevated; there was no evidence of residual pneumonia. On examination, he complained of fatigue, anxiety, a sense of futility, suicidal thoughts with no active plan or intent, decreased sleep, and anhedonia. He was determined to be intact cognitively with a Mini-Mental State Exam score of 27 out of 30. A diagnosis of major depressive disorder was made. A treatment plan was assembled that consisted of weekly individual therapy sessions and an antidepressant trial of the agent mirtazapine. He was also started on vitamin B12 replacement injections. In addition, he was encouraged to attend the facility's recreation sessions once per week, but, consistently refused to do so. Over the course of a few weeks, he transiently showed more animation and willingness to bathe. However, he continued to lose weight over the subsequent 4–6 weeks and remained confined to his room. An additional antidepressant agent, venlafaxine, was added as an augmentation strategy. Ultimately, Mr A stopped eating and drinking. Due to the severity of symptoms and continuing weight loss and nonresponse over 2 months, he was admitted to a psychiatric inpatient unit. He agreed to an acute course of ECT and responded robustly after the sixth treatment. He subsequently returned to the nursing home and continued to stay in remission on the antidepressant sertraline at 150 mg daily. He continued to receive weekly visits with a consulting psychologist and a recreation therapist.

ASSESSMENT OF DEMENTIA-ASSOCIATED BEHAVIORAL SYMPTOMS

Education of nursing home staff to recognize, assess, treat, and monitor behavioral symptoms is essential. The MDS cannot adequately identify all residents suffering from these symptoms. Behavioral symptoms, such as aggression, verbal agitation, or restlessness, should be described specifically in order to be consistently identified and quantified. Precipitants to the behaviors must also be identified. Verbal and nonverbal communication of unmet needs, such as hunger, thirst, micturition, warmth, sleep, and touch, should be assessed. New onset of symptoms or changes should prompt assessment for psychosis, depression, anxiety, insomnia, drug effects, and prescription drug such as benzodiazepine overuse or withdrawal. Assessment for hearing and visual problems must be considered when there is a possibility of sensory deprivation. New onset or changes in symptoms should prompt vital sign check and evaluation for infections, dehydration, pain or discomfort, delirium, fecal impaction and injury. Environmental, situational, social and psychological factors should be assessed. For residents who threaten or attempt harm to self or others or fail to respond to treatment within 30 days, referral to a mental health professional should be considered. An estimated one third of the elderly population develops psychiatric symptoms secondary to underlying medical disorders (Sutor, Rummans, & Glenn, 2001). Medical causes contributing to behavior symptoms could range from a wide array of conditions including dehydration, congestive heart failure, diabetes, hypothyroidism or hyperthyroidism, urinary tract infection, pneumonia, and cellulitis. Neurological conditions, such as stroke, subdural hematoma, and traumatic brain injury, can contribute to psychiatric symptoms. Drug effects can be a potential factor in causing anticholinergic-induced delirium.

Case vignette

Ms B was a 76–year-old female recently admitted to the nursing home four months previously. Her medical history included hypertension, congestive heart failure, and Alzheimer's disease, diagnosed 6 years previously. She had become physically aggressive toward another resident and had also attempted to strike her aide earlier in the morning during routine ADL care. Upon examination, she was found to be severely aphasic and unable to clearly express her ideas. However, when approached by the examiner, she seemed to be quite fearful, and was pacing across the hallway with a severely impaired attention span. Her speech appeared slurred. The staff reported that she appeared significantly more confused than upon admission and was prone to pointing to invisible objects in her vicinity. Her medication list included the recent addition of oxybutynin for urinary incontinence and an antihistamine, chlorpheniramine, as needed for sleep. This latter agent had been administered at bedtime during the prior 6 weeks. Recent laboratory results were unrevealing with the exception of a urinalysis that indicated a urinary tract infection. A delirium brought on by the combination of medications with anticholinergic side effects along with a urinary tract infection was thought to be contributory to the resident's deteriorated mental state. Both oxybutynin and chlorpheniramine were discontinued and Ms B was started on an antibiotic. For 2 weeks, she was also treated with an atypical antipsychotic agent, quetiapine. She was approached in a calm nonthreatening demeanor during ADL care. She gradually appeared to be calmer and was more easily understood when she conversed, and there were no more episodes of aggression or possible hallucinations noted.

TREATMENT OF MENTAL ILLNESS: GENERAL PRINCIPLES AND ISSUES

Once the case of nursing home resident is comprehensively evaluated, a clear, unambiguous definition of the symptoms and their frequency and severity should be documented. All patient-centered (e.g., dementia with aphasia, pain, hearing impairment) and milieu contributors (e.g., environmental overstimulation, personal ADL assistance) must be defined.

TABLE 4.1 Summary of OBRA Guidelines Where Antipsychotics Must *Not* Be Prescribed

- Wandering
- Restlessness
- Anxiety
- Poor self-care
- Insomnia
- Depression without psychosis
- Uncooperative behavior
- Agitation with no harm to self or others
- Impaired memory

Treatment is then directed at the dominant symptoms and should consist of interventions to minimize the impact of all patient-centered and milieu factors on the symptoms to be managed. Treatment goals need to be realistic and must aim at reducing the target symptoms and not to attempt to completely eliminate such behaviors (Sutor et al., 2001).

The OBRA 1987 (Omnibus Budget Reconciliation Act, 1990) enacted in 1990 provided guidelines for use of psychotropic medications and chemical–physical restraint use (Tables 4.1, 4.2).

The impact of OBRA on prescription of psychotropic drug reveals an overall decrease in the rates of antipsychotic use, increase in antidepressant use, decrease in hypnotic use, and anxiolytic use remaining more or less the same (Ryan, Kidder, Daiello, & Tariot, 2002) (Table 4.3). Since the enactment of OBRA, the use of psychotropic medication has decreased but there is scant evidence to indicate that the use of nonpharmacological interventions has increased (Cody, Beck, & Svarstad, 2002). The authors discuss various challenges to the use of nonpharmacological interventions. These include inadequate communication between the Medical Director and Staff Physicians and

TABLE 4.2 Acceptable Indications for Antipsychotic Use in Nursing Homes, OBRA Guidelines

- Schizophrenia
- Huntington's disease
- Schizo-affective disorder
- Psychotic and delusional disorders
- Tourette's syndrome
- Mood disorders with psychotic features
- Organic mental disorders (dementia and delirium) with associated psychotic/agitated behaviors with appropriate justification and documentation

TABLE 4.3 Guidelines for Antipsychotic Use, OBRA Guidelines

- Target behavior documented, permanent/persisting and causing danger to patient or others or severe functional impairment
- Routine orders preferred to "PRN" use
- Attempt dosage reduction twice a year
- If dosage reduction failed or a psychiatric diagnosis present and symptoms stable without side effects and written justification of effectiveness provided
- Monitor for side effects (emphasizing tardive dyskinesia, cognitive/behavioral impairment, hypotension, parkinsonism

the nursing home staff particularly about the residents' mental health needs. Often the nursing assistants have negative feelings when residents are aggressive. They may get overwhelmed and tend to avoid residents who display aggressive behaviors. Nursing assistants receive inadequate training in nonpharmacological interventions. When training does occur, it is rare that there is a system to provide feedback and reinforcement. Nursing assistants are often pressed for time to get their tasks done for the day, which might hinder their ability to provide nonpharmacological interventions.

PHARMACOLOGICAL TREATMENT OF DEPRESSION IN THE LONG-TERM CARE SETTING

Double-blind, placebo-controlled trials of antidepressants in the nursing home setting are quite limited (Table 4.4). Data suggest efficacy of selective serotonin reuptake inhibitors (SSRIs) in cognitively intact patients, but limited efficacy in those with severe dementia and depression. There are no studies that combine antidepressants with nonpharmacological interventions.

According to published expert consensus guidelines for the treatment of depression in the elderly (Alexopoulos et al., 1998a), SSRIs are considered the agents of first choice. In these guidelines, sertraline and citalopram are mentioned as first-line option as they have a low likelihood of drug–drug interactions. Always the adage of "start low and go slow" in using any medication intervention in the geriatric population must be followed, as the elderly often have comorbid medical illnesses and are receiving other medications, which increases the risk of developing side effects. There are no data on the use of serotonergic-noradrenergic agents in the nursing home; Venlafaxine, however, a drug in this class, is often a second-line option for the treatment of geriatric

TABLE 4.4 Overview of Antidepressant Trials in the Nursing Home

Study	Treatment	Method	Results	Issues
Katz (1999)	Nortriptyline, average dose 65 mg, major depression, HAMD 18	Randomized controlled trial, *n* = 30, 7 weeks	40% statistically significant change in HAMD scores with nortriptyline versus 11% with placebo	34% randomized to nortriptyline discontinued due to side effects
Rosen, Mulsant, and Pollock (2000)	Sertraline	6-week open-label, *n* = 12, minor depression	75% remission on HAMD and global assessment scale	
Trappler and Cohen (1998)	Fluoxetine, Paroxetine, Sertraline	12-week open-label, *n* = 50	42% response rate across all treatment groups	93% responders cognitively intact versus 7% in demented subjects
Roose, Nelson, Salzman, Hollander, and Rodrigues (2003)	Mirtazapine	Open-label 12 week, *n* = 127, AD with depression	54% improvement on CGI-I, 47% were HAMD responders	
Magai (2000)	Sertraline	8-week, placebo-controlled, *n* = 31, AD with depression	No significant difference between sertraline and placebo	

depression as it is also relatively well tolerated. Underlying vulnerabilities to the potential side effects of medication need to be kept in mind while selecting a particular antidepressant agent (Table 4.5). For example, a patient with chronic constipation, in addition to depression, can be given a trial of an agent, which is often associated with causing loose bowel movements, such as sertraline. Adverse effects of the SSRIs include

TABLE 4.5 Commonly Used Antidepressants, Recommended Dosage in the Elderly

Drug	Starting dose (mg)	Maximum dosage (mg)
Setraline	25	150–200
Citalopram	10	20–40
Duloxetine	20	40–60
Paroxetine	10	20–40
Fluoxetine	10	20–40
Mirtazapine	7.5–15	45
Buproprion SR	100	150 (twice daily)
Venlafaxine XR	37.5	150–225

gastrointestinal symptoms such as nausea, emesis, and diarrhea. In addition, these agents reportedly can also cause extrapyramidal symptoms and hyponatremia. Mirtazapine, a serotonergic agent with a mechanism of action distinct from the SSRIs, is associated with sedation and weight gain, so it is often used in the elderly when loss of appetite and insomnia are predominant symptoms of depression. Buproprion, a nonserotonergic compound, is contraindicated in individuals with seizure disorder as it lowers seizure threshold. Individuals with very severe depression, severe weight loss, persistent and active suicidal ideation and depression unresponsive to pharmacologic intervention may require electroconvulsive therapy (Peskind, 2003).

In AMDA-issued CPG to treat depression in the nursing home (American Medical Directors Association, 1996), it is recommended that nonpharmacologic interventions as well as drug therapy must be considered. In addition, treatment must be consistent with patient and family wishes or any existing advanced directives. A treatment plan must address symptoms, follow-up visit frequency, and objectives of treatment. In addition to being effective, treatment must address environmental, spiritual, cultural, family, and ethnic needs. These guidelines recommend the use of electroconvulsive therapy for patients who refuse to eat or drink in addition to the above-mentioned indicators. Patients must be monitored for 6 weeks after antidepressant medication is initiated. As patients with dementia or aphasia may have difficulty articulating their experience of medication side effects, they may require more frequent monitoring and more focused observation by nursing home staff. As per other consensus guidelines (American Geriatrics Society and American Association for Geriatric Psychiatry, 2003), patients who meet criteria for minor depression should be treated with nonpharmacological interventions and observation of response for up to 2 months. Depending upon symptom severity, these patients may need antidepressant treatment. Major depression should be treated with antidepressant medication and SSRIs are considered first-line interventions. Patients who meet criteria for major depression with psychotic features must be treated with an antidepressant and antipsychotic medication. Nonpharmacological interventions for major depression must include resident participation in structured activities, socialization, and activities that help to maintain previous role functioning. Patients with a first or second episode of major depression must be continued on the antidepressant medication they have responded to for at least 6 months after improvement is noted. Patients should be reassessed to monitor effectiveness and for evidence of adverse effects at 6 and 12 weeks of treatment.

PHARMACOLOGIC TREATMENT OF DEMENTIA-ASSOCIATED BEHAVIORAL SYMPTOMS

In the nursing home setting, a wealth of open-label data have emerged over the past few decades describing the use of antipsychotic and other agents for the treatment of dementia-associated behavioral symptoms (Table 4.6). A comprehensive review of the pertinent literature is beyond the scope of this chapter. However, several noteworthy observations can be made as a result of more recently published data related to placebo-controlled studies of psychotropic agents conducted in multicenter nursing home clinical trials.

Studies of the efficacy and tolerability of two of the newer atypical antipsychotics, aripiprazole, and ziprasidone, in nursing home residents have not yet appeared in the peer-reviewed literature. The available evidence suggests that overall, atypical neuroleptics are better tolerated than conventional neuroleptics and more efficacious than placebo, in decreasing agitation in patients with dementia. Importantly, it has been recently reported that agents in this class of medication may increase the risk of glucose intolerance and cerebrovascular adverse events in treated patients. Clozapine is occasionally recommended for treatment of refractory elderly patients with movement disorders such as parkinsonism or tardive dyskinesia and psychosis. One of the major drawbacks with clozapine use is a significantly increased risk of agranulocytosis and the need for standardized blood monitoring (Kasckow, Mulchahey, & Mohamed, 2004).

In addition to the emergence of atypical antipsychotic agents as commonly used agents for dementia-associated behavioral problems, the use of anticonvulsant medications, such as carbamazepine and sodium valproate, has commanded significant attention. One placebo-controlled

TABLE 4.6 Overview of Trials of Antipsychotics for Dementia-Associated Behavioral Symptoms in the Nursing Home

Study	Medication	Method	Results
Katz et al. (1999)	Risperidone versus placebo risperidone, daily doses of 0.5, 1.0, and 2.0 mg	Double-blind 12-week, *n* = 625	Significant reductions in some psychotic symptoms and aggression with risperidone 1 mg
DeDeyn et al. (1999)	Risperidone or haloperidol, versus placebo risperidone, mean daily dose 1.1 mg; haloperidol, mean daily dose 1.2 mg	Double-blind 13-week, *n* = 344	Risperidone caused reduction in some measures of aggression
Street et al. (2000)	Olanzapine versus placebo olanzapine, 5, 10, and 15 mg daily doses	Double-blind 6-week, *n* = 206	Agitation and psychosis improved with olanzapine 5 and 10 mg
Tariot, Schneider, and Katz (2002)	Quetiapine, mean daily dose 120 mg; haloperidol, mean daily dose 2 mg	Randomized placebo-controlled 10-week trial	Both treatment groups improved in severity of psychotic symptoms and agitation. Overall, quetiapine was better tolerated than haloperidol

study using an average dose of 300 mg per day of carbamazepine showed that the drug was well tolerated by patients and significantly decreased aggression and agitation (Tariot et al., 1998). Potential side effects of carbamazepine include drowsiness, gastrointestinal distress, ataxia, rash, elevated hepatic enzymes, and drug interactions with other agents. This agent has also been associated with aplastic anemia and agranulocytosis.

Sodium valproate has reportedly been effective in the treatment of behavioral disturbances in dementia and has fewer drug interactions than carbamazepine. Porteinsson, Tariot, and Erb (2001) reported on the use of sodium valproate in a randomized placebo-controlled 6-week study of 56 nursing home patients with dementia and agitation. The average dose of divalproex sodium used was 840 mg per day. The authors noted that their results suggested improvement in the agitation subscale of the Brief Psychiatric Rating Scale. Potential side effects of this agent include nausea, vomiting, sedation, diarrhea, ataxia, and tremor. Hepatotoxicity and pancreatitis have been noted to be rare complications of the use of sodium valproate. When this medication is administered, complete blood counts, hepatic enzymes, and serum drug concentrations need to be monitored regularly to prevent toxicity.

Gabapentin, lamotrigine, and topiramate are newer anticonvulsants whose efficacy and tolerability have not been systematically evaluated in the treatment of dementia-associated behavioral changes.

Benzodiazepines, such as lorazepam and oxazepam, are often used in the management of agitation, but their efficacy has not been comprehensively studied. These agents are generally safe when used in low doses, but with increasing doses, common side effects that emerge include oversedation, ataxia, confusion, and paradoxical agitation. In addition, with long-term use, tolerance and dependence is likely. Zolpidem, a hypnotic, was found to reduce night-time wandering in two patients (Shelton & Hocking, 1997).

The antianxiety agent buspirone has shown efficacy in case reports (Sakauye, Camp, & Ford, 1993) in reducing anxiety, aggression, and agitation in patients with dementia. The drug is generally well tolerated; however, if used in combination with SSRIs, the patient is at increased risk for the development of serotonin syndrome (confusion, tremors, hyperthermia, hypertension, and seizure).

Acetylcholinesterase inhibitors, such as tacrine, donepezil, rivastigmine, and galantamine, have been studied quite extensively in community settings for their presumed efficacy on cognition, behavior, and functioning in Alzheimer's dementia; they show modest benefit. However, there are very limited data on the use of these agents for treating or preventing agitation in dementia in nursing home settings. Tariot et al. (2001) reported on a 24-week double–blind, placebo-controlled study of donepezil with 208 nursing home patients who had Alzheimer's disease or Alzheimer's disease with cerebrovascular disease. The donepezil-treated group showed improved agitation and aggression as noted on the Neuropsychiatric Inventory–Nursing Home Version scale as compared with the placebo treated group. Agitation and aggression were the most common behavioral symptoms associated with Alzheimer's disease in this study. Of the 64% of patients who displayed these behaviors, 67% were noted to experience symptom relief with the use of donepezil.

In a 26-week-long open-label nursing home study, rivastigmine use was reportedly associated with stabilization or improvement in behavioral symptoms in the 59% of patients who completed the trial (Rabinowicz et al., 2003). McKeith et al. (2000) noted the efficacy of rivastigmine in improving behavior disturbances in patients with Lewy body dementia.

There are no studies to date with galantamine in the nursing home. Cummings, Schneider, Tariot, Kershaw, and Yuan (2004) noted in a double–blind, placebo-controlled study that galantamine was associated with reduced emergence of behavior disturbances and improvement in existing behavior problems in patients living at home.

Memantine, an NMDA antagonist, indicated for use in moderate-to-severe Alzheimer's disease, has proven to be effective and tolerable in monotherapy and in conjunction with donepezil with modest improvements in cognition, behavior, and function (Tariot et al., 2004).

As with the treatment of depression, expert consensus guidelines have been published regarding the treatment of agitation in older patients with dementia (Expert Consensus Guideline, 1998) (Table 4.7). The guidelines recommend initiating therapy with risperidone at low doses of 0.25–0.5 mg per day with an average maximum dose of 1–1.5 mg per day, if there is an evidence of psychosis. These guidelines also recommend the use of environmental interventions in addition to medication treatment. If agitation is due to depression and/or anxiety, an SSRI trial is also recommended. If insomnia is a contributing factor, trazodone use is indicated. Other consensus guidelines (American Geriatrics Society and American Association for Geriatric Psychiatry, 2003) recommend that nonpharmacological interventions alone are indicated if there is no threat to the resident or others, medical conditions are being addressed, and if no psychotic symptoms are evident. Atypical antipsychotics are the first-line agents of choice for severe behavioral symptoms with psychosis. When medications are used to manage behavior disturbances one must document the specific target symptoms being addressed. Combination therapy is indicated only after two different trials with two different classes of agents have proven unsuccessful. Taper or discontinuation of medications should be attempted and documented for 6 months following response and every 6 months, thereafter. There is no consensus on the choice of medication for nonpsychotic behavioral symptoms. There are no comparison studies between pharmacological and nonpharmacological interventions, making it difficult to prioritize a specific approach for most nonpsychotic behavioral symptoms.

TABLE 4.7 Commonly Prescribed Drugs, Dosage Guidelines in the Elderly

Drug (mg)	Starting dose (mg)	Maximum dose
Divalproex	125 (twice daily)	1000
Carbamazepine	50–100	500–800
Risperidone	0.25–0.5	1
Olanzapine	2.5	5–10
Quetiapine	25	200–250
Trazodone	25	100–150
Buspirone	5 (twice daily)	30–45
Lorazepam	0.5	2
Zolpidem	5–10	10

CONCLUSIONS

Today's nursing home resembles a long-term psychiatric hospital for the elderly. There is a high prevalence of psychiatric diagnoses and of psychotropic drug use among the resident population. Many facilities lack adequate staff expertise in identifying and treating psychiatric illness and have inadequate access to formal psychiatric consultation. Many nursing homes are environments in which the mental health and related feelings of residents with regard to personal competence, mastery, and well-being are undermined. When mental illness is apparent, there needs to be an integrated team approach to assist in maintaining the highest possible quality of care while restoring the resident's sense of well-being. Assessment of depression and behavioral symptoms must always include ruling out any contribution from environmental influences and an underlying medical condition. A comprehensive treatment plan must include nonpharmacological interventions and the fostering of a milieu in which strong mental health is encouraged and fostered.

REFERENCES

Alexopoulos, G., et al. (1998a). An expert consensus guideline for the treatment of depression in the elderly. Postgraduate Medicine Special Supplement.

Alexopoulos, G. S., Abrams, R. C., Young, R. C., & Shamoian, C. A. (1998b). Cornell scale for depression in dementia. *Biological Psychiatry, 23*, 271–284.

American Geriatrics Society and American Association for Geriatric Psychiatry. (2003). Consensus statement on improving the quality of mental health care in U.S. nursing homes: Management of depression and behavioral symptoms associated with dementia. *Journal of the Geriatric Society, 51*, 1287–1298.

American Medical Directors Association. (1996). *Depression clinical practice guideline*. Columbia, MD: American Medical Directors Association.

Bartels, S. J., Maok, G. S., & Dums, A. R. (2002). Models of mental health services in nursing homes: A review of the literature. *Psychiatric Services, 53*, 1390–1396.

Beck, A. T., Ward, C. H., Mendelson, M., Mock, J., & Erbaugh, J. 1961). An inventory for measuring depression. *Archives of General Psychiatry, 4*, 53–63.

Beck, A. T., Ward, C. H., Mendelson, M., Mock, J., & Erbaugh, J. (1961). An inventory for measuring depression. *Archives of General Psychiatry, 4*, 561–571.

Borson, S., Reichman, W. E., Coyne, A. C., Rovner, B., & Sakauye, K. (2000). Effectiveness of nursing home staff as managers of disruptive behavior: Perceptions of nursing directors. *American Journal of Geriatric Psychiatry, 8*(3), 251–253.

Borson, S., Reichman, W. E., Coyne, A. C., Rovner, B., & Sakauye, K. (2000). Effectiveness of nursing home staff as managers of disruptive behavior: Perceptions of nursing directors. *American Journal of Geriatric Psychiatry, 8*(3), 251–253.

Browne, C., Braun, K., Mokuau, N., & McLaughlin, L. (2002). Developing a multisite project in geriatric and/or gerontological education with emphasis in interdisciplinary practice and cultural competence. *Gerontologist, 42*, 698–704.

Burns, B. J., Wagner, H. R., Taube, J. E., & Magaziner, J. (1993). Mental health service use by the elderly in nursing homes. *American Journal of Public Health, 83*(3), 331–337.

Burrows, A. B., Satlin, A., Salzman, C., Nobel, K., & Lipsitz, L. (1995). Depression in a long-term care facility: Clinical features and discordance between nursing assessment and patient interviews. *Journal of the American Geriatrics Society, 43*, 1118–1122.

Cody, M., Beck, C., & Svarstad, B. (2002). Mental health services in nursing homes: Challenges to the use of nonpharmacologic interventions in nursing homes. *Psychiatric Services, 53*, 1402–1406.

Colenda, C., Streim, J., Greene, J., Meyers, N., Beckwith, E., & Rabins, P. (1999). The impact of OBRA 87 on psychiatric services in nursing homes. *American Journal of Geriatric Psychiatry, 7*, 12–17.

Cummings, J. L., Schneider, L., Tariot, P. N., Kershaw, P. R., & Yuan, W. (2004). Reduction of behavioral disturbances and caregiver distress by galantamine in patients with Alzheimer's disease. *American Journal of Psychiatry, 161*(3), 532–538.

Emerson, L. N. B., Fogel, B. S., Robinson, G. K., & Weiss, H. P. (1996). Achieving mental health of nursing home residents: Overcoming barriers to mental health care.

Engel, G. L. (1980). The clinical application of the biopsychosocial model. *American Journal of Psychiatry, 137*, 535.

Expert Consensus Guideline. (1998). Expert consensus guideline on the treatment of agitation in older persons with dementia. Postgraduate Medicine Special Report.

Fenton, J., Raskin, A., Gruber-Baldini, A., Menon, S., Zimmerman, S., Kaup, B., Loreck, D., Ruskin, P., & Magaziner, J. (2004). Some predictors of psychiatric consultation in nursing home residents. *American Journal of Geriatric Psychiatry, 12*, 297–304.

Kasckow, J. W., Mulchahey, J. J., & Mohamed, S. (2004). The use of novel antipsychotics in the older patient with neurodegenerative disorders in the long-term care setting. *Journal of American Medical Directors Association, 5*(4), 242–248.

Katz, I. R., Jeste, D. V., Mintzer, J. E., Clyde, C., Napolitano, J., Brecher, M., & Risperidone Study Group. (1999). Comparison of risperidone and placebo for psychosis and behavioral disturbances associated with dementia: A randomized, double-blind trial. *Journal of Clinical Psychiatry, 60*, 107–115.

Kim, E., & Rovner, B. (1996). The nursing home as a psychiatric hospital in psychiatric care in the nursing home. In W. E. Reichman, & P. R. Katz (1996). *Psychiatric care in the nursing home*. New York: Oxford University Press.

Katz, I. R., Simpson, G. M., Curlik, S. M., Parmelee, P. A., & Muhly, C. (1990). Pharmacologic treatment of major depression for elderly patients in residential care settings. *Journal of Clinical Psychiatry, 51 Suppl*, 41–47.

Long-Term Care Forum. (2002). Care of the psychiatric patient in the nursing home. *American Association of Geriatric Psychiatry: Challenges and Opportunities, 1*(3).

Magai, C., Kennedy, G., Cohen, C. I., & Gomberg, D. (2000). A controlled clinical trial of sertraline in the treatment of depression in nursing home patients with late-stage Alzheimer's disease. *The American journal of Geriatric Psychiatry, 8*(1), 66–74.

McKeith, I., Del Ser, T., Spano, P., Emre, M., Wesnes, K., Anand, R., Cicin-Sain, A., Ferrara, R., & Spiegel, R. (2000). Efficacy of rivastigmine in dementia with Lewy bodies: A randomized double-blind, placebo-controlled international study. *Lancet, 356*(9247), 2031–2036.

NIH. (1992). NIH consensus development panel on late-life depression. Diagnosis and treatment of depression in late life. *JAMA*, 268, 1018–1024.

Omnibus Budget Reconciliation Act. (1990). P.L. 101-508, Sections 4206 and 4751 (Medicare and Medicaid) 42 U.S.C. Section 135 cc (a)(I)(Q). 135 mm (c)(8), 1395 cc(f), 1396 a (a)(57), (58), 1396a(w).

Peskind, E. (2003). Management of depression in long-term care of patients with Alzheimer's disease. *Journal of American Medical Directors Association*, (November–December), S141–S145.

Porteinsson, A. P., Tariot, P., & Erb, R. (2001). Placebo-controlled study of divalproex sodium for agitation in dementia. *American Journal of Geriatric Psychiatry, 9*, 58–66.

Qualls, S. H., Segal, D., Norman, S., Niederehe, G., & Gallagher-Thompson, D. (2002). Psychologists in practice with older adults: Current patterns, sources of training and need for continuing education. *Professional Psychology: Research and Practice, 33*(5), 435–442.

Radloff, L. S. (1977). The CES-D scale: A self-report depression scale for research in the general population. *Journal of Applied Psychosocial measures, 1*, 385–401.

Reichman, W. E., Coyne, A., Borson, S., Negron, A., Rovner, B., Pelchat, R., Sakauye, K., Katz, P., Cantillon, M., & Hamer, R. (1998). Psychiatric consultation in the nursing home: A survey of six states. *American Journal of Geriatric Psychiatry, 6*, 320–327.

Roose, S., Nelson, C., Salzman, C., Hollander, S., & Rodrigues, H. (2003). Mirtazapine in the nursing home study group. Open-label study of mirtazapine orally disintegrating tablets in depressed patients in the nursing home. *Current Medical Research and Opinions, 19*(8), 737–746.

Rosen, J., Mulsant, B., & Pollock, B. (2000). Sertraline in the treatment of minor depression in nursing home residents: A pilot study. *International Journal of Geriatric Psychiatry, 15*, 177–180.

Rovner, B., Kafonek, S., Filipp, L., Lucas, M. J., & Folstein, M. (1986). Prevalence of mental illness in a community nursing home. *American Journal of Psychiatry, 143*, 1446–1449.

Ryan, M. J., Kidder, S., Daiello, L., & Tariot, P. (2002). Mental health services in nursing homes: Psychopharmacologic interventions in nursing homes: What do we know and where should we go? *Psychiatric Services, 53*, 1407–1413.

Sakauye, K. M., Camp, C. J., & Ford, P. A. (1993). Effects of buspirone on agitation associated with dementia. *American Journal of Geriatric Psychiatry, 1*, 82–84.

Shea, D. G., Clark, P., & Smyer, M. A. (1995). Treatment of persons with a mental illness in nursing homes after OBRA'87. *Gerontologist, 35*(1), Abstract #259, 308.

Shelton, P. S., & Hocking, L. B.(1997). Zolpidem for dementia-related insomnia and nighttime wandering. *Annals of Pharmacotherapy, 31*(3), 319–322.

Smyer, M. A., Shea, D. G., & Streit, A. (1994). The provision and use of mental health services in nursing homes: Results from the National Medical Expenditure Survey. *American Journal of Public Health, 84*(2), 284–287.

Snowden, M., Sato, K., & Roy-Byrne, P. (2003). Assessment and treatment of nursing home residents with depression or behavioral symptoms associated with dementia: A review of the literature. *Journal of the American Geriatrics Society, 51*, 1305–1317.

Street, J., Clark, S., Gannon, K., Cummings, J., Bymaster, F., Tamura, R., Mitan, S., Kadam, D., Sanger, T., Feldman, P., Tollefson, G., & Breier, A. (2000). Olanzapine treatment of psychotic and behavioral symptoms in patients with Alzheimer's disease in nursing care facilities. *Archives of General Psychiatry, 57*, 968–976.

Sutor, B., Rummans, T., & Glenn, S. (2001). Assessment and management of behavioral disturbances in nursing home patients with dementia. *Mayo Clinic Proceedings, 76*(5), 540–550.

Tariot, P. N., Podgorski, C. A., Blazina, L., & Leibovici, A. (1993). Mental disorders in the nursing home: another perspective. *American Journal of Psychiatry, 150*(7), 1063–1069.

Tariot, P. N., Cummings, J. L., Katz, I. R., Mintzer, J., Perdomo, C., Schwam, E., & Whalen, E. (2001). A randomized, double-blind, placebo-controlled study of the efficacy and safety of donepezil in patients with Alzheimer's disease in the nursing home setting. *Journal of American Geriatrics Society, 49*(12), 1590–1599.

Tariot, P. N., Farlow, M. R., Grossberg, G. T., Graham, S. M., McDonald, S., Gergel, I., & Memantine Study Group. (2004). Memantine treatment in patients with moderate to severe Alzheimer's disease already receiving donepezil, a randomized controlled trial. *JAMA, 291*(14), 1695.

Tariot, P. N., Rosemary, R. N., Podgorski, C. A., Cox, C., Patel, S., Jakimovich, L., & Irvine, C. (1998). Efficacy and tolerability of carbamazepine for agitation and aggression in dementia. *American Journal of Psychiatry, 155*(1), 54–61.

Tariot, P. N., Schneider, L., & Katz, I. (2002). Quetiapine in nursing home residents with Alzheimer's dementia and psychosis. *American Journal of geriatric Psychiatry, 10*(Suppl 1), 93.

Trappler, B., & Cohen, C. (1998). Use of SSRIs in "very old" depressed nursing home residents. *American Journal of Geriatric Psychiatry,* 6, 83–89.

Yesavage, J. A. (1998). Geriatric depression scale. *Psychopharmacology Bulletin, 24*, 709–710.

CHAPTER FIVE

Treating Depression in Nursing Homes

Beyond the Medical Model

Michael Duffy and Bradley Karlin

Depression causes considerable and at times excruciating pain, and yet is quite amenable to successful treatment. The prevalence of unipolar depression is estimated in the general population between 15 and 20% at any given time with the lifetime incidence of depression between 20 and 55% (Amenson & Lewinsohn, 1981; Kessler et al., 1994). Interestingly, the prevalence of depression among older adults is now thought to be essentially equivalent to the general population. This generally accepted conclusion comes after an extended period of debate in which it was assumed that older adults in general were more beset by depression. Indeed, it is probably accurate that older adults are more vulnerable to depression, especially with the increasing incidence of chronic medical disorders and environmental constraints such as long-term care settings. However, it is doubtless a testimony to the adaptability and resilience in later life that the incidence of geriatric depression remains at its current level. It is important to point out, however, that older adults with multiple chronic disorders, and especially those in nursing homes, probably do have a significantly higher incidence of depression. Psychology colleagues who work routinely in long-term care report that referrals for the treatment of depression represent 80–90% of all referrals for psychological services in the nursing home. Despite the single referral report, in many cases depression is accompanied by other comorbid problems such as personality disorders, severe psychiatric disorders, and dementia. In these latter cases especially, the psychological and behavioral treatment of depression takes on new challenges and alternate treatment forms that will be discussed later in this chapter.

LIMITATIONS OF PSYCHOPHARMACOLOGY

Within the medical model and medical treatment, depression has been largely identified as a biological and neurochemical problem. This has led to an almost exclusive reliance on medication in the treatment of depression, despite growing evidence that questions the effectiveness of medication in treating depression. In their overview of treatments, for depression, Antonuccio, Danton, and DeNelsky (1995) revealed a striking lack of clear and empirical evidence for the effectiveness of medications, either the older tricyclic or the newer SSRI varieties. Across many studies using randomized clinical trials, medication was often inferior to a variety of behavioral therapies. This is despite the much vaunted randomized clinical trials methodology, in which there are problems that complicate results. Because the placebo conditions use inert substances that show few clinical side effects compared to the depression medications, it is unclear whether treatment evaluators' judgments are truly blind to treatment versus control group differences. This methodological problem has been evident for some time, yet is rarely discussed in the conclusions and limitations of treatment studies. Apparently, there are also significant limitations in the newer SSRI depression medications. These were developed on the theory that depression is caused by a deficiency in serotonin in the brain even though this has not been shown clearly to lower depressive rates (Hallman & Oreland, 1989). In this model, the SSRIs increase the serotonin available to the brain by interfering and inhibiting the reuptake receptors. However, an interesting anomaly occurs in this situation; apparently, in as early as 2 days the brain compensates for this artificial intrusion of extra serotonin and reduces the number of serotonin receptors, effectively eliminating any therapeutic effect (Breggin, 1994). This is a curious affirmation of the adaptability and resilience of the human organism. Apparently, these induced compensatory receptor changes can become permanent and thus create unanticipated serious long-term problems. Science has encountered an unexpected foe in the very resilience of the body. We believe that a similar adaptability and resilience is a powerful asset in psychological life, especially in older adults.

Relatively little is known about the pharmacological treatment of depression in older adults with dementia that exceeds 50% of nursing home residents. Physicians and even psychiatrists routinely over and under prescribe medications for older adults, and there is little definitive guidance in the medical literature. Again, this is especially problematic in nursing homes where physicians are rarely involved directly. Slowing metabolism in late life extends the length of half-life side effects. In addition, a high number of daily medications and the danger of drug–drug and drug–food interactions all make this a pharmacological minefield. In a recent review of randomized clinical trials on the use of antidepressive medication for the treatment of depression in older adults with a diagnosis of dementia, a recent study found only eight published placebo-controlled trials. Significantly, five of these eight failed to demonstrate efficacy (Olin, Katz, & Meyers, 2002).

Behavioral Interventions

Clearly, depression in older adults is a biopsychological phenomenon and it would be unwise for behavioral professionals to underestimate the role of biochemistry in the diagnoses and treatment of depression. Despite recent findings on the comparability and even superiority of behavioral treatment, recent studies also suggest that in serious, chronic, and vegetative depressions, medication can enhance the effect of psychotherapy (Otto, Smits, & Reese, 2005). However, it is also unwise to overestimate the significance of physical elements, and other data (Gatz, Pedersen, Plomin, Nesselroade, & McClearn, 1992) which suggest that genetic influences account for approximately 16% of the variance in depression scores. Thus, environment and life experience, including trauma, are the larger elements in depression and therefore its treatment.

Consistent with this, applied and clinical psychology has developed a series of behavioral and psychological treatments that have consistently shown both efficacious and effective results in clinical trials and field studies. This body of information will be reviewed in a following section. Psychology and particularly clinical and applied psychology has also fallen under the influence of a medical and illness model of understanding and treating disorders and this has been especially reinforced in a managed care environment. These treatments can and have been viewed within an illness model as an answer to a managed care requirement of accountability within an illness/remedial model. However, contemporary behavioral treatments can also be viewed from within a preventive, growth, and potential-oriented philosophy engaging the older person's capacity for resilience (Baltes & Baltes, 1990), a perspective familiar in the SOC (selection, optimization, and compensation) model and in developmental, community, and counseling psychology traditions which have a strength-based appreciation of the adaptive capacity of older adults. This especially is pertinent in nursing homes where untreated depression can kill (without the spontaneous remission observed in younger persons) when we underaccess the adaptive capacity of residents.

A Paradigm Shift

These philosophical differences are highly pertinent in diagnosis and treatment strategy; the medical or illness model tends to be somewhat static versus dynamic, remedial versus preventive and, in diagnostic thinking, providing a categorical/symptomatic versus developmental understanding of disorder. The dominant empirical and positivist emphasis within psychology has perhaps led to an overly exclusive reliance on symptomatic aspects of disorders such as depression. Many of the researched treatments we will review focus primarily on treating the symptomatic profile of depression with minimal attention to the variety of dynamic patterns that may lead to the clinical portrayal. With this in mind, this chapter has several goals. We review the valuable current treatment methods for depression in older adults, beginning with successful current behavioral treatments dealing largely with the symptomatic profile. We then discuss emerging treatment emphases such as physical exercise in the treatment of depression and also strategies designed to treat depression in dementia, a growing concern in long-term care.

Throughout our discussion, we attempt to view depression through the prism of a growth, adaptability, and change model of behavior. We believe that the SOC model (Baltes, 1996; Baltes & Baltes, 1986, 1990) articulates this approach in a practical manner. It may seem counter-intuitive that a disorder such as depression can be viewed within an adaptive and growth model. However, we believe that a focus on adaptability and plasticity is helpful in treatment planning and that even, in some cases, disorders such as depression can in some ways be inherently health promoting versus health destroying. In the parallel case of obsessive compulsive disorder, this counter-intuitive pattern can be observed. Although obsessions and compulsions are a serious problem needing aggressive treatment, they can in themselves be a form of anxiety self management, holding off more serious levels of anxiety. In fact, we know that a treatment insistence on removing the more serious obsessive and compulsive behaviors can put a client at risk of decompensation. In a parallel way, the meaning of depression can be quite counter-intuitive. For a client who is manifesting a severe, self preoccupied somatic disorder, depression may actually result from increasing self-awareness that represents a progression on the trajectory to improved psychological health (Duffy, 2000). In the SOC model, clinical practice must involve a shrewd estimate of the person's available unused psychological and physical capacity and also a realistic testing of the upper limits of the person's ability in both cognitive, effective, and personality dimensions.

The SOC Model of Behavior

The SOC model of behavior (Baltes & Baltes 1986, 1996) offers a significant challenge to prevailing notions of understanding human behavior, to the traditional medical model, and, we believe, in understanding and treating depression in older adults. There is a focus on adaptability and plasticity and the concept of a latent and often unused reserve in older adults that offers an optimistic alternative to the somewhat static view of disorder implicit in the medical/illness model. The SOC model, developed largely by Paul and Margaret Baltes in Germany, is expressed in several critical propositions as follows: (a) there are major differences between normal, optimal, and pathological aging; (b) there is much heterogeneity in aging (and, we would say, in geriatric depression); (c) there is much latent reserve in older adults emphasizing the concept of plasticity in psychological and cognitive functions, and (d) there is an aging loss of function that occurs at the upper limits of the latent reserve. There is also the belief that knowledge and technology can offset age-related decline in cognitive life. This notion of the plasticity of human resources and behavior is very compatible with a developmental view of human behavior and of disorders. In this sense, depression can be an example of an arrested development and a failure to thrive. Such an adaptive viewpoint is especially pertinent in nursing homes where failure to thrive may be institutionally endemic.

The SOC acronym itself represents the concepts of selection, optimization, and compensation that take place naturalistically in the adaptable internal and external behavior of every human being, at least potentially. We know that there is loss in both physical and cognitive domains in human life that places upper limits on the possibility of change. This means within this realistic view of behavior that an older adult (and therefore a therapist) is wise to select among possible available resources and skills. This in turn allows a person (and therapist) to optimize existing potential and to capitalize on the adaptive and plastic nature of the human organism. In turn, then, a person is able to compensate for the age-related losses, maximize to the upper limits the available resources without imposing unnecessary limits, and therefore creating a lifestyle which is both realistic and optimistic and reaches the best of human potential in affective, cognitive, and physical domains. Note that the

SOC model was not specifically developed within the severe disabilities of long-term care, where maintenance rather than enhanced growth is frequently the modal expectation.

As applied to the process of therapy, specifically working with depression, the therapist will do well to acknowledge the need for realistic selection in both client cognitive capacity and also the related therapeutic methods. As indicated earlier, methods of working with depression in dementia will focus more on behavioral and relational methods than on cognitive change methods. By the same token, the potential latent reserve of cognitive capacity in older adults envisioned by SOC suggests alternate cognitive strategies in dealing with depression. In addition to using cognitive techniques such as restructuring, distraction, and thought stopping in dealing with depression, therapists will consider the use of intellectual stimulation as a hedge against geriatric depression. Therapists often note that many depressed nursing home residents benefit from the intellectual stimulation that occurs within the therapeutic relationship. Thus, treatment for depression might include not only cognitive restructuring but also organized and planned intellectual stimulation through conversation, reading, and group interaction techniques. In this example we see that a therapeutic technique designed explicitly to intervene in a particular manner, for example interpersonal therapy (IPT), may also contain a multidimensional impact. Thus, the therapeutic relationship, which is a critical part of the interpersonal approach to working with depression in older adults, also contains an implicit enhancement of cognitive and intellectual faculties that in turn reduce depression symptoms. This last comment points to the existence and importance of implicit or "common factors" that are seen now to be implicated in the outcome effectiveness of disparate intervention methods (Wampold, 2001).

Efficacy of Behavioral Treatments for Late-Life Depression—State of the Art

The limited treatment of depression in older adults is not due to questionable treatment efficacy. In fact, over the last couple of decades, a variety of psychological interventions for the treatment of depression in older adults have been developed and empirically examined. This research, although still in an incipient stage, indicates that psychological interventions have clearly established efficacy for treating depression in older adults; however, it is important to note that this research has focused overwhelmingly on relatively healthy and higher functioning older adults. There is considerable unmet mental health need in nursing homes and other long-term care settings throughout this country and in nations abroad. As many as 50% of nursing home residents have significant depressive symptoms (Randall, 1993; Rovner & Katz, 1993). However, less than 5% of nursing home residents with mental illness receive mental health treatment (Burns et al., 1993). The rate of mental health service use is also extremely low among community-dwelling older adults (Karlin, Duffy, & Gleaves, 2004; Karlin & Norris, in press; VandenBos, Stapp, & Kilburg, 1981).

The most widely investigated psychological treatments for geriatric depression are cognitive, behavioral, and combined cognitive-behavioral therapies (CBTs), although other forms of psychotherapy, including brief psychodynamic therapy, IPT, and life review therapy, have received limited empirical attention. Cognitive therapy, behavior therapy, CBT, and brief psychodynamic therapy have been shown to have consistent and similar levels of efficacy with depressed elders. IPT and life review therapy also appear to be efficacious for a variety of problems producing depression in older adults. Of course, treatment selection should be guided by careful ideographic assessment and consideration of the client's abilities and functional status. This is particularly important in nursing homes and other long-term care settings, given that 75% of nursing home residents have disturbances in three or more activities of daily living (Gabrel, 2000). Additional treatment outcome research in long-term care, and with more medically and demographically diverse older adults, is greatly needed.

In recent years, several meta-analyses have been conducted confirming the efficacy of psychological and psychosocial interventions for the treatment of depression in the elderly (Engels & Vermey, 1997; Gerson, Belin, Kaufman, Mintz, & Jarvik, 1999; Pinquart & Sorensen, 2001; Scogin & McElreath, 1994). Significantly, the mean effect size obtained by Scogin and McElreath was $d = 0.78$, which is equivalent to a high effect size according to Cohen's (1988) classifications. Similarly, in their meta-analytic review of 17 studies examining psychological treatments for geriatric depression, Engels and Vermey reported a mean effect size of $d = 0.63$, using a more conservative effect size estimation procedure than that used by Scogin and McElreath that involved correcting for pretest differences between treatment and control conditions in many of the studies included in the meta-analysis.

The efficacy of psychological interventions for the treatment of depression in older adults has also been examined in comparison to and in combination with pharmacotherapy. Compared to psychotropic medication, CBT and IPT have been found to be at least as efficacious in treating depression in elderly individuals (Beutler et al., 1987; Reynolds, Frank, Houck, & Mazumdar, 1997; Reynolds et al., 1999; Scocco & Frank, 2002; Thompson, Coon, Gallagher-Thompson, Sommer, & Koin, 2001). In addition, it has been demonstrated that, in both younger and older adults, psychotherapy in conjunction with pharmacotherapy is significantly more efficacious in treating depression and other mental health problems than is pharmacotherapy alone (Areán & Cook, 2002; de Jonghe, Kool, van Aalst, Dekker, & Peen, 2001). In the next section, we review each of the four major psychotherapeutic approaches for the treatment of late-life depression.

In the sections that follow, we review the state of the art in psychotherapy for late-life depression, describing each of the four major psychotherapeutic approaches—CBT, brief psychodynamic therapy, life review therapy/reminiscence, and IPT—as they are most appropriately and uniquely applied to older clients. It should be noted, however, that most of this research has been done with community-dwelling elderly. Much work is needed to "compare and transfer" this research to long-term care settings. Although much seems to apply, there are critical environmental and psychological differences in nursing homes.

Cognitive-Behavioral Therapy

CBT is a structured, time-limited, and collaborative form of psychotherapy that combines, to varying degrees, elements of behavioral and cognitive interventions. Behavior therapy, developed by Lewinsohn (1974), is based on operant learning principles and emphasizes the influence of environmental contingencies on emotions. According to this model, depression is more likely to develop in individuals that participate in minimal enjoyable or meaningful activities, especially important in nursing home activities planning. Consequently, the goal of behavior therapy is to increase the frequency of pleasant experience, as well as decrease unpleasant events. Behavioral checklists, such as the pleasant events schedule (PES; MacPhillamy & Lewinsohn, 1982) and the unpleasant events schedule (UES; Lewinsohn, Mermelstein, Alexander, & MacPhillamy, 1985), are commonly used in therapy to identify and alter the nature and frequency of individual behaviors (or lack thereof) that may be producing or maintaining depression. The PES and UES have been modified for use with older adults (Teri & Lewinsohn, 1982). Recently, a more sophisticated and clinically useful version of the PES for use with older adults, known as the California older persons pleasant events schedule (COPPES; Rider, Gallagher-Thompson, & Thompson, 2004) was developed. The COPPES covers 66 pleasant events potentially enjoyable to older adults. The items can be categorized into 24 event facets indicating the kinds of event the client finds pleasant and the frequency with which each is engaged. A computer scoring program accompanies the measure that facilitates scoring and interpretation. Meeks and Depp (2003) provide a pleasant events-based behavioral model for use in nursing homes.

Using a systems approach to behavior therapy, incorporating education to, and assistance from staff can yield significant benefits when working with depressed older patients in nursing homes or other institutional settings. Behavioral procedures involving staff involvement, including operant methods and environmental modifications, have particular utility in treating depressive symptoms associated with dementia (for a detailed discussion of these procedures and review of outcome research, see Cohen-Mansfield, 2001, and Snowden, Sato, & Roy-Byrne, 2003). Carpenter, Ruckdeschel, Ruckdeschel, and Van Haitsma (2002) recently developed a manualized, behaviorally oriented program for treating depression in long-term care residents with mild-to-moderate dementia.

Cognitive therapy, developed by Beck, Rush, Shaw, and Emery, (1979), focuses on the link between thoughts and emotions and generally retains the traditional CBT principles and precepts in dealing with older adults (Laidlaw, 2001; Zeiss & Steffen, 1996b). The aim of cognitive therapy is to change dysfunctional and irrational thought patterns and develop more realistic ways of perceiving oneself, the environment, and the future—termed by Beck (1976) the "cognitive triad." To achieve this, clients are first taught the link between thoughts and emotions and then how to identify, challenge, and change irrational or extreme thoughts.

Other techniques also can enhance the CBT method. It is important to recognize that older adults often develop remarkable coping strategies over the life-course from their years of experience (Zeiss & Lewinsohn, 1986). Accordingly, focused reminiscence can be a useful component of CBT with some older clients by helping to identify previously successful coping strategies, as well as improve self-esteem through the recognition of past accomplishments.

Relaxation techniques can provide older adults with not only physical relief but also secondary cognitive gains due to a new sense of mastery and self-control. However, progressive muscle relaxation (PMR) may not be appropriate or even possible with older clients with neurological or physical (e.g., arthritic) impairments. With such patients, imagery is often more appropriate. Imagining muscle relaxation, which has been found to be as effective as PMR with older adults, can be a good alternative to traditional PMR (Rickard, Scogin, & Keith, 1994; Zeiss & Steffen, 1996b).

Finally, termination with older adults should proceed slowly and final sessions spaced gradually farther apart (Dick, Gallagher-Thompson, & Thompson, 1999; Moberg & Lazarus, 1990). Rehearsals can be effective for reviewing how to apply newly learned therapeutic techniques to real-world problems. Dick et al. (1999) recommend creating a "maintenance guide" toward the end of therapy that can serve as a later resource and provide both the client and therapist a sense of closure. Lastly, booster sessions are often scheduled with older clients to help facilitate termination and prevent relapse (Dick et al., 1999; Thompson, Davies, Gallagher, & Krantz, 1986).

CBT has been the most widely investigated treatment of late-life depression. The efficacy of CBT with depressed older adults has been well established (see, e.g., Beutler et al., 1987; Engels & Vermey, 1997; Gerson et al., 1999; Pinquart & Sorenson, 2001; Scogin & McElreath, 1994; Thompson et al., 2001). In addition, there is evidence that behavior therapy can be effective in reducing depression in older adults with dementia (Teri, Logsdon, Uomoto, & McCurry, 1997). Indeed, in nursing homes, with a high incidence of cognitive impairment, behavioral approaches can be more helpful than traditional cognitive approaches. This finding also in other areas of practice is leading to an unraveling of the symbiotic customary bond between cognitive and behavioral (cognitive-behavioral). Some theorists are questioning the closeness of this association given the considerable disparity of theoretical basis, and are suggesting that in many cases behaviorist approaches account for an independent and superior effect in intervention outcomes (Jacobson et al., 2000).

Studies evaluating CBT with depressed older adults have identified several factors that suggest a less favorable outcome. These factors include endogenous (vs. exogenous) depression (Gallagher & Thompson, 1983), dysthymia (Leung & Orrell, 1993), presence of a comorbid personality disorder (Thompson, Gallagher, & Czirr, 1988), severe symptomatology (Becker, 1989; Teri & Lewinsohn, 1986), cognitive impairment (Church, 1983), limited self-insight and psychological mindedness (Kennedy, 2000), lack of motivation for and commitment to treatment (Marmar, Gatson, Gallagher, & Thompson, 1989), and the provision of treatment by less qualified therapists (Pinquart & Sorensen, 2001).

Psychodynamic Therapy

Advanced age has historically been viewed as a contraindication for dynamically oriented psychotherapy. Although the notion that old age precludes successful therapeutic change has long been ubiquitous in psychoanalytic and psychodynamic circles (Freud, 1905, 1953), the emergence of lifespan psychology and increased understanding of developmental processes in the areas of ego function and object relations has provided significant insight into the important and unique function of old age in the development and expression of late-life depression and the utility of geropsychodynamic interventions.

In contrast to more skills-based approaches, psychodynamic therapy focuses on internal psychological processes and the resolution of unresolved conflicts from earlier years. Considerable emphasis is placed on the relationship between the therapist and the client, especially early on with older patients (Moberg & Lazarus, 1990; Smyer & Qualls, 1999); (see Knight [2004] for an excellent discussion on developing a therapeutic alliance with older patients). It is through the therapeutic relationship that the client is able to gain self-insight and resolve unconscious conflicts.

Psychodynamic theory can be particularly useful for understanding and conceptualizing late-life depression, particularly due to the frequent losses experienced with advanced age. Although loss in and of itself is not sufficient in producing depression in late life, it may uncover deep-seated neuroses that, prior to the loss, the patient was able to compensate for. The humbling experience of old age, replete with numerous narcissistic assaults and ruptures of object relations, if met by an underdeveloped self can lend the older adult susceptible to depression or other psychological problems. Simply put, old age is the time when the precariousness of the self may become fully exposed and most vulnerable; further, consistent with object relations theory, late life may expose deficiencies in childhood attachments and uncover scars from early unmet emotional needs (Horner, 1979; Kohut, 1979). It might be assumed that this type of dynamic considerations would be less applicable with impaired nursing home elderly. We believe this is to misunderstand the nature of the dynamic therapies which do not essentially involve "talking about" dynamic patterns, but rather to use those patterns to develop pertinent and targeted strategic interventions, which may be often covert, implicit, and behavioral.

Helpfully, in recent years, brief or time-limited forms of psychodynamic therapy have been developed (see Hoyt [2003] for an excellent detailed description of different forms of brief psychodynamic therapy). Time-limited psychodynamic therapy is typically more problem-focused than is its traditional cousin and focuses on only one or two specific issues. Further, transference is not explicitly examined in brief psychodynamic therapy (Kennedy, 2000). The number of sessions in brief forms of psychodynamic therapy varies widely, but the treatment length with older adults is commonly held to 15–20 sessions (Gallagher-Thompson & Thompson, 1995; Kennedy, 2000). In virtually all forms of brief psychodynamic therapy, the therapist assumes a more active stance than is typical in more traditional forms of psychodynamic therapy. This is particularly encouraged with older patients (Gallagher-Thompson & Thompson, 1995).

Common themes addressed in psychodynamic therapy with older adults include dealing with loss, restoring positive sense of self, and enhancing autonomy and mastery. Reparative work, in the form of supportive therapy, is sometimes necessary with more psychologically unstable older patients before embarking on the insight-oriented therapy journey (Lazarus, Sadavoy, & Langsley, 1991; Smyer & Qualls, 1999). According to Horner (1979), one's readiness for insight-oriented therapy depends upon the quality and degree of cohesiveness, reality relatedness, and object relatedness. Supportive therapy is a particularly important consideration with older adults due to internal and external assaults to the ego associated with loss (e.g., loss of cognitive ability, youthfulness, employment, relationships) in late life. For older patients with significant cognitive impairment where direct insight-oriented therapy is contraindicated, dynamic treatment can also function through supportive therapy.

Specifically, supportive therapy can help older adults with an underdeveloped self or diminished ego shore up adaptive, mature defenses and gain cohesiveness. It can also help older patients recently confronted with an assault to a generally healthy sense of self find restitution. Notably, several authors have reported that defenses in old age are more malleable that in earlier life (Grotjahn, 1951; Meerloo, 1953; Myers, 1995). In supportive therapy work with older adults, the therapist serves as a surrogate primary self-object to the older patient. Thus, it is through the transference that the therapist does her reparative work. In the words of Horner (1979), the therapist at times acts as "parallel to that of the primary mothering person or persons of early infancy: that is, as the mediator of organization." There are three functions that the therapist provides to facilitate the formation of a cohesive sense of self. These functions include mirroring, idealizing, and twinship (Newton & Jacobowitz, 1999). Through mirroring transference, the therapist provides praise and veneration that serve to disconfirm negative views the patient may have of himself and allows the client to see often unseen strengths and resources. Through the idealizing transference, the patient identifies the therapist as an omnipotent self-object who provides the patient with a sense of security and protection. Finally, the twinship transference helps to repair the patient's damaged sense of self by providing the patient with the feeling of being understood by one with whom he closely identifies (Newton & Jacobowitz, 1999).

Few empirical outcome studies have been conducted examining the efficacy of psychodynamic therapy with older adults. Most of these studies compared the efficacy of brief psychodynamic therapy with cognitive-behavioral forms of therapy. Overall, this research found that psychodynamic therapy was generally effective in reducing depression in older adults, with little difference between psychodynamic and cognitive-behavioral treatment modalities (Gallagher & Thompson, 1982;

Gallagher-Thompson, Hanley-Peterson, & Thompson, 1990; Thompson, Gallagher, & Breckenridge, 1987). Lazarus et al. (1991) examined the efficacy of brief psychodynamic therapy for treating depression and resolving specific psychosocial problems in eight elderly patients. The researchers found that 10–15 sessions resulted in significant reduction in depressive symptomatology, resolution of the focal problem, improvement in self-esteem, and changes in defense mechanisms for a majority of participants. There is an increasing amount of data demonstrating the efficacy of brief psychodynamic therapy with younger adults (Crits-Christoph, 1992; Messer & Warren, 1995).

Furthermore, there are numerous clinical reports in the extant literature on the success of dynamically oriented psychotherapy in late life, as well as attestations that older adults are as likely to benefit as younger adults, from psychodynamic therapy (Myers, 1991; Silberschatz & Curtis, 1991). Additional guidelines and clinical vignettes for applying dynamically oriented psychotherapy to the treatment of older patients are available (Nemiroff, & Colarusso 1985; Lazarus et al., 1991; Moberg & Lazarus, 1990; Silberschatz & Curtis, 1991). Such approaches can also enhance the quality of intergenerational relations. Nursing homes are the "last chance" to mend hurt, broken, and unfulfilled relationships, and family dynamic interventions can be powerful (Duffy, 1987).

The psychodynamic approach to depression also suggests that depression may be a more complex disorder than is revealed in the traditional empirical analysis of depression. There is probably a variety of depressions in the internal forum that, in turn, lead to a more differentiated approach to treatment (Duffy & Zellner, 2002). From a symptomatic perspective, depression often appears to be a unitary disorder with straightforward treatments, which can often be manualized. Therapists, however, often report cases that are more complex where traditional psychological treatments seem to be ineffective, medications do not work, and usually helpful prescriptions for behavioral lifestyle change are ignored. These situations can lead to another level of diagnosis that reveals much greater diversity in the dynamic patterns that lead to depression such as, for example, complicated bereavement and sociopathic dejection. This viewpoint is captured in the concept that symptomatic depression is a "final common pathway" (Draper, MacCuspie-Moore, & Brodaty, 1998; Harris, 2001) eventuating from a varied series of problematic psychological experiences.

Life Review and Reminiscence

Life review and reminiscence are specific forms of psychodynamic therapy developed specifically for older adults in which the client psychologically revisits the past to resolve unfinished business and past regret, as well as to bring past positive experiences and coping successes into the psychological present. Butler (1963) declared that the process of taking stock of one's life is universal, especially as individuals wrestle with challenges of loss, transition, and mortality in late life. Life review therapy was spawned by the work of Butler and also Erikson's (1959) postulation of a final developmental stage occurring in late life that involves a struggle between ego integrity and despair. According to Erikson, the ability to look back on one's life without major regret yields ego integrity, whereas unsuccessful reflection brings depression and despair. Although "life review" and "reminiscence" are commonly used in the literature synonymously, life review differs from reminiscence in that the former is a structured process of reflection undertaken within a therapeutic context to "resolve, reorganize, and reintegrate what is troubling or preoccupying" (Lewis & Butler, 1974, p. 165). Life review is therefore an adaptive process used in response to challenges encountered in late life and, thus, often serves a very positive function (Nemiroff & Colarusso, 1985b). In contrast, reminiscence is a typically more unstructured recollection of the past. As Molinari (1999) cogently states, life review is "a special form of reminiscence with an evaluative component—it is not the simple remembering of past events, but an active grappling with the past for the sake of settling unresolved tensions" and is a process that is "both intrapersonal and interpersonal" (p. 155). This can be particularly impactful for nursing home residents where short-term memory storage is compromised while often leaving vivid and detailed early recollections. Both the memory and the fact of remembering can be highly gratifying. Life review and reminiscence are not suitable, however, for all individuals, as the recollection of disturbing events and unresolved or unfinished business may yield negative results (e.g., ruminative obsessions) with lower functioning individuals (Butler, 1963).

There has been relatively limited outcome research on the use of life review and reminiscence therapy for the treatment of depression. The existing research has yielded somewhat mixed results. Haight (1988, 1992) found that life review was not superior to a friendly visit or no-treatment control group for treating depression in homebound older adults at post-treatment (8 weeks) or follow-up, although it did increase life satisfaction. In contrast, Fry (1983) found that life review significantly reduced depression in employed, community-dwelling older adults. The large effects found by Fry, in comparison to other studies involving forms of life review, were likely impacted by the nature of the sample and a more structured approach that was employed. Areán et al. (1993) examined the efficacy of group reminiscence therapy versus problem-solving therapy and a waiting list control group in treating major depression in older adults.

Both the reminiscence therapy and problem-solving therapy were superior to the control group at post-treatment (12 weeks) and 3-month follow-up. However, problem-solving therapy was superior to the reminiscence therapy at post-treatment and 3-month follow-up.

A few studies have examined the use of life review and reminiscence in nursing homes. Goldwasser, Auerbach, and Harkins (1987) found that reminiscence was superior to a control group in reducing depression in a small group of nursing home residents. However, as Knight (1996) notes, this finding may be due to random variation in the small sample. Rattenbury and Stones (1989) found no difference between reminiscence and a control group in reducing depression within a nursing home sample. Youssef (1990) found life-review to reduce depression in young-old (65–74 years old) nursing home residents, but not in old-old (75 and older) residents.

On the whole, the available data suggest that life review can be an effective treatment for depression in somewhat higher functioning and introspective older adults with the cognitive and psychological capacity to revisit the past. Moreover, structured, theoretically based life review work appears to be clearly superior to unstructured reminiscence. Specific recommendations on conducting life review work are available (Molinari, 1999; Watt & Cappeliez, 1995).

Interpersonal Therapy

IPT is a time-limited form of psychotherapy that emphasizes the role of relationships on psychological well-being, developed specifically for the treatment of depression (Klerman, Weissman, Rounsaville, & Chevron, 1984). Rather than acquisition of self-insight or resolution of internal psychological conflicts, the goal of IPT is on changing present-day interpersonal behaviors. IPT focuses on one or two specific problems within one or more of the following four interpersonal areas: interpersonal conflicts, interpersonal deficits, relationship loss, and role changes. During the therapy course, clients gain interpersonal insight and skills to improve personal relationships and reactions to interpersonal events. For a detailed approach to each of the four problem areas, the interested reader is referred to Klerman et al. (1984). IPT typically lasts from 12 to 20 sessions (Miller & Silberman, 1996).

Given the important role that loss and role transition play in the graying years, IPT is often well suited for older adults suffering from depressive symptomatology, although there is a paucity of empirical research on IPT for latelife depression; nonetheless, existing data are promising (Mossey, Knott, Higgins, & Talerico, 1996; Reynolds et al., 1997, 1999; Scocco & Frank, 2002; Sloane, Staples, & Schneider, 1985).

IPT has consistently been shown to have considerable efficacy in the treatment of depression in younger adults (see, e.g., Markowitz & Weissman, 1995; Weissman & Markowitz, 1994). Our review of the literature and clinical experience suggest that very few changes are needed when using IPT with older adults (Miller & Silberman, 1996; Sholomskas, Chevron, Prusoff, & Berry, 1983; Hinrichsen, 1999). Specific guidelines and clinical reports on the use of IPT with older adults are available (Frank et al., 1993; Hinrichsen, 1997; Sholomskas et al., 1983).

EMERGING TREATMENT EMPHASES

Treating Depression with Physical Exercise

In recent years, there has been mounting clinical and empirical evidence of the role of physical exercise in treating the affective aspects of depression. In the last few years of clinical literature, we traced 12 studies that showed that physical exercise had an efficacious or effective impact on the symptoms of depression (Arent, Landers, & Etnier, 2000; Babyak et al., 2000; Doyne, Chambless, & Beutler, 1983; Fukukawa et al., 2004; Mather et al., 2002; McNeil LeBlanc, & Joyner, 1991; Palleschi et al., 1998; Singh Clements, & Fiatarone Singh, 2001; Stathi, Fox, & McKenna, 2002; Timonen, Rantanen, Timonen, & Sulkava, 2002; Watanabe, Takeshima, Okada, & Inomata, 2001). Exercise consisted of both aerobic and anaerobic regimens with a variety of exercise routines, including walking, swimming, and lifting weights, and delivered in both individual and group formats. Some results showed the superiority of group exercise regimes versus individual exercise regimes. Many showed positive outcomes, not only in remission of affective symptoms, but also in cognitive skills enhancement, life satisfaction, and interpersonal activity and satisfaction. Although this was not long-term care research, there has been a growing practice of modified exercise regimens in nursing homes that seems to echo the positive general research findings. Exercise is also consistent with the positive adaptive, health-oriented approach to treatment in SOC and other similar viewpoints, focusing less on disease entities and more on health and mental health enhancement. It is interesting that most of these studies came from and were published in the gerontology and psychiatric literature. Only three studies were published in psychology, namely in the *Perceptual and Motor Skills*, *Behavior Therapy*, and the *Journal of Psychology and Aging* which might be considered of more traditional disposition. Recent literature has included several methodological critiques of these data—including concerns with control group subject attendance rates and statistical analyses. A comprehensive review in a British medical journal (Lawlor & Hopker, 2001) examined 14 studies and concluded that many had methodological weaknesses; randomization was adequately concealed (see our earlier discussion) in only three studies, and assessment of outcome was blinded in only one. Studies were judged to be of poor quality, had brief follow-up, and were undertaken on non-clinical volunteers. Even this study however acknowledged that exercise at least might be efficacious in reducing the symptoms of the depression in some volunteers in the short term. This modest praise is counterbalanced by the growing number of studies that seem to be implicating exercise in the effective treatment of depression. Although methodological flaws exist, it is hard not to conclude that the clinical researchers were "on to something" in their conclusion that physical exercise is an important facet of psychological health especially in the case of depression. Many clinicians, convinced of the importance of "moving one's body," routinely assign physical exercise in their treatment planning for older persons with depression. Exercise must be undertaken within the limits of physical ability and sensitive to special medical needs (Burns, 2002). Older adults, however, despite the often painful experience of physical exercise, seem to respond well and gain considerably. Clearly, these intervention methods and research finds need to be extended to nursing homes where group exercise (including such methods as Tai Chi) is an almost universal feature, perhaps with a more general goal of remotivation and health enhancement.

Depression in Dementia

The clearly demonstrated effectiveness of a series of cognitive behavioral and interpersonal techniques in alleviating depression in older adults must be filtered through the complication that occurs when depression coexists with dementia; acerbated in long-term care settings where in excess of 50% of residents have a dementing disorder at some level, and where traditional verbal and cognitive methods have diminishing impact. Dementia is a generic term signifying disturbances (of various etiologies) in cognition that include short- and long-term memory, executive function, and logical language. In these situations, the therapist obviously has little access to the traditional vehicles of cognitive therapy or verbal IPT because cognition is often massively deteriorated. The question then is how to impact depressive feelings in a person who cannot "think their way out" of a depression. Although a relatively small number of studies, as we have seen, deal with behavioral strategies with depression in older adults, an even smaller corpus of material relates to depression in patients who also have a dementing illness. A recent survey identified

11 randomized control clinical trials conducted on older adults where depression-related outcomes were reported. This is an important area of inquiry because we know that dementia and depression frequently coexist in elderly persons. It is quite common to find comorbid depression among demented older residents of nursing homes where attending nursing home staff and family members often effectively "emotionally abandon" such persons upon losing the intuitively needed ability to communicate verbally with each other. This often results in a total cognitive and emotional isolation of older adults in nursing homes, which inevitably produces the affective symptoms of depression. Parenthetically, this same relational dynamic frequently happens with elderly nursing home residents who survive strokes. Although the cognitive effects of strokes are more variable and do not necessarily include dementia, the frequent loss of verbal communication often leads to an emotional disconnection of the patient from other significant persons in their life.

A small number of clinical studies have been conducted to investigate the effectiveness of a series of behavioral treatments for depression in dementia. These can be divided into behavioral approaches (Teri et al., 1997), social engagement approaches, and sensory environmental stimulation approaches. These approaches clearly bypass cognitive interventions. Behavior therapy approaches, based on a social-learning model, view depression as a series of behaviors that are learned and then changed through positive and negative contingencies (Lewinsohn, Sullivan, & Grosscup, 1980). Therapeutic approaches focus on increasing pleasant interactions and decreasing unpleasant interactions as well as developing the skills to alter the environment when possible (Teri & Truax, 1994). This involves an intensive application of pleasant stimulation in the patient's life. For example, in a poststroke depressed client that we were recently treating, we found that moving the therapy outdoors seemed to improve the client's mood and cognitive status. Behavioral problem solving also would include environmental modification, distraction, and communication. Within the social engagement model, the older demented patient is encouraged to interact, often nonverbally, with staff therapists and peers within the family or institution. Also involved in this area would be validation therapy which uses a counter-intuitive approach in dealing with disturbed cognitions and delusions. It is assumed, and often noted by clinicians, that disturbed cognitions and language can be understood as surrogates for emotions of various kinds including unfinished family relationships, etc. Instead of a reality orientation to delusional behavior, the validation therapist accepts and validates the disturbed cognitive behavior thus assuring an anxiety-free and supportive relationship with the client while exploring the emotional connotation of the confused cognitions. This approach has been controversial and atypical within the dominant empirical tradition of psychology, but receives much validation itself in the work of many practicing clinicians. These various cited studies generally have shown effectiveness in a variety of outcome indices and must be considered seriously in the attempt to provide psychotherapeutic services to depressed older persons who have a dementia.

CONCLUSIONS

Depression is a significant mental health problem for older adults, especially for those suffering from chronic medical problems and those who reside in nursing homes. Although medication may prove to be effective, the evidence to date is less than compelling. Behavioral and psychological treatments are clearly effective and need to target internal psychological differences. As there is a psychological component in most depressions, medication-only prescriptions seem highly questionable.

It is also the case that aggressive treatment for depression is especially necessary for older persons because depression can more easily be life-threatening. It is also the conclusion of this chapter that older as well as younger adults have the adaptive resiliency to restore health. Therapists will do well to incorporate this awareness into treatment planning because underestimation of capacity will impede maximum possible change.

REFERENCES

Amenson, C. S., & Lewinsohn, P. M. (1981). An investigation into the observed sex difference in prevalence of unipolar depression. *Journal of Abnormal Psychology, 90*, 1–13.

Antonuccio, D. O., Danton, W. G., & DeNelsky, G. Y. (1995). Psychotherapy versus medication for depression: Challenging the conventional wisdom with data. *Professional Psychology: Research and Practice, 26*(6), 574–585.

Areán, P. A., & Cook, B. L. (2002). Psychotherapy and combined psychotherapy/pharmacotherapy for late life depression. *Biological Psychiatry, 52*, 293–303.

Areán, P. A., Perri, M. G., Nezu, A. M., Schein, R. L., Christopher, F., & Joseph, T. X. (1993). Comparative effectiveness of social problem-solving therapy and reminiscence therapy as treatments for depression in older adults. *Journal of Consulting and Clinical Psychology, 61*, 1003–1010.

Arent, S. M., Landers, D. M., & Etnier, J. L. (2000). The effects of exercise on mood in older adults: A meta-analytic review. *Journal of Aging and Physical Activity, 8*(4), 407–430.

Babyak, M. A., Blumenthal, J. A., Herman, S., Khatri, P., Doraiswamy, P. M., Moore, K. A., Craighead, W. E., Baldewicz, T. T., & Krishnan, K. R. (2000). Exercise treatment for major depression: Maintenance of therapeutic benefit at 10 months. *Psychosomatic Medicine, 62*, 633–638.

Baltes, M. (1996). *The many faces of dependency in old age.* New York: Cambridge University Press.

Baltes, M. M., & Baltes, P. B. (Eds.). (1986). *The psychology of control and aging.* New Jersey: Lawrence Erlbaum Associates.

Baltes, M. M., & Baltes, P. B. (Eds.). (1990). *Successful aging: Perspectives from the behavioral sciences.* New York: Cambridge University Press.

Beck, A. T. (1976). *Cognitive therapy and the emotional disorders.* New York: Meridian.

Beck, A. T., Rush, A. J., Shaw, B. F., & Emery, G. (1979). *Cognitive therapy of depression.* New York: Guilford Press.

Becker, D. (1989). Lithium and propranolol: Possible synergism? *Journal of Clinical Psychiatry, 50*(12), 473.

Beutler, L. E., Scogin, F., Kirkish, P., Schretlen, D., Corbishley, A., Hamblin, D., Meredith, K., Potter, R., Bamford, C. R., Levenson, A. I. (1987). Group cognitive therapy and alprazolam in the treatment of depression in older adults. *Journal of Consulting and Clinical Psychology, 55*(4), 550–556.

Breggin, P. (1994). *Talking back to Prozac.* New York: St. Martin's Press.

Burns, E. A. (2002). Commentary: Challenges to using exercise interventions in older adults. In K. W. Schaie, H. Leventhal & S. L. Willis(Eds.), *Effective health behavior in older adults. Societal impact on aging* (pp. 179–189). New York: Springer Publishing Company.

Burns, B., Wagner, R., Taube, J., Magaziner, J., Purmutt, T., & Landerman, L. (1993). Mental health service use by the elderly in nursing homes. *American Journal of Public Health, 83*, 331–337.

Butler, R. (1963). The life review: An interpretation of reminiscence in the aged. *Psychiatry, 26*, 65–76.

Carpenter, B. D., Ruckdeschel, K., Ruckdeschel, H., & Van Haitsma, K. (2002). R-E-M psychotherapy: A manualized approach for long-term care residents with depression and dementia. *Clinical Gerontologist, 25*, 25–50.

Church, M. (1983). Psychological therapy with elderly people. *Bulletin of the British Psychological Society, 36*, 110–112.

Cohen, J. (1988). *Statistical power analysis for the behavioral sciences* (2nd ed.). Hillsdale, NJ: Erlbaum.

Cohen-Mansfield, J. (2001). Nonpharmacologic interventions for inappropriate behaviors in dementia: A review, summary, and critique. *American Journal of Geriatric Psychiatry, 9*, 361–381.

Crits-Christoph, P. (1992). The efficacy of brief dynamic psychotherapy: A meta-analysis. *American Journal of Psychiatry, 149*, 151–158.

de Jonghe, F., Kool, S., van Aalst, G., Dekker, J., & Peen, J. (2001). Combining psychotherapy and antidepressants in the treatment of depression. *Journal of Affective Disorders, 64*, 217–229.

Dick, L. P., Gallagher-Thompson, D., & Thompson, L. (1999). Cognitive-behavioural therapy. In R. T. Woods (Ed.), *Psychological problems of ageing:*

Assessment, treatment and care (pp. 253–291). New York: John Wiley & Sons.

Doyne, E. J., Chambless, D. L., & Beutler, L. E. (1983). Aerobic exercise as a treatment for depression in women. *Behavior Therapy, 14*(3), 434–440.

Draper, B., MacCuspie-Moore, C., & Brodaty, H. (1998). Suicidal ideation and the 'wish to die' in dementia patients: The role of depression. *Age and Ageing, 27*(4), 502–507.

Duffy, M. (1987). The techniques and contexts of multigenerational therapy. *Clinical Gerontologist, 5*(3/4), 347–362.

Duffy, M. (2000). Individual therapy in long term care. In V. Molinari (Ed.), *Professional psychology in long term care: A comprehensive guide* (pp. 73–89). New York: Hatherleigh Press.

Duffy, M., & Zellner, R. (2002). Varieties of depression: Differential dynamics and techniques. *Proceedings of the British Psychological Society, Division of Counselling Psychology Annual Conference*, Torquay, England.

Engels, G. I., & Vermey, M. (1997). Efficacy of nonmedical treatments of depression in elders: A qualitative analysis. *Journal of Clinical Geropsychology, 3*, 17–35.

Erikson, E. H. (1959). *Identity and the life cycle: Selected papers.* Oxford: International Universities Press.

Frank, E., Frank, N., Cornes, C., Imber, S. D., Miller, M. D., & Morris, S. (1993). Interpersonal psychotherapy in the treatment of late-life depression. In G. L. Klerman, & M. M. Weissman (Eds.), *New applications of interpersonal psychotherapy* (pp. 167–198). Washington, DC: American Psychiatric Association.

Freud, S. (1905, 1953). On psychotherapy. In J. Strachey (Ed), *The complete psychological works of Sigmund Freud* (Vol. 6). London: Hogarth.

Fry, P. S. (1983). Structured and unstructured reminiscence training and depression among the elderly. *Clinical Gerontologist, 1*, 15–37.

Fukukawa, Y., Nakashima, C., Tsuboi, S., Kozakai, R., Doyo, W., Niino, N., Ando, F., & Shimokata, H. (2004). Age differences in the effect of physical activity on depressive symptoms. *Psychology and Aging, 19*(2), 346–351.

Gabrel, C. S. (2000). *Characteristics of elderly nursing home current residents and discharges: Data from the 1997 National Nursing Home Survey.* Advance data from vital and health statistics no. 312. Hyattsville, MD: National Center for Health Statistics.

Gallagher, D. E., & Thompson, L. W. (1982). Treatment of major depressive disorder in older adult outpatients with brief psychotherapies. *Psychotherapy: Theory, Research & Practice, 19*(4), 482–490.

Gallagher, D. E., & Thompson, L. W. (1983). Effectiveness of psychotherapy for both endogenous and nonendogenous depression in older adult outpatients. *Journal of Gerontology, 38*(6), 707–712.

Gallagher-Thompson, D., Hanley-Peterson, P., & Thompson, L. W. (1990). Maintenance of gains versus relapse following brief psychotherapy for depression. *Journal of Consulting & Clinical Psychology, 58*, 371–374.

Gallagher-Thompson, D., & Thompson, L. W. (1995). Psychotherapy with older adults in theory and practice. In B. M. Bongar, & L. E. Beutler (Eds.),

Comprehensive textbook of psychotherapy: Theory and practice. Oxford textbooks in clinical psychology (Vol. 1, pp. 359–379). London: Oxford University Press.

Gatz, M., Pederson, N. S., Plomin, R., Nesselroade, J. R., & McClearn, G. E. (1992). Importance of shared genes and shared environments for symptoms of depression in older adults. *Journal of Abnormal Psychology, 101*, 701–708.

Gerson, S., Belin, T. R., Kaufman, A., Mintz, J., & Jarvik, L. (1999). Pharmacological and psychological treatments for depressed older patients: A meta-analysis and overview of recent findings. *Harvard Review of Psychiatry, 7*, 1–28.

Goldwasser, A. N., Auerbach, S. M., & Harkins, S. W. (1987). Cognitive, affective, and behavioral effects of reminiscence group therapy on demented elderly. *International Journal of Aging & Human Development, 25*, 209–222.

Grotjahn, M. (1951). Some analytic observations about the process of growing old. In G. Roheim (Ed.), *Psychoanalysis and the social sciences* (Vol. III, pp. 301–312). Oxford: International Universities Press.

Haight, B. K. (1988). The therapeutic role of a structured life review process in homebound elderly subjects. *Journals of Gerontology, 43*, P40–P44.

Haight, B. K. (1992). Long-term effects of a structured life review process. *Journals of Gerontology, 47*, P312–P315.

Hallman, J., & Oreland, L. (1989). Serotonergic mechanisms and psychiatric disorders. *Nordisk Psykiatrisk Tidsskrift, 43*, 53–59.

Harris, T. (2001). Recent developments in understanding the psychosocial aspects of depression. *British Medical Bulletin, 57*, 17–32.

Hinrichsen, G. A. (1997). Interpersonal psychotherapy for depressed older adults. *Journal of Geriatric Psychiatry, 30*, 239–257.

Hinrichsen, G. A. (1999). Interpersonal psychotherapy for late-life depression. In M. Duffy (Ed.), *Handbook of counseling and psychotherapy for older adults*. New York: John Wiley & Sons.

Horner, A. (1979). Object relations defined. *Object relations in therapy, 25*, 3–22.

Hoyt, M. F. (2003). Brief psychotherapies. In A. S. Gurman, & S. B. Messer (Eds.), *Essential psychotherapies: Theory and practice theory and practice (2nd ed.): Guilford Press.* (pp. 350–399).

Jacobson, N. S., Dobson, K. S., Truax, P. A., Addis, M. E., Koerner, J. K., Gortner, E., & Prince, S. E. (2000). A component analysis of cognitive-behavioral treatment for depression. *Journal of Consulting and Clinical Psychology, 64*(2), 295–304.

Karlin, B. E., Duffy, M., & Gleaves, D. H. (2004). *Mental health care utilization by community-dwelling elderly: Identifying service use and predictors of care.* Paper presented at the 57th Annual Scientific Meeting of the Gerontological Society of America, Washington, DC.

Karlin, B. E., & Norris, M. P. (in press). Public mental health care utilization by older adults. *Administration and Policy in Mental Health.*

Kennedy, G. J. (2000). *Geriatric mental health care: A treatment guide for health professionals*. New York: Guilford Press.

Kessler, R. C., McGonagle, K. A., Zhao, S., Nelson, C. B., Hughes, M., Eshleman, S., Wttchen, H., & Kendler, K. S. (1994). Lifetime and 12-month prevalence of DSM-III-R psychiatric disorders in the United States. *Archives of General Psychiatry, 51*, 8–19.

Klerman, G. L., Weissman M. M., Rounsaville B. J, & Chevron R. S. (1984). *Interpersonal psychotherapy of depression*. New York: Basic Books.

Knight, B. G. (1996). Psychodynamic therapy with older adults: Lessons from scientific gerontology. In R. T. Woods (Ed.), *Handbook of the clinical psychology of ageing* (pp. 545–560). Oxford: John Wiley & Sons.

Knight, B. G. (2004). *Psychotherapy with older adults* (3rd ed.). Thousand Oaks, CA: Sage.

Kohut, H. (1979). The two analyses of Mr. Z. *International Journal of Psycho-Analysis, 60*, 3–27.

Laidlaw, K. (2001). Cognitive therapy for late life depression: Does research evidence suggest adaptations are necessary for cognitive therapy with older adults? *Clinical Psychology & Psychotherapy: An International Journal of Theory & Practice, 8*, 1–14.

Lawlor, D. A., & Hopker, S. W. (2001). The effectiveness of exercise as an intervention in the management of depression: Systematic review and meta-regression analysis of randomized controlled trials. *British Medical Journal, 322*(7289), 763–766.

Lazarus, L. W., Sadavoy, J., & Langsley, P. R. (1991). Individual psychotherapy. In J. Sadavoy, L. W. Lazarus, & L. F. & Jarvik, al. (Eds.), *Comprehensive review of geriatric psychiatry* (pp. 487–512). Washington, DC: American Psychiatric Association.

Leung, S. N., & Orrell, M. W. (1993). A brief cognitive behavioural therapy group for the elderly: Who benefits? *International Journal of Geriatric Psychiatry, 8*, 593–598.

Lewinsohn, P. M. (1974). A behavioral approach to depression. In R. J. Friedman, & M. M. Katz (Eds.), *The psychology of depression: Contemporary theory and research* (pp. 157–178). Washington, DC: Winston-Wiley.

Lewinsohn, P. M., Mermelstein, R. M., Alexander, C., & MacPhillamy, D. J. (1985). The unpleasant events schedule: A scale for the measurement of aversive events. *Journal of Clinical Psychology, 41*, 483–498.

Lewinsohn, P. M., Sullivan, J. M., & Grosscup, S. J. (1980). Changing reinforcing events: An approach to the treatment of depression. *Psychotherapy: Theory, Research and Practice, 17*, 322–334.

Lewis, M., & Butler, R. (1974). Life-review therapy: Putting memories to work in individual and group psychotherapy. *Geriatrics, 29*, 165–173.

MacPhillamy, D., & Lewinsohn, P. M. (1982). The pleasant events schedule: Studies on reliability, validity, and scale intercorrelation. *Journal of Consulting & Clinical Psychology, 50*, 363–380.

Markowitz, J. C., & Weissman, M. M. (1995). Interpersonal psychotherapy. In E. E. Beckham, & W. R. Leber (Eds.), *Handbook of depression* (2nd ed., pp. 376–390). New York: Guilford Press.

Marmar, C. R., Gaston, L., Gallagher, D., & Thompson, L. W. (1989). Alliance and outcome in late-life depression. *Journal of Nervous & Mental Disease, 177*, 464–472.

Mather, A. S., Rodriguez, C., Guthrie, M. F., McHarg, A. M., Reid, I. C., & McMurdo, M. E. T. (2002). Effects of exercise on depressive symptoms in older adults with poorly responsive depressive disorder: Randomized controlled trial. *British Journal of Psychiatry, 180*(5), 411–415.

McNeil, J. K., LeBlanc, E. M., & Joyner, M. (1991). The effects of exercise on depressive symptoms in the moderately depressed elderly. *Psychology and Aging, 6*(3), 487–488.

Meeks, S., & Depp, C. A. (2003). Pleasant-events based behavioral intervention for depression in nursing home residents: A conceptual and empirical foundation. *Clinical Geropsychologist, 25*, 125–148.

Meerloo, J. (1953). Contributions of psychoanalysis to problems of the aged. In M. Heiman (Ed.), *Psychoanalysis and social work* (Vol. I, pp. 321–337). Oxford: International Universities Press.

Messer, S. B., & Warren, C. S. (1995). *Models of brief psychodynamic therapy: A comparative approach*: Guilford Press.

Miller, M. D., & Silberman, R. L. (1996). Using interpersonal psychotherapy with depressed elders. In H. Zarit, & B. G. Knight (Eds.), *A guide to psychotherapy and aging: Effective clinical interventions in a life-stage context* (pp. 83–99). Washington, DC: American Psychological Association.

Moberg, P. J., & Lazarus, L. W. (1990). Psychotherapy of depression in the elderly. *Psychiatric Annals, 20*, 92–96.

Molinari, V. (1999). Using reminiscence and life review as natural therapeutic strategies in group therapy. In M. Duffy (Ed.), *Handbook of counseling and psychotherapy with older adults* (pp. 154–165). New York: John Wiley & Sons.

Mossey, J. M., Knott, K. A., Higgins, M., & Talerico, K. (1996). Effectiveness of a psychosocial intervention, interpersonal counseling, for subdysthymic depression in medically ill elderly. *Journals of Gerontology, 51A*, M172–M178.

Myers, W. A. (1991). Psychoanalytic psychotherapy and psychoanalysis with older patients. In W. A. Myers (Ed.), *New techniques in the psychotherapy of older patients* (pp. 265–279). Washington, DC: American Psychiatric Association.

Myers, W. A. (1995). The depressed geriatric patient. In H. J. Schwartz, E. Bleiberg, & S. H. Weissman, (et al. (Eds.), *Psychodynamic concepts in general psychiatry* (pp. 383–397). Washington, DC: American Psychiatric Association.

Nemiroff, R. A., & Colarusso, C. A. (1985). The literature on psychotherapy and psychoanalysis in the second half of life. In R. A. Nemiroff, & C. A. Colarusso (Eds.), *The race against time: Psychotherapy and psychoanalysis in the second half of life* (pp. 25–43). New York: Plenum.

Newton, N. A, & Jacobowitz, J. (1999). Transferential and countertransferential processes in therapy with older adults. In M. Duffy (Ed.), *Handbook of counseling and psychotherapy with older adults* (pp. 21–40). New York: John Wiley & Sons.

Olin, J. T., Katz, I. R., Meyers, B. S. (2002). Provisional diagnostic criteria for depression of Alzheimer disease: Rational and background. *American Journal of Geriatric Psychiatry, 10*, 129–141.

Otto, M. C., Smits, J. A., & Reese, H. E. (2005). Combined psychotherapy and pharmacotherapy for mood and anxiety disorders in adults: Review and analysis. *Clinical Psychology: Science and Practice, 12*(1), 72–86.

Palleschi, L., De Gennaro, E., Sottosanti, G., Vetta, F., Ronzoni, S., Lato, P. F. A., Marigliano, V. (1998). The role of exercise training in aged subjects with anxiety-depression syndrome. *Archives of Gerontology & Geriatrics, 6*, 381–384.

Pinquart, M., & Sorensen, S. (2001). How effective are psychotherapeutic and other psychosocial interventions with older adults? A meta-analysis. *Journal of Mental Health & Aging, 7*, 207–243.

Randall, T. (1993). Demographers ponder the aging of the aged and await unprecedented looming elder boom. *Journal of the American Medical Association, 269*, 2331–2332.

Rattenbury, C., & Stones, M. J. (1989). A controlled evaluation of reminiscence and current topics discussion groups in a nursing home context. *Gerontologist, 29*, 768–771.

Reynolds, C. F., Frank, E., Houck, P. R., & Mazumdar, S. (1997). Which elderly patients with remitted depression remain well with continued interpersonal psychotherapy after discontinuation of antidepressant medication? *American Journal of Psychiatry, 54*, 958–962.

Reynolds, C. F., III, Perel, J. M., Frank, E., Cornes, C., Miller, M. D., Houck, P. R., et al. (1999). Three-year outcomes of maintenance nortriptyline treatment in late-life depression: A study of two fixed plasma levels. *American Journal of Psychiatry, 156*(8), 1177–1181.

Rickard, H. C., Scogin, F., & Keith, S. (1994). A one-year follow-up of relaxation training for elders with subjective anxiety. *Gerontologist, 34*, 121–122.

Rider, K. L., Gallagher-Thompson, D., & Thompson, L. W. (2004). *California older persons pleasant events schedule: Manual (beta version)*. Palo Alto, CA: Older Adult and Family Center, Veterans Affairs Palo Alto Health Care System.

Rovner, B. W., & Katz, I. R. (1993). Psychiatric disorders in the nursing home: A selective review of studies related to clinical care. *International Journal of Geriatric Psychiatry, 8*, 75–87.

Scocco, P., & Frank, E. (2002). Interpersonal psychotherapy as augmentation treatment in depressed elderly responding poorly to antidepressant drugs: A case series. *Psychotherapy & Psychosomatics, 71*, 357–361.

Scogin, F., & McElreath, L. (1994). Efficacy of psychosocial treatments for geriatric depression: A quantitative review. *Journal of Consulting & Clinical Psychology, 62*, 29–73.

Sholomskas, A. J., Chevron, E. S., Prusoff, B. A., & Berry, C. (1983). Short-term interpersonal therapy (IPT) with the depressed elderly: Case reports and discussion. *American Journal of Psychotherapy, 37*, 552–566.

Silberschatz, G., & Curtis, J. T. (1991). Time-limited psychodynamic therapy with older adults. In W. A. Myers (Ed.), *New techniques in the psychotherapy of older patients* (pp. 95–108). Washington, DC: American Psychiatric Association.

Singh, N. A., Clements, K. M., & Fiatarone Singh, M. A. (2001). The efficacy of exercise as a long-term antidepressant in elderly subjects: A randomized, controlled trial. *Journals of Gerontology: Series A: Biological Sciences & Medical Sciences, 56A*(8), M497–M504.

Sloane, R. B., Staples, F. R., & Schneider, L. S. (1985). Interpersonal therapy vs. nortriptyline for depression in the elderly. In G. D. Burrows, T. R. Norman, & L. Denerstein (Eds.), *Clinical and pharmacological studies in psychiatric disorders* (pp. 344–346). London: John Libby.

Smyer, M. A., & Qualls, S. H. (1999). *Aging and mental health*. Oxford: Blackwell.

Snowden, M., Sato, K., & Roy-Byrne, P. (2003). Assessment and treatment of nursing home residents with depression or behavioral symptoms associated with dementia: A review of the literature. *Journal of the American Geriatrics Society, 51*, 1305–1317.

Stathi, A., Fox, K. R., & McKenna, J. (2002). Physical activity and dimensions of subjective well-being in older adults. *Journal of Aging and Physical Activity, 10*(1), 76–92.

Teri, L., & Lewinsohn, P. M. (1982). Modification of the pleasant and unpleasant events schedules for use with the elderly. *Journal of Consulting & Clinical Psychology, 50*, 444–445.

Teri, L., & Lewinsohn, P. M. (1986). Individual and group treatment of unipolar depression: Comparison of treatment outcome and identification of predictors of successful treatment outcome. *Behavior Therapy, 17*, 215–228.

Teri, L., Logsdon, R., G., Uomoto, J., & McCurry, S. M. (1997). Behavioral treatment of depression in dementia patients: A controlled clinical trial. *Journals of Gerontology, 52B*, P159–P166.

Teri, L., & Truax, P. (1994). Assessment of depression in dementia patients: Association of caregiver mood with depression ratings. *Gerontologist, 34*(2), 231–234.

Thompson, L. W., Coon, D. W., Gallagher-Thompson, D., Sommer, B. R., & Koin, D. (2001). Comparison of desipramine and cognitive/behavioral therapy in the treatment of elderly outpatients with mild-to-moderate depression. *American Journal of Geriatric Psychiatry, 9*, 225–240.

Thompson, L. W., Davies, R., Gallagher, D., & Krantz, S. E. (1986). Cognitive therapy with older adults. *Clinical Gerontologist, 5*, 245–279.

Thompson, L. W., Gallagher, D., & Breckenridge, J. S. (1987). Comparative effectiveness of psychotherapies for depressed elders. *Journal of Consulting and Clinical Psychology, 55*, 385–390.

Thompson, L. W., Gallagher, D., & Czirr, R. (1988). Personality disorder and outcome in the treatment of late-life depression. *Journal of Geriatric Psychiatry, 21*, 133–146.

Timonen, L., Rantanen, T., Timonen, T. E., & Sulkava, R. (2002). Effects of a group-based exercise program on the mood state of frail older women after discharge from hospital. *International Journal of Geriatric Psychiatry, 17*(12), 1106–1111.

VandenBos, G. R., Stapp, J., & Kilburg, R. R. (1981). Health services providers in psychology: Results of the 1978 APA human resources survey. *American Psychologist, 36*, 1395–1418.

Wampold, B. E. (2001). *The great psychotherapy debate: Models, methods and findings*. Hillsdale, NJ: Lawrence Erlbaum.

Watanabe, E., Takeshima, N., Okada, A., & Inomata, K. (2001). Effects of increasing expenditure of energy during exercise on psychological wellbeing in older adults. *Perceptual and Motor Skills, 92*(1), 288–298.

Watt, L. M., & Cappeliez, P. (1995). Reminiscence interventions for the treatment of depression in older adults. In B. K. Haight, & J. D. Webster (Eds.), *The art and science of reminiscing: Theory, research, methods, and applications* (pp. 221–232). Philadelphia: Taylor & Francis.

Weissman, M. M., & Markowitz, J. C. (1994). Interpersonal psychotherapy: Current status. *Archives of General Psychiatry, 51*(8), 599–606.

Youssef, F. A. (1990). The impact of group reminiscence counseling on a depressed elderly population. *Nurse Practitioner, 15*, 32–38.

Zeiss, A., & Lewinsohn, P. (1986). Adapting behavioral treatment for depression to meet the needs of the elderly. *Clinical Psychologist, 39*, 98–100.

Zeiss, A. M., & Steffen, A. (1996b). Behavioral and cognitive-behavioral treatments: An overview of social learning. In S. H. Zarit, & B. G. Knight (Eds.), *A guide to psychotherapy and aging: Effective clinical interventions in a life-stage context* (pp. 35–60). Washington, DC, US: American Psychological Association.

PART III

"There Is Still a Person in There"

CHAPTER SIX

SOC, Personality, and Long-Term Care

Victor Molinari, Frederick J. Kier, and Erlene Rosowsky

Millon (1981) defines personality as "ingrained and habitual ways of psychological functioning that emerge from the individual's entire developmental history . . . distinctive ways of coping with others and relating to ourselves" (pp. 4, 5). Given this definition, the average older adult, with a longer "developmental history," could be said to have more "depth" of personality, one based upon a larger range of life experiences, than a typical younger person. Cross-sectional and cross-national research indicates that, despite the "psychological maturing" of the personality that comes with age, the core aspects of a personality, for the majority of persons, remain relatively constant throughout the lifespan (McCrae et al., 1999). However, researchers also find that a fair minority of individuals show significant changes in at least some personality domains (Small, Hertzog, Hultsch, & Dixon, 2003; Valliant, 2002) probably as a result of life-changing nodal points and transitions such as divorce, job promotion, or death(s) of loved ones.

Personality dictates, to a large degree, how a person copes with stressors; and personality factors should thereby take center stage in understanding how older adults manage the vicissitudes of late life. An older adult faces significant life events entailing profound losses (e.g., death of a spouse, retirement, illness), and these events have been theorized to play a more significant role in development as one ages (Baltes, Reese, & Lipsitt, 1980). This may be especially true for residents in long-term care (LTC) settings who have sustained life events that have precipitated dependence on others for assistance in daily living requiring institutional placement.

We will first briefly examine personality vis-a-vis the SOC model, and examine the research that has been conducted on SOC and personality factors. We next evaluate how the SOC model meshes with personality factors in the LTC environment. We then discuss the practical implications of the SOC model for enhancing the quality of life of LTC residents, and present a clinical vignette to illustrate these ideas. Finally, we identify areas for future research.

PERSONALITY AND THE SOC MODEL—THEORETICAL CONSIDERATIONS

The Baltes' SOC model posits that, as one ages, the means of social compensation (often referred to as "culture" in the SOC model) for the mental and physical decline associated with aging becomes less and less available, even as the need for such compensation increases (Baltes, 1991, 1997; Baltes & Baltes, 1990). As noted by Baltes (1991), feelings of self-esteem and self-worth typically do not reflect the numerous losses faced by older adults, and may even counteract them. Personality thus appears to be one of the few resources that older adults can utilize to buffer the frailties of aging. In Ryff's (1987) words, ". . . personality is the realm compensating for loss in other spheres" (p. 210).

Baltes (1991) addresses the durability of older adults' personality, and their ability to handle the heightened demands of aging, vis-a-vis the SOC model. Older adults become more selective in goals, altering or changing them as needed by circumstances. Flowing from the SOC model, socioemotional selectivity theory (Carstensen, Isaacowitz, & Charles, 1999) argues that as individuals age, they become less concerned with gaining new information and forming new friendships, and more interested in nurturing close family ties. These changes may be reflected in declining openness and extraversion, and increasing agreeableness (Srivastava, John, Gosling, & Potter, 2003). Such selectivity may define character and reflect sage experience, not necessarily rigidity (Vaillant, 2002).

Smith and Fruend (2002) discuss the theory of "possible selves" which are "highly personalized hoped for and feared images of the self that function as incentives for action," (p. 492) and thus can be useful in considering the process of selection in the SOC model (Baltes & Carstensen, 1991; Freund & Baltes, 2002; Smith & Fruend, 2002). In coping with the demands of aging, these images can be accentuated or discarded when goals need to be modified. Older adults in LTC settings who have possible selves that are overly focused on health matters coupled with "feared self-images" (picturing themselves having bad outcomes and becoming more disabled) exhibit less feelings of well-being; those with more varied, balanced (between positive and negative) "future possible selves" report enhanced feelings of well-being (Smith & Fruend, 2002).

Personality can be defined behaviorally as a system of strategies by which the individual achieves personal, social, and material goals. It may thus be posited that the flexibility of a personality to alter goals and expectations, in light of flagging capacity due to aging, can yield positive results for the individual. But this occurs only if the person has an array of personal options to draw from. Optimization of resources requires development over time of inner strengths, insight, adaptability, and openness to experience.

In addition to selection and optimization, compensation is also an active strategy, in that older persons can change the comparison group by which they "measure themselves" against (Baltes, 1991; Baltes & Baltes, 1990), for example, by choosing a group that has impairments, stressors, or life experiences similar to their own. Feeling like one is an integral part of such a group, however, appears to be critical. Bailes and Chipperfield (2002) theorize that collective self-esteem, i.e., one's perception of worth in a social group, may compensate for individual losses.

In describing the importance of personality on how adults deal with aging, Baltes (1991) states "we have remarkable resiliency and adaptive capacity for reorganization and maintaining integrity. . . . It seems possible for most older persons to continue to use this dynamic and adaptive feature of the self as a kind of protective shield against the adversities associated with becoming old" (p. 849).

RESEARCH ON PERSONALITY AND THE SOC MODEL

Research on stress and coping styles in older adults is congruent with the outcomes of studies on variables in the SOC model. Older adults have been shown to be more selective and use more adaptive, mature, efficient coping mechanisms (Diehl, Coyle, & Labouvie-Vief, 1996; Irion & Blanchard-Fields, 1987), and fewer immature coping mechanisms such as avoidance and escapist fantasy than younger adults (Feifel & Strack, 1989; McCrae, 1982). The reason could be that older adults, despite accruing losses, subject themselves to less general stress (Aldwin, 1991) due to narrowing of life focus or due to developing a more philosophical outlook (Cavanaugh & Blanchard-Fields, 2002). However, this body of research on diminished stress may not necessarily hold in LTC settings.

Given the importance of personality in the SOC model, in terms of its ability to moderate the deleterious effects of growing older via choice of coping styles, one would expect SOC research to emphasize personality factors. Much of the research involving the SOC model, however, only appears to indirectly deal with characterological traits. This may be because the SOC model itself can be viewed as an overarching framework for how individuals can (and do) successfully age, i.e., via selectivity of goals, optimizing strengths, and compensating for weaknesses.

Fruend and Baltes (1998) found that, in a sample of 206 German older adults, those who utilized SOC-style approaches scored higher on measures of successful aging than those who did not. It can be assumed that successful agers' personality styles have allowed them, via their cumulative life experiences, to incorporate SOC elements into their coping styles. Some research suggests that a majority of normally functioning individuals, both young and old, discover that strategies congruent with the SOC model are appealing in terms of managing problems in their lives (Freund & Baltes, 2002).

Other studies have also investigated the relationship between positive aging and the incorporation of SOC strategies into one's personality style. Abraham and Hansson (1995) examined a sample of 224 employed, successful adults between the ages of 40 and 69 and found that, in general, they utilized SOC strategies to maintain their competence in the workplace. These authors suggest that job context and individual characteristics may mediate SOC behaviors. Baltes and Lang (1997) found that older adults with greater social and personality resources exhibit fewer aging problems than those older adults with less social and personality resources. This makes some sense, given that those individuals who have more social skills at their disposal are more apt to engage in social relationships, and would be expected, on average, to have greater social networks and resources than those with personality types which render them less socially active and more isolative. In an extension of this study, Lang, Rieckmann, and Baltes (2002) concluded that older adults who have more social and personality resources are more likely to utilize SOC-style strategies in their daily lives. It appears that older adults who have the most need of using SOC-style strategies, i.e., those with fewer social and personality resources, are the ones who are the least likely to use them.

PERSONALITY, SOC, AND LTC

Placement in an LTC facility is often a highly stressful event and is usually the consequence of an individual having deficits in physical, mental, and/or, in some cases, social resources. Coupled with the stigma that LTC facilities convey in our culture, the depersonalization of institutionalization, and the reliance on others for well-being, an older person in an LTC site is likely to face a severe personal crisis.

Research bears this out. The transition to LTC facilities requires a major adjustment with frequent negative emotional sequelae (Yawney & Slover, 1973), which may contribute to the high rate of mental disorders (Burns et al., 1993). Brooke (1989) and Mikhail (1992) postulate that new residents of LTC settings undergo a discrete set of stages of adjustment to their new surroundings: disorientation (feelings of abandonment and vulnerability), reorientation (reasons for placement begin to be identified), relationship building (emotional tie-forming), and stabilization (acceptance). Extrapolating from SOC theory (Baltes, 1997), those individuals entering LTC facilities will negotiate these stages by selecting very specific goals that they will attempt to achieve by optimizing their personal strengths and offsetting their weaknesses. For most, this will mean slowly but surely finding some kind of inner peace and meaning with the new life situation by mustering their unique abilities to achieve this end.

Under the circumstances of such novel surroundings, personality styles may be construed as moderating factors across the specific stages of adjustment to an LTC facility. For example, in the disorientation stage, the depression, anxiety, and insecurity accompanying the personality trait of neuroticism may adversely affect the person's ability to adjust, while the openness to experience personality trait may assist in managing the initial shock of relocation and thereby reduce the time it takes for the person to reorganize. If a person is disagreeable and "acts out," she/he may be unable to listen to family and LTC staff so that misunderstanding of reasons for placement may continue, thwarting reorganization. Extraverted people, those who are likely to have greater sociocultural resources according to the SOC model, may have it easier in the relationship-building stage where new relationships with staff and roommates are forged. Finally, those who are open to experience and conscientious may more quickly recognize LTC living as a necessity for which they must accept.

However, personality characteristics may also become greatly intensified under the acute stress of relocation. In particular, two groups of older adults entering LTC settings may not fare so well. Those individuals with longstanding exaggerated personality characteristics (i.e., those with a personality disorder [PD]) are frequently described as having poor personal insight. They may view themselves in grandiose (narcissistic) or demeaning (dependent) ways, and may be unable to accurately evaluate their strengths or limitations.

In a series of studies on the prevalence of PD in older adults, Molinari and his associates found that older adults are much less likely to meet the criteria for more than one PD than are younger adults in inpatient (Molinari, Ames, & Essa, 1994), outpatient (Molinari & Marmion, 1993), and community (Ames & Molinari, 1994) settings. Older adults with PD finally appear to adhere to just one strategy to manage their relationships. However, it is unclear whether the PD strategy chosen is always the most optimal and effective one in their dysfunctional repertoire, given the lack of insight and already restricted behavioral range of those with PD. As Schulz and Heckhausen (1996) have noted, diversity provides the raw material for developmental advances and reduces the risk of narrow specialization. The lack of variability in PD older adults' interpersonal armamentarium may put them at a distinct disadvantage in the transition to new living arrangements. With only a narrow band of personal strengths to sustain them, they may thereby further inappropriately amplify their "tried and true" personality style to satisfy their needs.

The second group consists of "normal" individuals whose transitional stress is compounded by cognitive impairment, medical frailty, and/or lack of social support. Those personality traits which may have once served them well (unlike those individuals with PD) now become overutilized and thereby liabilities for successful adjustment. In terms of identity process theory (Whitbourne, 2001), individuals in both of these groups are unable to interpret their experiences in ways that are congruent with their fragile self-identities. Rather than accomodating new self-schemas into their identity, they twist and skew their perceptions to preserve a now atavistic view of themselves.

Research suggests, however, that even well-adjusted older adults may have certain personality characteristics encouraged or extinguished in the LTC facility environment. Probably the most studied personality characteristic in the field of geropsychology is dependency. Baltes (1996) referred to it as "one of the most pressing problems of old age" (p. 1). Dependency was theorized by the Baltes' and their colleagues to be due to ageism and a culture that values independence, rather than due to any true character deficits, or personality factors, intrinsic to older adults (Baltes, 1996; Baltes & Zerbe, 1976).

To illustrate the effects of the environment and social factors, Lester and Baltes (1978) examined the behavioral interactions between staff and residents of a nursing home facility. They found that staff typically respond to dependency behaviors, but ignore behaviors that reflect independence. Baltes, Honn, Barton, Orzech, and Lago (1983) performed a similar study on a slightly larger sample and found comparable results. These studies looked not only at nursing home staff, but also the interactions of every person that the individual nursing home residents in the sample encountered in their daily lives. Regardless of many factors (types of behavior, staff vs. visitor, length of institutionalization), it appears that the nursing home social environment itself rewards dependency and ignores behaviors consistent with independence.

The environment of an LTC facility could conceivably change a person's behavioral strategy for attaining social and instrumental rewards, encourage those elements of personality that incorporate dependency, and, given enough time, alter personality. One could easily imagine how different personality styles may react to the dependency-fostering nursing home environment. A dependent personality, one who seeks positive reinforcement for dependent behaviors, could be theorized to actually function reasonably well in a nursing home environment. More independent personality styles might be expected to react more poorly, act out, or become depressed.

PRACTICAL IMPLICATIONS

One way of adding conceptual clarity to the older adult personality literature is to view the "selectivity of goals" and "optimization of means" factors as potentials for promoting remaining *internal* positive personality traits, and the "compensation for decline" factor as a potential for keeping negative personality features from being expressed by modifying and "containing" the LTC *external* environment. Extrapolations from SOC theory yield recommendations into how to assist LTC residents into realistically accommodating to their new living environment. Practical applications include the following factors:

1. During the transition period assessment should be considered a process, thus preventing premature pessimistic conclusions. On-going personality evaluation should offer updated formulations that identify weaknesses to be compensated for and strengths to be drawn from.
2. The SOC model draws attention to the limitations of focusing on deficits and impairments, particularly with frail older adults in crisis.
3. There is a tendency for mental health professionals to assist new LTC residents by only tapping external resources. All older adults, even frail ones (except perhaps those with severe dementia) also have internal strengths.
4. External sources of emotional support (e.g., friends, relatives) should be utilized only after an assessment of the history of the LTC residents' introverted/extraverted tendencies, family members' relationships with the LTC individual, and the emotional burden on former caregivers. Highly emotionally expressive

relationships may do more harm than good (Ingersoll-Dayton, Morgan, & Antonucci, 1997), even if the person is extraverted and socially isolated.

5. Use of environmental planning (e.g., allowing LTC residents the freedom to choose their diet or to sleep late in the morning) may be a powerful means of assisting individuals in gaining mastery over their environment. Kahana and Kahana's (1983) congruence model suggests that personal factors must be taken into account when designing environments for older adults. An exact/inexact fit between person and environment can either restore feelings of competence or increase stress levels (Cavanaugh & Blanchard-Fields, 2002). Some inner-directed individuals may simply desire to "do their own thing." Conscientious people may do well in managing their own medication regimens. Dependent persons may have improved feelings of mastery and control if "powerful" staff members consistently interact with them on a regular basis; an individual high on "openness to experience," on the other hand, may need to engage in more "risky" stimulating activities to promote self-continuity and self-efficacy. Achieving mastery via SOC therefore means ongoing reappraisal of the person's goals, strengths, and weaknesses.
6. As suggested above, it would appear that there are certain 5-factor model (McCrae & Costa, 1987) personality traits that facilitate an easier transition to LTC living. Those older adults who are extraverted and agreeable may readily adjust to a communal living situation. Risk takers may initially do well when facing such a novel challenge, but may easily become bored with LTC routine. Those who are high in neuroticism will do poorly in most transitional situations, and perhaps should be flagged for more intensive evaluation and follow up.
7. Evaluation of personality traits upon LTC admission should be guided by the SOC model. To promote the modified and realistic goals of frail older adults, what are the constellation of personality trait strengths to draw from and limitations to avoid, and which in combination with social supports and LTC environmental flexibility achieve this desired end?

CASE VIGNETTE

Mr C—The Patient

Mr C is an 83-year-old resident of an LTC facility where he has been living for the past 7 years. He has multiple physical health conditions requiring that he live in a skilled nursing setting. These include hypertension, sequelae of cerebrovascular accidents (CVAs), hyperlipidemia, and osteroarthritis. His psychiatric history includes an episode of major depression without psychotic features on Axis I, and a diagnosis of narcissistic PD (NPD) on Axis II.

The LTC facility requested a mental health consultation because of the resident's increasingly "impossible" behaviors. Mr C, by their report, has progressively changed for the worse. He is angry, hostile to staff, has been physically aggressive at times, and refuses to be involved in his prescribed physical therapy (PT) program or to participate in group activities.

History

Mr C had been living independently in the community until age 74. For the next approximately 2 years he had several hospitalizations, including two stays in a rehabilitation facility following CVAs. His hypertension has been severe at times and difficult to control, requiring close monitoring, a number of medication changes, and strict attention to diet. Mr C had been a cigarette smoker—a habit he gave up following his first CVA. He experiences some shortness of breath, particularly when he becomes agitated. Always a gregarious person, he enjoyed social drinking, but there is no history of frank alcohol abuse.

Mr C was raised in NYC, the only son of immigrant parents. He was the favorite child, and his mother's "golden boy." He was very good looking, and comfortable in social situations. While not an exceptionally good student, he was one of the most "popular" in high school. He attended City College for a year or two, and then left because he was offered "a job I couldn't refuse" with a manufacturing company. He was an early "swinger" in the off hours, but apparently a responsible worker at his job, which he kept for over 20 years. He developed a gambling habit and was a clear womanizer. Both of these conditions led to the break-up of his marriage. He loved to travel, and knew many people "everywhere." He appears to have no regrets for how he lived his life. Indeed he had been fond of telling stories suggesting pride in the high life he led, frequently testing the boundaries of conventional definitions of "moral" and "legal."

Mr C has been divorced for more than 40 years. He has had a number of partners since then, but none whom he married or with whom he lived. He has two adult sons from his marriage. One of his sons lives in the area, and had been a fairly regular visitor to the LTC facility. However, as his father's condition deteriorated, so has the father–son relationship. Mr C became increasingly hostile toward his son with the result that visits became briefer and further apart. While Mr C proclaims he would like to see more of his family, he states, "They don't care about me, anyhow. They put me out like a pile of old rags."

For the first years, Mr C was a favorite resident. Historically "a real charmer," Mr C was generally liked by the facility staff, and even his more dramatic outbursts and demanding behaviors were well tolerated. People enjoyed being around him because of his outgoing nature and colorful stories. He did not develop close relationships with other residents, as his style was not to dialog but rather to monolog. When his physical condition deteriorated and his anger became more overt, the residents shied away from him.

As he became more reliant on the physical care of aides, his old style began to wear thin. At first, he began to passively receive their ministrations, but later would begin to lash out, mostly verbally, but occasionally physically as well. On other occasions, Mr C has been inappropriate with female aides, resulting in incident reports being filed for "sexual acting out." He is often extremely rude to staff, using rage-fueled expletives liberally. At other times, he refuses to participate in therapies or social activities.

Premise

The hallmark features of NPD include a grandiose sense of self, lack of empathy, and hypersensitivity to the attention of others. This does not change with age, but clearly the inflated self-image and the positive regard of others becomes markedly more difficult to secure and maintain.

Mr C's 5-Factor Personality Profile

High N

Suggests vulnerability to stress and exaggerated self-consciousness.

High E

Suggests extreme extraversion; high need for feedback from others.

Low O

Suggests low ability to consider options; a limited coping repertoire.

Low A

Consistent with limited regard for others; very low trust, honesty, modesty.

Low C

Consistent with a history of impulsiveness and poor self-discipline.

Core Concepts and Themes as They Relate to the SOC Framework

Mr C has suffered more narcissistic insults than he can bear. His usual ways of being, his coping strategies, have become increasingly less effective. In the past, they enabled him to engage the positive feedback of others, reflecting back to him his belief in his unique, exceptional status.

Those with NPD depend heavily upon feedback from others to reconfirm the self, the feeling of "me"-ness. There is little in Mr C's life now to provide the continuity of whom he was/is: a man who is special, vital, engaging, a bit of a rogue, and charmer. For someone with his personality structure, if not acknowledged and appreciated, his life has no meaning, purpose, or future. Mr C has become depleted and defeated. He alternates feeling empty and abandoned, leading to withdrawal and depression, or feeling cheated and enraged, leading to acting-out.

What he lacks most, consistent with a PD, is flexibility and a range of coping responses. Those with PD tend to rely on a limited repertoire of responses, often inadequate or inappropriate to the situation or interaction (Rosowsky, 1999). When challenged, the PD individual will tend to apply the (maladaptive) response even louder, harder, stronger, or suffer psychiatric consequences, such as depression and anxiety, which are highly comorbid with PD (Zweig, 2003).

The SOC model describes a framework for an expanded vision of positive selves. The special challenge with Mr C is to identify goals that will support healthy narcissism, expand coping options, and optimize personal resources. Goals must be selected from a repertoire lined by his own constellation of personality traits and the LTC facility's regulations. They would ideally lead to not only a better quality of life for Mr C but also the continued development of future stage and context-relevant aspirations. Interventions could be directed toward achieving the following goals: (a) positive (at least nonabusive) contact with nurses and aides during their care services; (b) participation in the PT regimen; (c) participation in some group activities; and (d) increased time with family.

The antecedents of his negative behaviors should be identified and used to inform interventions. Triggers that reflect personal weaknesses of Mr C include:

1. Boredom. For the narcissistic character, high stimulation is ego-syntonic.
2. Lack of attention. Attention and positive feedback are lifelong nutrients for the narcissistic character.
3. Ordinary status in a group. Special status or a unique role is required to engage this character type in a group or community.

Examples of Interventions

1. Mr C's history of "charming the ladies" can be put to use with the female aides by their being coached to communicate with him like the gentleman he believes himself to be. Since he can no longer "wine and dine" them, he can be encouraged to regale them with the stories of times when he could, which they might appreciate anew.
2. His PT program should be individualized and made one-on-one if possible, so that he receives the undivided attention of the therapist. The goals within the program need to have real meaning for him. For example, his "walking" could be for the purpose of choosing a tie to wear at dinner from a "closet" set a reasonable walking distance away as prescribed in his program.
3. It is usually wise to put the dominant personality features to positive use (compensation). Consider that Mr C had been a leader, but has now lost an audience for his stories, so his most positive way of being is now denied him. Allow him to be special in a group activity by leading it, starting first, and recalling with/for him prior experiences that "fit" with the group's activity. For example, in a group with the purpose of promoting reminiscence and executive functioning, the activity might be to "plan" a trip: what is needed, sequencing, anticipating consequences, etc. Mr C could be asked to start off because "You've traveled so much and had so many experiences." He could be invited to share an adventure or two. This is loss-based restoration using the auxiliary help of the facilitator and the group. Group identity and some sense of community can compensate for lost or diminished self-resources.
4. One success promotes another. It is very likely that as his healthy narcissism becomes strengthened, negative behaviors will diminish and positive ones will re-emerge. The whole system will thereby

change. When his son or other family members visit, interactions will be less toxic, more pleasant, because of changes not only with Mr C, but also between the facility and the family. In anticipation of the visits, Mr C would also be coached about "what to remember to tell your son when he comes the next time." This will serve to compensate for memory slippage, to decide on specific topics and themes, to encourage the pleasure to be extended through anticipation, and to organize the encounter to maximize the probability of its being successful, that is, meeting his goal of more family contact.

RESEARCH DIRECTIONS

Reviewing the literature, we found surprisingly few studies on resilience and LTC residents. Research has just begun to address issues of self-efficacy, mastery, and control in LTC settings (see Jang, Haley, Small, & Mortimer, 2003). In order for health care professionals to promote adjustment, positive personality variables must be further explored.

Researchers should also turn their attention to those older adults with psychopathology, and how their personality and coping styles contrast with healthier SOC stratagems. Studies should be conducted to determine if the selectivity and optimization strategies of older adults with PD are consistent with the adaptive maturity of most older adults or reflect more specialized but continued ineffective coping. Investigators should integrate basic and applied research findings to determine how mental health professionals can transform the SOC strategies of well-functioning older adults into guides for clinical interventions.

We must recognize that the personality styles of the spouses and adult children of LTC residents will also play a significant role in the residents' adjustment, and should therefore be explored in more detail vis-a-vis the SOC model. The stages of adjustment for the LTC resident might be extrapolated to family members as well. For example, family caregivers who are open to the idea of placement and are outgoing in their interactions with staff may more quickly accept the inevitable and promote stabilization of their loved one by carving out a new relationship-building "care manager" role for themselves.

Research on personality dimensions other than dependency, and how they affect adjustment to the culture(s) of LTC settings should be conducted. Is the openness to experience variable stifled in some LTC facilities, thus preventing the individual from drawing from a range of personal strengths to handle the challenges of their new environment? On a broader scale, how can LTC environments be planned to allow residents to optimize personal assets and compensate for weaknesses? Are there certain "better fits" between personality traits (e.g., extraversion, neuroticism) and particular LTC settings (e.g., assisted living facilities, nursing homes) that should be considered in hospital discharge planning?

Perhaps most importantly, quantitative and qualitative findings should be integrated and put to practical use in guiding public policy decisions. Baltes (1997) has recently expressed concern that there may be limits to what can be achieved by very old adults utilizing SOC-style coping mechanisms. Research-based advocacy by professional organizations must be conducted to promote societal and environmental compensatory systemic changes in the way LTC housing and health services are organized and financed.

CONCLUSIONS

The overarching premise of the SOC model as applied to the LTC resident is the acknowledgment of reciprocal adaptation and accommodation between the resident and the facility. Selection, optimization, and compensation occur in a specialized social context. If an individual optimizes internal resources, and the LTC setting compensates for coping limitations, modified selected goals can be achieved. The resident's changing competencies and self-resources, as well as modifications within the system itself, need periodic reassessment for a continued proper fit.

The SOC model provides a theoretical framework for conceptualizing research findings on personality and adjustment in LTC settings, and directing avenues of future research. For example, quality-of-life research may need to focus on individual factors that support adaptive selection and optimization strategies, and on family/environmental factors that support compensation strategies.

The SOC model also yields practical mental health and quality of life implications. Only by a thorough bio-psycho-social assessment of the individual, including an inventory of personality features and an evaluation of family support encompassing each resident and family members' own internal and external characteristics, can a treatment plan be forged within the context of a specific LTC site reflecting its own unique management style and dedication to the mission of caring for our frailest population.

REFERENCES

Abraham, J. D., & Hansson, R. O. (1995). Successful aging at work: An applied study of selection, optimization, and compensation through impression management. *Journal of Gerontology: Psychological Sciences, 50B*(2), P94–P103.

Aldwin, C. M. (1991). Does age affect the stress and coping process? Implications of age differences in perceived control. *Journal of Gerontology: Psychological Sciences, 46*, P174–P180.

Ames, A., & Molinari, V. (1994). Prevalence of personality disorders in community-living elderly. *Journal of Geriatric Psychiatry and Neurology, 7*(3), 189–194.

Bailes, D. S., & Chipperfield, J. G. (2002). Compensating for losses in perceived personal control over health: A role for collective self-esteem in healthy aging. *Journal of Gerontology: Psychological Sciences, 57B*, P531–P539.

Baltes, P. (1991). The many faces of human aging: Toward a psychological culture of old age. *Psychological Medicine, 21*, 837–854.

Baltes, M. M. (1996). *The many faces of dependency in old age.* Melbourne, Australia: Cambridge.

Baltes, P. (1997). On the incomplete architecture of human ontogeny: Selection, optimization, and compensation as foundation of developmental theory. *American Psychologist, 52*(4), 366–380.

Baltes, P. B., & Baltes, M. M. (Eds.). (1990). *Successful aging: Perspectives from the behavioral sciences.* Cambridge: Cambridge University Press

Baltes, M. M., & Carstensen, L. L. (1991). Possible selves across the life span. *Human-Development, 34*(4), 256–260.

Baltes, M. M., Honn, S., Barton, E. M., Orzech, M., & Lago, D. (1983). On the social ecology of dependence and independence in elderly nursing home residents: A replication and extension. *Journal of Gerontology, 38*(5), 556–564.

Baltes, M. M., & Lang, F. R. (1997). Everyday functioning and successful aging: The impact of resources. *Psychology & Aging, 12*(3), 433–443.

Baltes, P. B., Reese, H. W., & Lipsitt, L. P. (1980). Life-span developmental psychology. *Annual Review of Psychology, 31*, 65–110.

Baltes, M. M., & Zerbe, M. B. (1976). Independence training in nursing home residents. *Gerontologist, 16*(5), 428–432.

Brooke, V. (1989). How elders adjust. *Geriatric Nursing, 10*, 66–68, 126–128.

Burns, B. J., Wagner, H. R., Taube, J. E., Magaziner, J., Permyutt, T., & Landerman, L. R. (1993). Mental health service use by the elderly in nursing homes. *American Journal of Public Health, 83*, 331–337.

Carstensen, L. L., Isaacowitz, D. M., & Charles, S. T. (1999). Taking time seriously: A theory of socialemotional selectivity. *American Psychologist, 54*, 165–181.

Cavanaugh, J. C., & Blanchard-Fields, F. (2002). *Adult development and aging* (4th ed.). Belmont, CA: Wadsworth.

Diehl, M., Coyle, N., & Labouvie-Vief, G. (1996). Age and sex differences in strategies of coping and defense across the life span. *Psychology and Aging, 11*(1), 127–139.

Feifel, H., & Strack, S. (1989). Coping with conflict situations: Middle-aged and elderly men. *Psychology and Aging, 4*(1), 26–33.
Fruend, A. M., & Baltes, P. B. (1998). Selection, optimization, and compensation as strategies of life management: Correlations with subjective indicators of successful aging. *Psychology and Aging, 13*(4), 531–543.
Freund, A. M., & Baltes, P. B. (2002). The adaptiveness of selection, optimization, and compensation as strategies of life management: Evidence from a preference study on proverbs. *Journal of Gerontology: Psychological Sciences, 57B*, P426–P434.
Ingersoll-Dayton, B., Morgan, D., & Antonucci, T. (1997). The effects of positive and negative social exchanges on aging adults. *Journals of Gerontology Social Sciences, 52*(4), S167–S169.
Irion, J. C., & Blanchard-Fields, F. (1987). A cross-sectional comparison of adaptive coping in adulthood. *Journal of Gerontology, 42*, 502–504.
Jang, Y., Haley, W. E., Small, B. J., & Mortimer, J. A. (2002). The role of mastery and social resources in the associations between disability and depression in later life. *Gerontologist, 42*(6), 807–813.
Kahana, E., & Kahana, B. (1983). Environmental continuity, futurity, and adaptation to the aged. In G. D. Rowles, & R. J. Ohta (Eds.), *Aging and milieu: Environmental perspectives on growing old* (pp. 205–230). New York: Academic Press.
Lang, F. R., Rieckmann, N., & Baltes, M. M. (2002). Adapting to aging losses: Do resources facilitate strategies of selection, compensation and optimization in everyday functioning? *Journal of Gerontology: Psychological Sciences, 57B*, P501–P509.
Lester, P. B., & Baltes, M. M. (1978). Functional interdependence of the social environment and the behavior of the institutionalized aged. *Journal of Gerontological Nursing, 4*(2), 22–27.
McCrae, R. R. (1982). Age differences in the use of coping mechanisms. *Journal of Gerontology, 37*(4), 454–460.
McCrae, R. R., & Costa, P. T. Jr. (1987). Validation of the five-factor model of personality across instruments and observers. *Journal of Personality and Social Psychology, 52*(1), 81–90.
McCrae, R. R., Costa, P. T., Jr., de Lima, M. P., Simoes, A., Ostendorf, F., Angleitner, A., Marusic, I., Bratko, D., Caprara, G. V., Barbaranelli, C., Chae, J. H., & Piedmont, R. L. (1999). Age differences in personality across the adult life span: Parallels in five cultures. *Developmental Psychology, 35*, 466–477.
Mikhail, M. L. (1992). Psychological responses to relocation to a nursing home. *Journal of Gerontological Nursing, 18*(3), 35–39.
Millon, T. (1981). *Disorders of personality, DSM-III, Axis II*. New York: Wiley & Sons.
Molinari, V., Ames, A., & Essa, M. (1994). Prevalence of personality disorders in two geropsychiatric inpatient units. *Journal of Geriatric Psychiatry and* Neurology, 7(4), 209–215.
Molinari, V., & Marmion, J. (1993). Personality disorders in geropsychiatric outpatients. *Psychological Reports, 73*, 256–258.

Rosowsky, E. (1999). The patient-therapist relationship and the psychotherapy of the older adult with personality disorder. In E. Rosowsky, R. Abrams, & R. Zweig (Eds.), *Personality disorders in older adults: Emerging issues in diagnosis and treatment* (pp. 153–174). New Jersey: Lawrence Erlbaum Associates.

Ryff, C. D. (1987). Successful aging: A developmental approach. *Gerontologist, 22*, 209–214.

Schulz, R., & Heckhausen, J. (1996). A life span model of successful aging. *American Psychologist, 51*(7), 702–714.

Small, B. J., Hertzog, C., Hultsch, D. F., & Dixon, R. A. (2003). Stability and change in adult personality over 6 years: Findings from the Victoria Longitudinal Study. *Journal of Gerontology: Psychological Sciences, 58B*(3), P166–P176.

Smith, J., & Freund, A. M. (2002). The dynamics of possible selves in old age. *Journal of Gerontology: Psychological Sciences, 57B*, P492–P500.

Srivastava, S., John, O. P. Gosling, S. D., Potter, J. (2003). Development of personality in early and middle adulthood: Set like plaster or persistent change. *Journal of Personality and Social Psychology, 84*(5), 1041–1053.

Vaillant, G. E. (2002). *Aging well.* Boston: Little, Brown.

Whitbourne, S. K. (2001). *Adult development and aging: Biopsychosocial perspectives* (pp. 45–48). New York: John Wiley & Sons.

Yawney, B. A., & Slover, D. L. (1973). Relocation of the elderly. *Social Work,* (May), 86–93. *Social Work; 18*(3), 86–95.

Zweig, R. (2003). Personality disorders in older adults: Managing the difficult patient. *Clinical Geriatrics, 11*, 22–25.

CHAPTER SEVEN

Utilization of Self-Identity Roles in Individualized Activities Designed to Enhance Well-Being in Persons with Dementia*

Aleksandra Parpura-Gill and Jiska Cohen-Mansfield

In recent years, the framework for examining dementia has shifted from a medical model to a psychosocial model, and interventions have thus expanded to include nonbiological domains, highlighting the importance of psychosocial activities. Nevertheless, the provision of activities in long-term care facilities has often remained inadequate or inappropriate for the functional status and interest of residents (Buettner & Fitzsimmons, 2003). The reality of daily clinical practice is such that activities are planned without significant attention to their effects on individuals with dementia. Group activities are often based on general templates for a range of cognitive abilities, while activities for one-on-one interactions are mostly based on trial and error. Additionally, these activities frequently fail to recognize the person's continuing awareness of self, possibly due to the paucity of guidance for such individualized care (Perrin, 1997).

*This study was funded by Alzheimer's Association grant IIRG-99-1558

TAILORING INTERVENTIONS FOR THE INDIVIDUAL

The majority of interventions individualized for persons with dementia have been designed with regard to functional status or condition rather than personal preferences, as in the case of individualized interventions designed for providing ADL care in accordance with persons' functional abilities (Beck et al., 1997; Rogers et al., 1999; Wells, Dawson, Sidani, Craig, & Pringle, 2000) and interventions for improving the sleep of persons with dementia (Alessi, Yoon, Schnelle, Al-Samarrai, & Cruise, 1999; Schnelle, Alessi, Al-Samarrai, Fricker, & Ouslander, 1999). The results of these studies have been promising, suggesting that individualized care can successfully improve the quality of life of persons with dementia.

Less common than interventions based on functional status are those that accommodate the preferences of individual persons. One example of such an intervention is a program called individualized positive psychosocial intervention (IPPI), which aims to improve the quality of life of persons with dementia by matching an individual's past and present leisure interests with an activity that is then provided by nursing assistants (see Van Haitsma & Ruckdeschel, 2001 for a review). This individualized program was more successful at improving emotional quality of life and affecting resident behavior than was one-on-one attention, and helped CNAs better understand residents' identities.

SELF-IDENTITY

Our definition of self-identity refers to roles that people assume throughout their lifetimes as they are defined by peoples' attitudes toward those roles and manifested by enactment of the roles (e.g., demonstration in talk and behavior). Knowledge of such roles has practical value for the design of interventions. Because this operationalization focuses on assumed roles, we interchangeably use the terms self-identity and role-identity.

The literature on self-identity has focused on two domains: the persistence or changes in self over the course of dementia, and the mechanisms for enhancement of self in persons with dementia.

The Persistence of Self in Dementia

Dementia has been identified as the loss of self (Cohen & Eisdorfer, 1986). Many persons with advanced dementia experience great and frequent distress as they feel their sense of identity slipping away

(McGowin, 1993). Family members and other loved ones experience their own unique painful reactions. They suffer in attempts to "hang on" to their loved ones as they once knew them and often despair that the ailing relative is not the person they knew, grew up with, or married.

Despite the tremendous loss of identity that takes place over the course of dementia, a remarkable sense of self can survive (McGregor & Bell, 1993). Sabat and Harre (1992) suggest that because persons with dementia are often poorly understood, social identity can diminish and disappear over the course of dementia, but personal identity persists far into the end stages of the disease. Tappen, Williams, Fishman, and Touhy (1999) explored the persistence of personal identity through conversational analysis of 23 persons with Alzheimer's disease and found clear indices of personal identity, such as responding to one's name and referring to oneself in the first person during conversation. Yet, the persistence of self-identity in persons with dementia may depend on interactions with others that allow the identity to be expressed (Golander and Raz, 1996; Li & Orleans, 2002; Sabat & Harre, 1992; Small, Geldart, Gutman, & Scott, 1998; Vittoria, 1998).

While people with dementia do retain a sense of personal identity, the functional losses they experience, such as deterioration of language and speech, often prevent them from clearly expressing this identity. Hubbard, Cook, Tester, and Downs (2002) observed nonverbal communicative behaviors occurring in senior day care centers as well as the interpretation of these behaviors by other persons with dementia, and found that older people with dementia use nonverbal communication in meaningful ways. Usita, Hyman, and Herman (1998) analyzed narrative life stories of six persons with dementia and found that the participants were able to retrieve and share such stories as well as update their sense of selves to include the present.

In an exploratory study, Cohen-Mansfield, Golander, and Arnheim (2000) examined a systematic approach for the assessment of self-identity. Four domains of role-identity were investigated (professional, family, leisure activities, and personal attributes) through information obtained from the persons themselves, their family members, and their formal caregivers. The familial role was found most likely to be remembered even during advanced stages of progressive dementia, possibly because stronger past roles and connections are more likely to be maintained.

Mechanisms for the Enhancement of Self

Several studies point to the potential benefit of enhancing self-identity in persons with dementia. Small, Geldart, Gutman, and Scott (1998) concluded that personalized interactions between staff members and residents elicited more cooperative responses by residents than did nonpersonalized interactions. Reminiscence therapy and encouraging personal narratives and fostering life stories may also be effective in promoting and expressing self-identity (Basting, 2003; Usita et al., 1998). Golander and Raz (1996) demonstrated the importance of caregivers' reminding, constructing, and re-editing past biographies of residents with dementia in a nursing home in Israel. In a previous study by Cohen-Mansfield et al. (2000), family members and staff caregivers believed that most participants could achieve an enhanced sense of identity that would improve their well-being.

Surprisingly, no research has systematically examined whether interventions aimed at enhancing self-identity have an effect on the well-being of persons with dementia. The literature is still in the early stages of exploring the phenomenon of selfhood in dementia, and outcome measurement interventions are, therefore, still in their infancy. In this chapter, we describe how we have utilized self-identity roles of nursing home residents with dementia in order to provide these persons with psychosocial activities for enhancing their well-being.

OUR METHODOLOGY

Overview

In order to obtain a complete profile for each nursing home resident who will be receiving the interventions (i.e., the study participants), our protocol is to interview not only the participants but also staff members and family caregivers. In addition, background data (e.g., demographics, medical history) are recorded from participants' charts at the nursing home. We rely on multiple sources for a variety of reasons, such as—one source may not be knowledgeable enough about the participant (e.g., staff members may not be familiar with the participant's role identities prior to nursing home entry), or it could also be the case that the participant is not able to communicate with us (due to physical or cognitive decline). The information obtained from the interviews is then used to design personalized interventions for each participant.

Instruments

Our primary assessment tool is the *Self-Identity Questionnaire,* which taps self-identity roles, their retention, importance, and attitudes

(Cohen-Mansfield et al., 2000). This is a detailed questionnaire that explores four self-identity domains (professional, family/social, leisure time/hobbies activities, and attributes/achievements/traits) with regard to the participant's past and present. Through this questionnaire, we gain insight as to the participant's most important identity role and also obtain suggestions for activities that may have positive effects on the participant in the present.

Questionnaire items are close-ended (list of options or yes/no answers), with an option to elaborate on responses. Participants and staff are interviewed in-person. While staff questionnaires are completed in one session, participants sometimes need multiple sessions to complete the questionnaire as they can become fatigued. Because of scheduling difficulties and time constraints, family members are generally interviewed over the phone. Interview sessions typically last 30–45 min. As to the internal consistency of the questionnaire, Cronbach alphas for family informants were 0.82, 0.83, 0.82, and 0.84, for professional, family, hobbies/leisure time, and achievements role-identity scales, respectively; for staff informants, the corresponding values were 0.85, 0.67, 0.84, and 0.87. At first glance, the value of 0.67 seems low, but is understandable when we consider that staff members would not be expected to be particularly knowledgeable about items pertaining to the family domain of the participants. Test–retest reliability of the questionnaire was performed for a subset of family members (n = 10) and the exact agreement rate averaged 86.2%.

In addition to examining self-identity, we tapped participants' quality of life through two assessments. For both, systematic observations are recorded directly onto a Palm pilot. In the first, we capture five emotional responses (pleasure, interest, sadness, anxiety, and anger) using *Lawton's Modified Behavior Stream* (LMBS; Lawton, Van Haitsma, & Klapper, 1996). In the second, we measure agitated behaviors and their frequency using the *Agitation Behavior Mapping Instrument* (ABMI; Cohen-Mansfield, Werner, & Marx, 1989).

Participants' cognitive performance is assessed by the *Mini-Mental State Exam* (MMSE; Folstein, Folstein, & McHugh, 1975) and the *Brief Cognitive Rating Scale* (BCRS; Reisberg, Schneck, Ferris, Schwartz, & deLeon, 1983).

Design of Interventions

Interventions are designed with consideration of the salience of participants' identity roles, cognitive status, and physical and sensory abilities. The steps that we utilize for designing the interventions are as follows.

DETERMINATION OF ROLE-IDENTITY SALIENCE

This involves reviewing the answers to the Self-Identity Questionnaire from all informants, and prioritizing role identities with respect to both the past and present (e.g., an identity that was very important in both the past and present would receive a higher priority than one that was important in only one time frame). When there is a discrepancy among informants, we consider the participant's level of cognitive functioning.

Sometimes informants do not identify which of the roles were most important. When this occurs we look for an overlap between role-identity domains, as was the case for our selecting the family-identity for a woman whose data revealed an overlapping of the professional domain (for homemakers) with the achievement domain (success of the family).

DETERMINATION OF THE INTERVENTION

We tailor our interventions according to the data obtained through the Self-Identity Questionnaire, such as the particular job that was important to the participant, the particular family member who is the most important to the participant, specific activities/hobbies the participant enjoyed, etc. In our experience, we find that the choice of an intervention is affected by a variety of factors:

- In general, we tailor an intervention so that its content is directly related to the role-identity (e.g., folding towels or baking for a former homemaker). However, we sometimes tailor an intervention with respect to the context rather than the content. For example, for a participant who once held a high official/executive position, our intervention could be the manner in which we engage the participant in conversation, soliciting his advice and putting him in an authoritative position.
- We find that the cognitive abilities of the participant determine the level of complexity of the intervention. Of course, it is critical not to oversimplify the intervention and, in turn, infantilize the participant. Along these lines, we always consider the physical and sensory abilities of the participant when designing an intervention. Although dancing is not a possibility for a wheelchair user, similar effects can be achieved with an intervention of movement to music.
- We pay attention to participant's demographics such as gender, ethnicity, religion, educational background, and primary language. For example, a blind Spanish-speaking participant received much pleasure from an intervention of Spanish Bible audiotapes. Similarly, male participants, who are less likely to

engage in traditional craft projects, find alternatives such as mechanical crafts (assembly of bridge and airplane models) or family tree development to be quite acceptable.
- We find that having an activity that involves helping or providing something valuable to others is often a motivator for engagement (e.g., making an album for a favorite family member, stamping envelopes to help office workers, etc).

Sometimes two roles can be accommodated (e.g., when a participant's interests include crafts, a family role-identity could be addressed through a craft project centered on a family theme). The interventions are therefore designed considering individuals' preferences and available physical and emotional resources. The choice of interventions can be performed within the context of the SOC (selection, optimization, and compensation) model that describes the losses and gains that occur with the aging process, as well as adaptation to those changes (Baltes & Baltes, 1990). According to the SOC model, as loss of function occurs, a person focuses energy on the goals and tasks that are more important or salient (*selection*), and uses new and alternative means of achieving these goals (*compensation*) as well as finding means of maximizing remaining resources (*optimization*).

Therefore, designing an intervention by selecting the individual's most salient roles and adjusting the intervention based on personal preferences and available sensory and physical abilities increases the likelihood of the intervention's success. Additionally, in doing so, the intervention itself becomes an external source of optimization by providing alternative means for achievement of the selected goals.

Case Studies

Below are findings from three case studies that demonstrate our methodology and the outcomes of our interventions. These case studies were part of a larger randomized controlled trial study, the results of which are discussed elsewhere (Cohen-Mansfield, Parpura-Gill, & Golander under review). In order to provide as much description as possible, we present qualitative data of the interventions (i.e., narratives of informal participant observation and staff impressions) as well as quantitative outcome data (i.e., systematic observations of well-being).

Participant A

This participant was an 89-year-old Caucasian male who had worked as a lawyer for many years. He had resided in the nursing home for

5 years. He had various medical conditions (cardiovascular, pulmonary, endocrine) as well as depression and was a wheelchair user. He had been diagnosed with dementia, with an MMSE score of 11 and a BCRS score of 6.5. Observations performed on the days prior to the intervention (i.e., baseline) found him to be agitated, manifesting primarily physical nonaggressive behaviors such as pacing (in his wheelchair), and showing no pleasure and little interest.

Intervention design

In order to devise appropriate interventions for this participant, we examined responses supplied by all three sources to the Self-Identity Questionnaire, the main findings of which are outlined in Table 7.1. We were not able to discern which role was most important to Participant A. The family role was unclear because the participant had indicated his parental role, while the family member felt that being a son had been very important in the past but not at all important in the present. Of the other domains, only the achievement domain held some importance in the present (and only according to the participant), while others, such as professional (being a lawyer) and leisure roles (reading and playing golf), had been rated as very important only in the past. After much discussion, we developed interventions that overlapped between role-identity domains, addressing his professional and intellectual achievements as well as hobbies and leisure time activities. The specific activities planned for Participant A are listed below, in order of our "best" idea for an intervention, "second best" idea, and so on.

- Reading newspaper articles on elections and sports—in order to preserve his identity from his hobbies.
- Asking for his expert opinion during a discussion of political, ethical, and legal issues (e.g., the recent presidential election, a news story about separating conjoined twins)—he enjoys "doing work."
- Looking at and reading *Golf* magazine—golf had been a much enjoyed leisure activity.
- Listening to music—Participant A's son told us that his father seems to enjoy hearing songs by Frank Sinatra while attending weekly music nights at his facility.

Obtaining items for these interventions was relatively simple and inexpensive. Preparation for the first three involved purchasing the *Washington Post* and *New York Times*, preparing current event scenarios, and purchasing a magazine dedicated to golf. As to the intervention of listening to music, all that was necessary was to purchase a

TABLE 7.1 Summary of the Most Salient Role Identities, from Three Informants
Participant A

Role-identity	Professional		Family		Leisure time/hobbies		Achievements/traits		Activities that could enhance identity
informant	Past	Present	Past	Present	Past	Present	Past	Present	
Participant	Lawyer		Being a father		Reading, painting, politics, cards, traveling		Family heritage, devotion to work and family, academic achievement		
	Very important	Not at all important	Very important	Important	Very important	Not at all important	Important	Important	
Family	Lawyer		Being a son		Reading, golf, sports fan		Work, contribution to his country, golfing achievement, honesty, determination, devotion to family		Music—seems to enjoy music night (with Sinatra songs) at his facility, reading newspapers, recalling memories
	Very important	Not at all important	Very impor-tant	Not at all important	Very impor-tant	Not at all important	Very impor-tant	Not at all important	
Staff	Do not know		Being a father		Reading about religion		Do not know		Talking about family, visits with children and pets
		Do not know		Very important		Not at all important		Do not know	

TABLE 7.1 *(Cont.)*
Participant B

Role-identity	Professional		Family		Leisure time/hobbies		Achievements/traits		Activities that could enhance
informant	Past	Present	Past	Present	Past	Present	Past	Present	identity
Participant	Clerical/secretarial		Mother		Bridge, socializing, reading, traveling, cooking, politics, music, dancing, and religious activities		Devotion to family, academic achievement, honesty, and fairness		
	Very impor-tant	Not at all important	Very impor-tant	Slightly important	Important	Slightly important	Important	Slightly important	
Family	Homemaker		Mother		Bridge, craft, cooking		Volunteering		Looking at pictures of friends and family, eating foods she likes
	Very impor-tant	Do not know	Very impor-tant	Not at all important	Moderately important	Do not know	Very important	Not at all important	
Staff	Do not know		Mother to family		Bridge, reading, TV		Family heritage, devotion		Playing bridge, clothing, getting a manicure
		Do not know		Very important		Slightly important		Important	

TABLE 7.1 *(Cont.)*
Participant C

Participant	Office work		Husband		Reading, traveling, TV, politics, music, physical and religious activities		Proud of the success of his children		Something related to being productive
	Very important	Very important	Important	Important	Very important	Very important	Very important	Very important	
Family	Economist, high position		Husband, parent		Reading, traveling, socializing, politics, music, tennis, and bridge		Contribution to country as military officer, success of children, devotion to work, he wrote a book about the economy		A task with a purpose (e.g., reading a book about finance)
	Very important	Slightly important	Important	Important	Slightly important	Not at all important	Important	Not at all important	
Staff	Professor with a PhD		Do not know		Do not know		Do not know		Talking about family, pictures of family, socializing, painting
		Do not know		Do not know		Do not know		Do not know	

Sinatra CD and make sure that we had a working CD player. We brought the materials for all activities to each intervention session in order to provide options.

The interventions

Day 1. Interventions—reading about the election in time and answering questions about politics; listening to the Frank Sinatra CD. The nursing staff member warned us that this participant had been grumpy all day and had slapped her. During the intervention, he answered questions about the election with monosyllabic responses, staying fairly alert. When we played the Sinatra CD (by his request), he fell asleep.

Day 2. Intervention—reading Golf. This participant was interested in Tiger Woods and articles about his golf swing, and responded with appropriate answers, such as, "Yeah, that would be hard to do."

Day 3. Intervention—listening to the Frank Sinatra CD. After hearing the list of song choices on the CD, Participant A requested "America the Beautiful." He sang along, recalling almost all of the words. He listened to the song for a total of three times—it was the only one that held his attention.

Day 4. Interventions—listening to the Frank Sinatra CD; political discussion; asking for his opinion while looking at Golf. At first, he said he was not interested in "America the Beautiful" but he ended up choosing it anyway. He listened to the song repeatedly, laughing and smiling as it played, and telling a nursing assistant that he was happy. The nursing assistant was amazed, saying that it was the first time that she had seen Participant A smiling or singing, and further remarking that the activities coordinator had not been able to evoke this type of response from him. Participant A was then engaged in a conversation during which he offered suggestions for improving one's golf swing and another in which he discussed his choice of candidate for the upcoming presidential election.

Day 5. Interventions—listening to the Frank Sinatra CD. Participant A was very responsive on this day, not only singing to "America the Beautiful" but also responding fully to questions about his job as a lawyer, his sons' careers, and playing golf with his sons. When asked if he had always liked "America the Beautiful" so much, he said that he had not and was not sure why he did so much now. When asked if the song brought back memories, he said it made him think of Russia and the United States during the Cold War.

Outcomes

From the qualitative data, it is clear that the personalized interventions served to engage this participant. Moreover, his engagement increased across the days of the interventions, from one-syllable responses during the first intervention day to reciprocal discussions on the final 2 days of interventions. In addition, he sang, smiled, and said that he was happy during the intervention with "America the Beautiful," to the amazement of a nursing assistant.

Analysis of the quantitative data revealed findings consistent with those just described for the qualitative data. Remarkable decreases in observed agitation were seen during our interventions (days 6–10, see Figure 7.1), relative to the amount of agitation observed at baseline (baseline was assessed on each of the 5 days prior to the interventions, Figure 7.1). Specifically, baseline levels of agitation ranged from 7.3 (quantified as a mean of 7.3 times during a 3-min period of observation) to 1.7, while the amount of agitation was observed to be 0 on 3 days and less than 2.0 during the other 2 days of our interventions. It is also

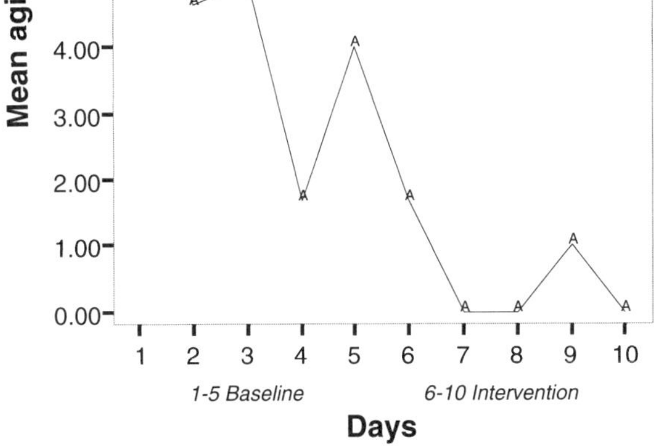

FIGURE 7.1 Daily changes in agitation for Participant A.

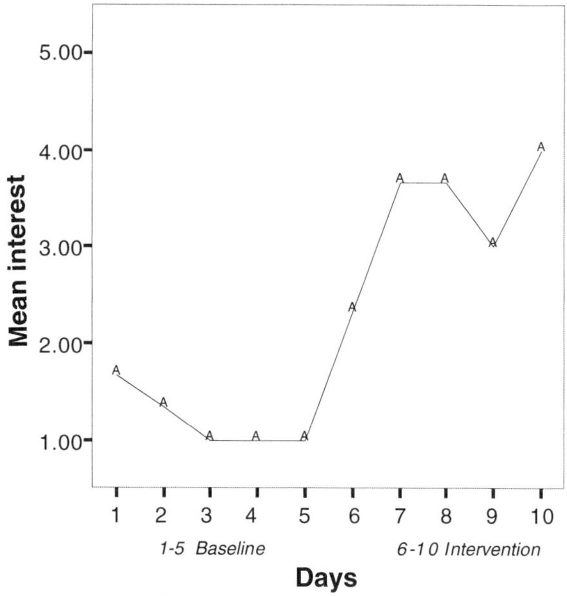

FIGURE 7.2 Daily changes in interest for Participant A.

noteworthy that Participant A's level of agitation was comparatively higher on the first day of the interventions (relative to subsequent intervention days), corresponding to a comment by a nursing staff member that he had been grumpy and hit her on that day. As to the other measures of well-being, there were no changes in levels of anger, anxiety, or sadness across the baseline and intervention days (all of which did not occur throughout the period) and slight pleasure was seen only on day 10 (i.e., one observation for less than 16s). However, interest increased during the interventions (see Figure 7.2). During baseline, mean interest values for Participant A were below 2.0 (quantified as being interested for less than 16s during a 3-min observation) on days 1 and 2, and he showed no interest during the latter 3 days of baseline. Yet, an increase in interest was seen on the first day of the interventions, with the level of interest climbing steadily through the final day of the interventions when the mean value equaled 4.0 (quantified as interested for more than half of the time).

In summary, the well-being of this participant was positively influenced by self-identity interventions, as demonstrated by the qualitative narrative as well as by the observed increase in interest and the decrease in agitation. Although "America the Beautiful" seemed to be his most preferred intervention, he clearly enjoyed the interventions that provided reading and discussions, highlighting the importance of offering choices in interventions.

Participant B

This participant was a Caucasian woman who had lived in the nursing home for 6 years. She was 94 years old, and had been described to us as a recluse who usually preferred to stay in her room rather than participate in activities. She used a wheelchair. She had been diagnosed with paranoia as well as a variety of medical conditions (cardiovascular, peripheral neurological and endocrine). She carried a diagnosis of dementia and had an MMSE score of 8 and a BCRS score of 6. Observations performed during baseline yielded no agitation, no pleasure, and slight interest.

Intervention design

As had been the case with Participant A, our first step was to evaluate the main findings from the Self-Identity Questionnaire for this participant (see Table 7.1). Family-identity emerged as important, spanning several domains including achievements and professional, as the participant had been a homemaker for most of her life. Her leisure time activity of Bridge still held some importance in the present, and according to her daughter, her extensive volunteer work had been very important in the past. With these role-identities in mind, the following interventions were designed for Participant B:

- Listening to an audiotape about her family—to preserve her identity as a mother. We asked her daughter to prepare this.
- Looking at a scrapbook of her achievements and family—to connect with her past achievements as well as her parental role. Again, we asked her daughter to provide this.
- Making get-well cards for people—to preserve her volunteering role.
- Playing Bridge—to tap into her leisure and hobbies role.

As was the case with the first two interventions just listed, it is sometimes necessary to enlist the help of family members when putting together an intervention. We were fortunate to be working with a family member who was eager to be of assistance, but it should be kept in mind that family members may not be willing or able to help prepare an intervention. As to specific items needed to prepare for the interventions for Participant B, these were simple to get: a Walkman, craft materials (for making the cards), and a deck of cards (for Bridge). Finally, while an initial time investment was required for arranging the production of the audiotape, we consider this acceptable, as the time investment was minimal during the actual intervention.

The interventions

Day 1. Intervention—Bridge. This intervention was conducted with a small group of nursing home residents. Participant B appeared very interested and talked a lot about the game, giving examples of hands, scoring, and general game rules. Participant B was obviously very proficient at Bridge, refusing to play a simpler game, such as Go Fish, because it was "baby stuff."

An interesting note is that when we greeted Participant B prior to the start of the intervention, she told us that she was not doing well. At the end of the intervention, her demeanor had changed for the better.

Day 2. Intervention—listening to the family audiotape. Participant B seemed to very much enjoy the tape made by her daughter. When we asked if everything was going well, she replied, "Yes, but I'd like to hear what comes next if you don't mind." She listened to the tape for a second time, remarking, "Isn't this wonderful!" She wanted to continue listening to the "trip down memory lane," quoting things that she remembered hearing her daughter say on the tape.

As we had seen on day 1, when we first arrived and asked Participant B how she was doing, she said, "I'm not feeling well. I'm tired. I'm doing terrible." Once we started to play the tape however, she smiled while listening, and became talkative and positive.

Day 3. Intervention—listening to the family audiotape. Participant B enjoyed hearing the tape again, not seeming to remember it from the previous day. She repeated some of the things that her daughter had said on the tape.

Day 4. Interventions—listening to the family audiotape; looking at a family scrapbook. For the first time, Participant B did not say she was feeling poorly when we arrived to do the intervention. She again enjoyed hearing the tape and talking about it. She also responded well to the family pictures, but was confused as to who the people were.

Day 5. Intervention—listening to the family audiotape. She wanted to hear the tape again on this day, and started to smile as soon as she heard her daughter's recorded voice. She seemed very content, listening to the tape multiple times.

Outcomes

Evaluation of the narrative data suggests that the Bridge intervention and the scrapbook intervention were both successful in that these engaged the participant. However, the family audiotape not only engaged Participant B but also made her very happy. She wanted to hear the tape over and over again, preferring to listen to it rather than participate in other recreational activities on her unit. In fact, she enjoyed the audiotape so much that we never had an opportunity to try the intervention of making get-well cards.

As had been the case with Participant A, the quantitative data are consistent with the qualitative findings. Participant B showed no pleasure during the baseline observations (days 1–5), displayed no pleasure during the first day of the interventions (day 6), and then showed increasing pleasure during the successive days of the interventions, with mean pleasure values above 4.0 (i.e., showing pleasure more than half of the time) on the last 2 days (see Figure 7.3). Taken with the narrative data, we know that although the Bridge intervention kept her involved on day 6, she did not enjoy it as much as she did the family audiotape intervention on days 7–10. Along these lines, interest increased

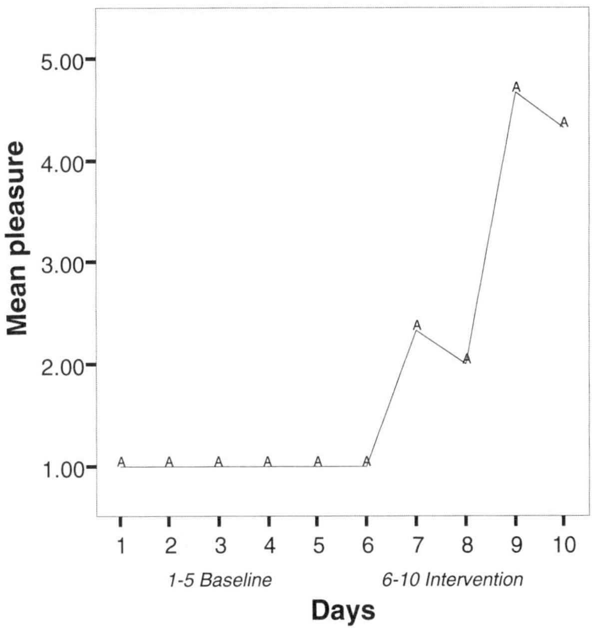

FIGURE 7.3 Daily changes in pleasure for Participant B.

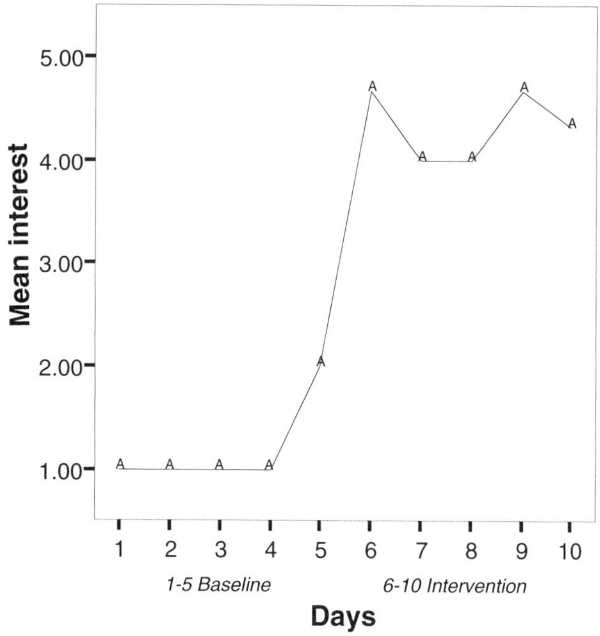

FIGURE 7.4 Daily changes in interest for Participant B.

remarkably from baseline days to intervention days (see Figure 7.4). While she displayed no interest during the first four baseline days and a mean interest of 2 (i.e., less than 16s) on day 5, the mean level of interest equaled 4.0 or greater (i.e., at least half of the time) during all of the intervention days. Occurrences of anger, sadness, and agitation were low during the baseline and intervention days. As to anxiety, this was not observed on days 1–9, and a small amount (less than 16s) was observed on day 10.

The documented increases in interest and pleasure suggest that our interventions were successful in improving the well-being of this participant. The differences seen in observed pleasure during the Bridge intervention and the family audiotape intervention illustrate the point that one should try multiple interventions in order to determine which will provide the resident with the maximum benefits. Another point to be made is that individualized interventions can sometimes be tailored for a small group setting. Small groups can be successful if all the participants are matched according to their interests and role-identities as well as their cognitive abilities and those physical abilities utilized in the intervention. And finally, Participant B's daughter was very appreciative of our work because she very much wanted to help her mother but did not know what to do. We need to develop better avenues for assisting family members with finding ways to communicate with and help their relatives.

Participant C

The third case study involved an 83-year-old Caucasian male who had been residing in a nursing home for 2 years. He had a PhD in economics and held a high position at a federal agency. His medical diagnoses included hypertension, prostate cancer, and Parkinson's disease. His MMSE score was 9 and his BCRS score was 5.5. He was ambulatory with a Merry-walker™. At the time of the baseline observations, he was intermittently agitated (mostly manifesting physical nonaggressive behavior, such as repetitive movements), sometimes showed interest, and never showed pleasure or sadness.

Intervention design

The summary of all sources on the Self-Identity Questionnaire is shown in Table 7.1. As can be seen, Participant C's role in the family was rated as important in the past and present by himself and by his family member. Although the informants were not able to define the most important role identity, his professional role was given a very high level of importance by the participant and given some level of importance by his family member. As both of these role identities overlap with achievement roles, the interventions were designed to address these two identities. The interventions planned were:

- Reading, discussing, and looking into the book on economics that he wrote and got published—as his professional work is an important role-identity.
- Reading the newspaper or magazines, especially articles related to his previous positions—to preserve his professional role-identity.
- Looking at family pictures—to tap the importance of his role in the family.
- Listening to an audiotape of his wife discussing their travels and his job—because his family role-identity is important, and this activity combines three of his role identities.

As had been the case for Participant B, we asked for the help of a family member (his wife) in order to get a copy of the book authored by the participant, family pictures, and to prepare an audiotape. His wife gave us a copy of the book, but was unable to supply the other two items, so we focused our attention on the first two interventions on our list. We had no difficulties in obtaining the necessary items, such as the *Washington Post* and magazines.

The Interventions

Day 1. Intervention—reading, discussing, and looking at the book he wrote. The participant was consistently interested in the book, and thanked us for bringing it. He flipped through the pages and said he would like to go through the whole book. He recognized the names of the people on the acknowledgments page and spoke of their contributions to the book. He laughed at the mention of his wife, and then seemed to get sad. Compliments and the mention of his children were also upsetting to him. He cried, seemingly because of his recognition of past abilities that he has lost.

Day 2. Intervention—reading a magazine and discussing politics. On this day, Participant C was engaged in discussing politics and asked relevant questions. Being asked for his opinions on specific matters seemed to boost his confidence, and he asked to look through a magazine so that he could give more informed opinions. Although it did not appear that he was actually reading the magazine, he did concentrate on the pages.

Day 3. Intervention—Reading, discussing, and looking at the book he wrote. He recognized his book immediately by his name on the cover, and said he did not write much of it. The book kept his interest, and he said it was not as good as he hoped it would be. He asked for our opinion on the issues discussed. At one point, he referred to himself as an economist. He mentioned something about going to his office when asked if he wanted to stay sitting where he was. He laughed, but also seemed sad for brief periods.

It is also noteworthy that Participant C was holding a newspaper when we arrived for the intervention. Several persons noticed that he had been carrying around a newspaper after the previous intervention.

Day 4. Intervention—reading, discussing, and looking at the book he wrote. Again, he was very interested in his book, and answered our questions with relevant but general comments.

Day 5. Intervention—reading, discussing, and looking at the book he wrote; reading and discussing an article from the Washington Post. Participant C seemed very quiet today but showed interest in looking at his book and in discussing an article from the newspaper.

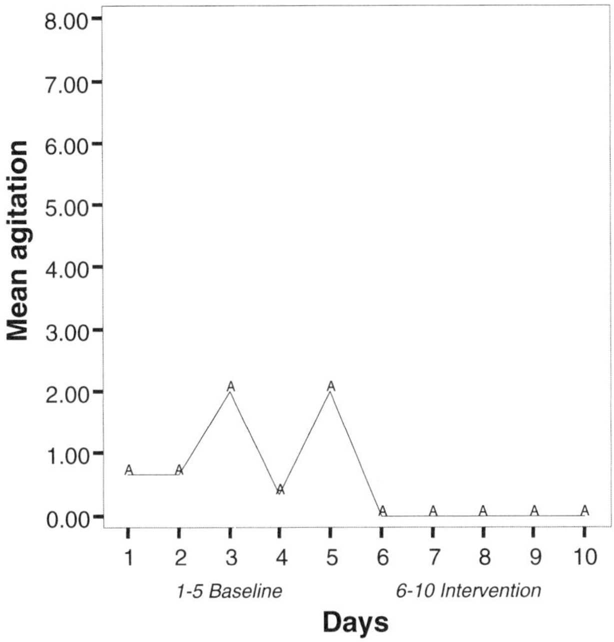

FIGURE 7.5 Daily changes in agitation for Participant C.

Outcomes

Our impressions from the qualitative data are that this participant was engaged during the interventions but that the link to past role identities was a source of sadness to him. We saw that he became upset by questions about his wife, children, and past abilities. In addition, it appears that the impact of the intervention for his professional role-identity was felt beyond the actual intervention, as the participant was observed carrying around and looking at a newspaper during nonintervention times.

As to the quantitative indicators of well-being, we observed that the mean level of agitation fluctuated during the baseline days, but that Participant C exhibited no agitation during the observations recorded during the interventions (see Figure 7.5). We also observed changes in interest when comparing baseline with intervention days (see Figure 7.6). Specifically, mean levels of interest during the baseline days fluctuated with a peak of 3.0 (where 3.0 = less than half of the time), while mean levels of interest peaked at 5.0 (where 5.0 = most or all of the time) during the interventions on days 8 and 9, dropping down to a level around 3.0 on day 10. It is noteworthy that

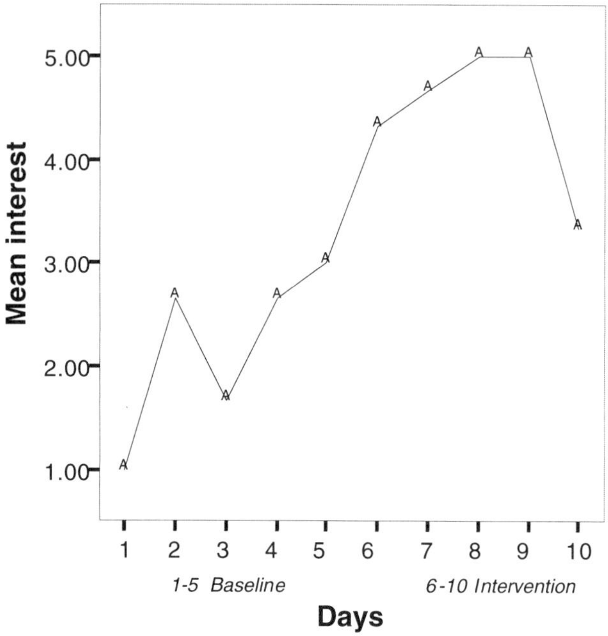

FIGURE 7.6 Daily changes in interest for Participant C.

according to the narrative data, the participant was very quiet although still interested on the last day of the interventions (i.e., day 10 on Figure 7.6). As to pleasure and sadness, neither was observed during the baseline days, while small amounts of each were observed during the interventions.

Our interventions were successful in decreasing agitation and increasing interest at the time of the intervention. Furthermore, it seems that these interventions had a longer term effect as the participant was observed looking at a newspaper outside the times of the interventions. This supports the position that these interventions may actually enhance the self-identity of a person with dementia. Yet, while getting in touch with identity roles may induce increased interest and pleasure, this may also increase sadness, which at first glance seems counterproductive for an intervention aimed at enhancing well-being. However, for people who focus on the loss of their abilities, negative affect may be an integral component of connecting with self-identity. Clearly, more research is warranted to develop a better understanding of this topic.

DISCUSSION

Although scientific evidence and theoretical concepts of care delivery have made advances over the past decade, less has been achieved in clinical practice for the design of activity programs and other psychosocial interventions. Until now, individualization of interventions for persons with dementia has been limited, with treatment designs individualized to address a particular person's needs or preferences without considering self-identity. Notwithstanding, researchers have broadly defined individualized treatments for a variety of conditions, including physical and mental disabilities, agitated behaviors, and sleep disturbances. For example, individualized treatments aimed at addressing various medical conditions, and taking into consideration a person's disabilities, have resulted in significant improvements of targeted disabilities (Kleban, Lawton, Brody, Moss, 1975). Music activities, for example, individualized to match personal preferences have been more effective than general relaxing music in reducing agitated behaviors of elderly people with dementia (Gerdner, 2000). An individualized approach to addressing unmet needs is also available (Cohen-Mansfield, 2000).

The self-identity methodology described in this chapter is a departure from the methodologies currently available in the literature in that it focuses on general well-being while simultaneously individualizing the interventions on the basis of the person's role-identity. This approach relates to the SOC model in that the methodology can be superimposed on all three aspects of the model (selection, optimization, and compensation). Interventions designed based on the salience of the self-identity roles are directly relevant to an individual's selection of the areas in life that are most meaningful (Carstensen, Isaacowitz, & Charles, 1999) (e.g., family relationships as identified in saliency of family role). Similarly, individualizing interventions for current physical, mental, and psychological resources has direct bearing on the optimization and compensation domains of the SOC model. In a separate report, we evaluate the utility of this methodology for elderly persons with dementia, and show that individualizing interventions can indeed contribute to well-being (Cohen-Mansfield et al., under review). However, when we examine the effect of our self-identity interventions at the individual level, we see that there are negative as well as positive results. For example, in our case study of Participant C, we saw that he sometimes became somewhat sad during an intervention (although he simultaneously showed positive results, such as decreased agitation, increased interest, and a small increase in pleasure). We feel that the participant's awareness of his previous roles led to the realization of his current roles and loss of functional abilities, which in turn caused the sadness. Notwithstanding, we hypothesize that reactions like these may be an expression of otherwise covert emotional states, which can then be addressed through various psychosocial interventions.

We faced a variety of challenges in providing self-identity interventions, including those arising from regular daily fluctuations of the mood and behaviors of persons with dementia, the consequences of changing the residents' usual routine through our interventions, and finally, insuring that we had sufficient time for residents and research staff (who provided the interventions) to familiarize themselves with one another, as there were no prior relationships. Our advice for other practitioners who institute self-identity interventions is that when challenges arise, it is necessary to persevere with an intervention until either success or failure is evident.

The self-identity methodology serves as confirmation of the feasibility of Kitwood (1997) vision of the "virtuous circle" for dementia care. Kitwood considers maintaining personhood to be the prime task of dementia care in the face of cognitive decline, and acknowledges the caregiver's significant role, stating, "if identity is to be maintained—then it will be very largely on the basis of what others provide" (p. 20). He has encouraged care providers to expand dementia interventions into person-centered care (Kitwood, 1997). Thus, an individualization of care could break down the vicious circle of "malignant social psychology," and revert it into a desired "virtuous circle" promoting the well-being of individuals with dementia as well as reducing agitation and distress.

Throughout the development of our methodology, family members have played an important role by providing both information and specific personal intervention materials. This methodology can be taught to family caregivers who can then use it to enhance the lives of persons with dementia in any setting, whether they are the primary caregivers at home or are supporting staff members' efforts in an institutional setting. Indeed, we have found that family members are sometimes so impressed with the effects of the intervention on their relatives that they become inspired to start other activities based on their relative's role identities.

Additionally, family members have anecdotally reported longer term effects of the interventions, but we have no data available on the duration of these effects. Future studies are warranted to explore the long-term effects of such interventions. More research is also needed to explore the various factors influencing success and individualized evaluation of success. Several relatives noted that their family members had experienced greater positive effects than they had ever thought possible.

In one case we considered an intervention to be unsuccessful, as the participant did not appear to respond. However, feedback from the spouse revealed that, given the person's current level of functioning, it was a great achievement that he sat and participated in the intervention.

Advances in scientific literature about the design and individualization of psychosocial interventions have generally not been followed in clinical practice. The gap between scientific advances and clinical applications may be due to a lack of knowledge and lack of adequate staffing for such interventions. The first step toward addressing this gap is a clearer identification of the barriers to translation of the research including educational and staffing issues.

The methodology presented in this chapter is a systematic approach to utilization of information that is often at least partially collected but seldom utilized in clinical practice. Although trial and error is not completely eradicated with this methodology, it is significantly reduced through our process of designing individualized interventions. This methodology can be used to optimize currently provided services. As we have shown, planning and successfully implementing individualized role-identity interventions do not necessarily involve significant staff time. Some of the interventions (e.g., discussing past roles) could take place while staff members interact with residents for other reasons (e.g., arranging the bed or preparing the person for sleep). The planning of these interventions (e.g., acquiring knowledge of the past identity roles of residents, obtaining activity-related materials) or the planning involved in matching residents by common interests, language, and functional ability would take additional staff time, yet should be an integral part of care of persons with dementia. Furthermore, such preparations could involve the family member who could be enlisted to prepare some of the activity materials, thereby involving his/herself in the relative's care plan, which in turn could help to form an alliance between family and staff caregivers.

Based on our own experiences, individualized interventions that provide an awareness of self do not need to involve greater costs than current interventions. While some interventions must be provided as one-on-one, others can be conducted in small groups based on the participants' extent of cognitive decline as well as the interventions designed for each person. In addition, some interventions require minimal staff involvement (e.g., listening to an audiotape of a family member reminiscing about past times). Finally, the benefits of individualized activities in reducing problem behaviors need to be acknowledged as cost-saving. Indeed, given that reimbursement is available for alternative methods for decreasing behavior problems (i.e., the administration of pharmaceutical agents), policy makers must consider reimbursement for individualized activities. The bottom line is that personalized interventions based on role-identity need not be cost-prohibitive, and should be incorporated into the care plans of all nursing home residents with dementia.

REFERENCES

Alessi, C. A., Yoon, E. J., Schnelle, J. F., Al-Samarrai, N. R., & Cruise, P. A. (1999). A randomized trial of a combined physical activity and environmental intervention in nursing home residents: Do sleep and agitation improve? *Journal of the American Geriatrics Society, 47*, 784–791.

Baltes, P. B., & Baltes, M. M. (1990). Psychological perspectives on successful aging: The model of selective optimization with compensation. In P. B. Baltes, & M. M. Baltes (Eds.), *Successful aging: Perspectives from the behavioral sciences* (pp. 1–34). New York: Cambridge University Press.

Basting, A. D. (2003). Looking back from loss: Views of the self in Alzheimer's disease. *Journal of Aging Studies, 17*, 87–99.

Beck, C., Heacock, P., Mercer, S. O., Walls, R. C., Rapp, C. G., & Vogelpohl, T. S. (1997). Improving dressing behavior in cognitively impaired nursing home residents. *Nursing Research, 46*(3), 126–132.

Buettner, L. L., & Fitzsimmons, S. (2003). Activity calendars for older adults with dementia: What you see is not what you get. *American Journal of Recreational Therapy, 2*(3), 9–22.

Carstensen, L. L., Isaacowitz, D. M., & Charles, S. T. (1999). Taking time seriously: A theory of socioemotional selectivity. *American Psychologist, 54*, 165–181.

Cohen, D., & Eisdorfer, C. (1986). *The loss of self.* New York: W.W. Norton.

Cohen-Mansfield, J. (2000). Nonpharmacological management of behavioral problems in persons with dementia: The TREA model. *Alzheimer's Care Quarterly, 1*(4), 22–34.

Cohen-Mansfield, J., Golander, H., & Arnheim, G. (2000). Self-identity in older persons suffering from dementia: Preliminary results. *Social Science & Medicine, 51*, 381–394.

Cohen-Mansfield, J., Parpura-Gill, A., & Golander, H. *Utilization of self-identity roles for designing interventions for persons with dementia*, under review.

Cohen-Mansfield, J., Werner, P., & Marx, M. S. (1989). An observational study of agitation in agitated nursing home residents. *International Psychogeriatrics, 1*(2), 153–165.

Folstein, M. F., Folstein, S. E., & McHugh, P. R. (1975). Mini-mental state: A practical method for grading the cognitive state of patients for the clinician. *Journal of Psychiatric Research, 12*, 189–198.

Gerdner, L. A. (2000). Effects of individualized versus classical "relaxation" music on the frequency of agitation in elderly persons with Alzheimer's disease and related disorders. *International Psychogeriatrics, 12*(1), 49–65.

Golander, H., & Raz, A. (1996). The mask of 'demented residents' in a nursing home. *Ageing and Society, 16*, 269–285.

Hubbard, G., Cook, A., Tester, S., & Downs, M. (2002). Beyond words: Older people with dementia using and interpreting nonverbal behaviour. *Journal of Aging Studies*, *16*, 155–167.

Kitwood, T. (1997). The experience of dementia. *Aging and Mental Health, 1*(1), 13–22.

Kleban, M. H., Lawton, M. P., Brody, E. M., & Moss, M. (1975). Characteristics of mentally-impaired aged profiting from individualized treatment. *Journal of Gerontology, 30*(1), 90–96.

Lawton, M. P., Van Haitsma, K., & Klapper, J. (1996). Observed affect in nursing home residents with Alzheimer's disease. *Journals of Gerontology, 51B*(1), 3–14.

Li, R., & Orleans, M. (2002). Personhood in a world of forgetfulness: An Ethnography of the self-process among Alzheimer's patients. *Journal of Aging and Identity, 7*(4), 227–244.

McGowin, D. F. (1993). *Living in the labyrinth: A personal journey through the maze of Alzheimer's.* San Francisco, CA: Elder Books.

McGregor, I., & Bell, J. (1993). Voyage of discovery. *Nursing Times, 89*(36), 29–31.

Perrin, T. (1997). Occupational need in severe dementia: A descriptive study. *Journal of Advanced Nursing, 25*, 934–941.

Reisberg, B., Schneck, M. K., Ferris, S. H., Schwartz, G. E., & deLeon, M. J. (1983). The brief cognitive rating scale (BCRS): Findings in primary degenerative dementia (PDD). *Psychopharmacological Bulletin, 19*, 47–50.

Rogers, J. C., Holm, M. B., Burgio, L. D., Granieri, E., Hsu, C., Hardin, J. M., & McDowell, B. J. et al. (1999). Improving morning care routines of nursing home residents with dementia. *Journal of the American Geriatrics Society, 47*(9), 1049–1057.

Sabat, S. R., & Harre, R. (1992). Construction and deconstruction of self in Alzheimer's disease. *Aging and Society, 12*, 443–461.

Schnelle, J. F., Alessi, C. A., Al-Samarrai, N. R., Fricker, R. D., & Ouslander, J. G. (1999). The nursing home at night: Effects of an intervention on noise, light, and sleep. *Journal of the American Geriatrics Society, 47*, 430–438.

Small, J. A., Geldart, K., Gutman, G., & Scott, M. A. C. (1998). The discourse of self in dementia. *Ageing and Society, 18*, 291–316.

Tappen, R. M., Williams, C., Fishman, S., & Touhy, T. (1999). Persistence of self in advanced Alzheimer's disease. *Image—Journal of Nursing Scholarship, 31*(2), 121–125.

Usita, PM., Hyman, I. E., & Herman, K. C. (1998). Narrative intentions: Listening to life stories in Alzheimer's disease. *Journal of Aging Studies, 12*(2), 185–197.

Van Haitsma, K., & Ruckdeschel, K. (2001). Special care for dementia in nursing homes: Overview of innovations in programs and activities. *Alzheimer's Care Quarterly, 2*(3), 49–56.

Vittoria, A. K. (1998). Preserving selves: Identity work and dementia. *Research on Aging, 20*(1), 91–136.

Wells, D. L., Dawson, P., Sidani, S., Craig, D., & Pringle, D. (2000). Effects of an abilities-focused program of morning care on residents who have dementia and on caregivers. *Journal of the American Geriatrics Society, 48*, 442–449.

CHAPTER EIGHT

The Influence of Changing Emotional Goals on the Psychological Well-Being of Nursing Home Residents

Paige E. Goodwin and Robert C. Intrieri

Over the years, a number of authors have considered the quality of life of long-term care (LTC) residents. For the most part, theorists have focused on the external environment of the nursing home, typically addressing how institutions structure or alter the environment to improve resident well-being. With the notable exceptions of Lawton (1983, 1985, 1989, 1996) and Baltes (Baltes & Carstensen, 1996; Baltes, Wahl, & Reichert, 1991), few have considered the role that residents might play in the shaping of their environmental context and maintenance of psychological well-being.

The present chapter hypothesizes that LTC residents maintain psychological well-being by actively shaping their environmental context via emotion regulation or affect management. Before focusing on issues of emotion management in LTC, we will review the general concept of emotion and/or affect. Once establishing definitions, we will briefly consider the prospect of change with age in the key components of emotional experience. In the second section we will introduce the concept of emotion regulation and explore the influence of age on the regulatory goals of the individual. Having firmly established the boundaries of our discussion, we will move toward a review of the very limited literature related to emotion in the nursing home. We will pay particular attention to the concept of person–environment transactions and affective experience (Baltes et al., 1991; Lawton, 1985, 1989). The absence of data means much of our discussion will be speculative, with the goal of presenting a slightly altered view of the emotional profile of nursing home residents.

EMOTION, AFFECT, AND AGE

Despite a long tradition of research and theory-building, the field of emotion remains characterized by continuing debate. Most of this dialog relates to the neurophysiological structure and regulatory function(s) of emotions (Izard & Ackerman, 1998). A perusal of the literature also suggests continuing debate regarding the definition of emotion and why terms like emotion, mood, and affect are often used interchangeably. Russell and Snodgrass (1987) provide perhaps the best overview of what we see as a fundamental source of confusion in the emotion literature, what we are referring to as definitional confusion, by arguing that emotion "lacks a set of necessary and sufficient features" (p. 246).

Emotion has typically been examined from a psychophysiological perspective that highlights the link between neuroanatomical structures and the subjective experience of emotion. An early example is the work of Schachter and Singer (1962), who hypothesized that emotion begins with the awareness of arousal, which precipitates an evaluation of the immediate environment in order to identify the contextual trigger. More recent theories reflect a discrete or differential emotions perspective (Ekman, Levenson, & Friesen, 1983; Izard, 1977; Malatesta & Kalnok, 1984), which argues that the experience of emotion is triggered by sensory feedback from the face. In general, emotions are seen as biologically based reactions that guide an individual's response to environmental stimuli. Further, emotions are seen as multidimensional, involving not only physiological responsiveness, but also expressive behavior and subjective experience (Cacioppo, Berntson, Klein, & Poehlmann, 1998; Carstensen, Charles, Isaacowitz, & Kennedy, 2003; Diener & Larsen, 1993; Ekman et al., 1983; Gross & Levenson, 1993; Gross & Munoz, 1995; Izard & Ackerman, 1998; Malatesta & Kalnok, 1984).

Gross and colleagues (Gross, 1998; Gross & Levenson, 1993; Gross & Munoz, 1995) suggest the process of emotion begins with an assessment of environmental cues (internal or external). Where appropriate, this assessment produces a systematic array of "emotional response tendencies" that assist the individual in responding adaptively to environmental challenges and opportunities (Gross & Munoz, 1995). Implicit within this model is a belief that the influence of any specific stimulus or event depends upon how the individual defines or represents the event. From this perspective, emotion is the individual's response when a specific stimulus is evaluated as significant (Gross & Levenson, 1993). This is similar to Plutchik's (1984) conceptualization of emotion as the individual's multidimensional cascading reaction to a stimulus, including neuroanatomical arousal, verbal and nonverbal expressive behavior, subjective experience, cognitive appraisal processes, and coping behaviors (Plutchik, 1984).

Embedded within the literature are a number of theoretically related concepts (Russell & Snodgrass, 1987). For example, one important distinction is between emotion, mood, and affect, terms that Schulz (1982, 1985) argues are virtually interchangeable. The facility with which theorists and researchers apply these terms may reflect the practical implications of Schachter and Singer's (1962) early conceptualization of emotion as a two-step process. As described by Cacioppo et al. (1998), when the individual identifies a change in level of arousal they also perceive a need to identify the source of the change. From this perspective, initial feelings of arousal are ill-defined, becoming emotion only when the appropriate cognitive label is found. Arousal is an affect (Cacioppo et al., 1998) and cannot be practically separated from its cognitive label (i.e., emotion). In other words, affect and emotion cannot be discussed independently of each other.

The Influence of Age on Emotion

At the time of birth, research suggests humans are genetically predisposed to experience emotion with individual differences in emotion programming in place (Izard & Ackerman, 1998). Research suggests the emotion system is regulated via subcortical processes located in the limbic system (Davidson, 1992), with involvement of both the sympathetic and parasympathetic systems (Schulz, 1982, 1985). The emotion system appears to be activated by sensory awareness, which then proceeds through the thalamus before reaching the amgydala (Izard & Ackerman, 1998). Additional research suggests the emotion system is characterized by hemispheric specificity (Davidson, 1992). In general, positive affect is linked to activation of the left hemisphere while negative affect is linked to activation of the right hemisphere.

The dependence of the emotion system on the physiological structures of the brain suggests a number of possible age-related changes in emotion functioning. Since Tomkins' (1962) classic work identifying a link between emotion and facial expression, a large body of research has emerged related to the role of the somatic system in emotion. The emphasis on expressive behavior like facial movement reflects its dual-function nature: facial expression not only provides feedback to the individual, but it also alerts others in the environment to the individual's emotional state (Magai & Passman, 1998). Ekman et al. (1983) found a directed facial action task that produced emotion-specific autonomic activity, suggesting facial expression(s) may influence specific emotional experiences. For a number of reasons, age may influence the link between facial expression and the experience of emotion (Levenson, Carstensen, Friesen, & Ekman, 1991; Malatesta, Fiore, & Messina, 1987; Malatesta & Kalnok, 1984). Greater experience with the display rules associated with emotion may lead older adults to engage in more suppression of facial expression, suppression that may alter feedback mechanisms (Izard & Ackerman, 1998; Malatesta & Kalnok, 1984). Further, age-related changes in facial musculature and skin elasticity may influence the somatic aspects of emotion. Levenson confirmed a link between facial expression and autonomic activity in a sample of older adults (Levenson, Carstensen, Friesen, & Ekman, 1991). However, the magnitude of the autonomic response was smaller in the older sample and the quality of facial expressions produced by older adults was judged to be lower. This finding is supported by Malatesta, Fiore, & Messina (1987), who found older adults' facial expressions were often incorrectly interpreted by younger decoders.

Age-related changes in the intensity of emotional experience have also been explored. Affect intensity is typically conceptualized as the strength of the individual's response to emotional stimuli (Larsen, Diener, & Emmons, 1986). Diener has found negative correlations between age and self-reported intensity for both positive and negative affects (Diener, Sandvik, & Larsen, 1985). Lawton, Kleban, Rajagopal, and Dean (1992) also reported that older adults were more likely to indicate others experience more intense moods. On the other hand, when asked to recall an intense emotional episode, older adults generally report levels of subjective intensity similar to younger adults (Levenson et al., 1991). In other words, the capacity to experience intense emotion remains stable with age although the self-report of intense emotions experienced on a daily basis declines, suggesting that while older adults are able to control the frequency of emotional events, once initiated subjective intensity does not decline with age (Carstensen, Pasupathi, Mayr, & Nesselroade, 2000; Gross et al., 1997).

Early stereotypes suggested an age-related increase in frequency of negative mood states with a corresponding age-related decrease in frequency of positive mood states (Schulz, 1982, 1985). Despite the assumptions, most data do not support this hypothesis (Cameron, 1975;

Carstensen et al., 2000; Diener et al., 1985; Malatesta & Kalnok, 1984; Mroczek & Kolarz, 1998; Ryff, 1989; Smith & Baltes, 1993). Early research by Malatesta and Kalnok (1984) found older adults reported no change in frequency of positive or negative affect. Smith and Baltes (1993) found that compared to young-old participants, very old participants experienced some decline in frequency of positive mood states but no change in negative affect. Ryff (1989) explored age differences in affect balance, depression, and morale, finding that younger adults reported lower levels of affect balance and morale while older adults reported higher levels of depression. Mroczek and Kolarz (1998) identified linear relationships between age and positive and negative affects. Similar to Ryff (1989), younger participants reported the highest level of negative affect while older participants reported the lowest level. Utilizing an experience sampling design, Carstensen et al. (2000) found no age differences for the frequency of positive emotional experiences while the relationship between age and negative affect was described as curvilinear.

In summary, emotion is generally understood to refer to the biologically based multichannel (physiological responses, subjective experience, and expressive behavior) response to environmental stimuli. Referencing the work of Zajonc (1984), a distinction is made between the concepts of affect (arousal) and emotion (the cognitive label applied to the affect state). Research typically finds the emotion system maintains itself into old age, with the capacity to experience and express emotions (both positive and negative) intact. Further, research indicates older adults experience better emotional well-being than younger adults in that the incidence of negative emotional events and moods appears to decline with age while positive mood states appear to be either stable or increased.

THE REGULATION OF EMOTION

As a general statement, the individual regulates emotion with the objective of maximizing positive affect and/or minimizing negative affect. As Magai and Passman (1998) point out, these goals would be easily achievable if the individual lived in a vacuum. However, the nature of being human is that we are, to a greater or lesser degree, social beings whose moods and emotions are frequently influenced by a social context that includes not only places but other people (with goals of their own). Magai and Passman (1998) argue that when it comes to the pursuit of positive and/or the avoidance of negative, we are influenced by our social context, an assertion supported by the research of Malatesta and Kalnok (1984) exploring the frequency of affect states. In an analysis examining the source of affect states, Malatesta and Kalnok (1984) found affect experiences were most frequently caused by another individual in the environmental context.

With the social context of emotion in mind, how does the individual achieve emotional goals? Theorists suggest goals are achieved through the regulation of emotion (Campos et al., 1989; Carstensen et al., 2000; Gross, 1998; Gross & Levenson, 1993; Gross & Munoz, 1995; Gross et al., 1997; Labouvie-Vief, Hakim-Larson, DeVoe, & Schoeberlein, 1989; Magai & Passman, 1998). Definitions of emotion regulation generally stress the individual's monitoring of their own affective state. Magai and Passman (1998) conceptualize emotion regulation as the individual's attention to, and adaptation of, affective response, similar to Campos et al.'s (1989) definition of regulation as the management of emotional expression. Gross and Levenson (1993) stress active manipulation by the individual is essential for the regulation of emotion. Implied within this definition is a distinction between strategies of emotion regulation. Antecedent-focused regulation refers to actions taken by the individual before a specific emotion starts that influence and whether the emotion actually occurs. According to Gross and Munoz (1995), this style of regulation typically involves some modification of the environmental context. Response-focused regulation occurs once an emotion program has been initiated and involves some modification of the response tendency (Gross, 1998; Gross & Munoz, 1995). A common form of response-focused regulation is suppression (e.g., suppression of facial expression) in which the individual consciously attempts to inhibit the display of emotional behavior.

Age differences in emotion regulation have been used to explain the favorable emotional profile of older adults. Labouvie-Vief et al. (1989) suggest a strong developmental explanation for the positive emotional profile of older adults (i.e., higher levels of positive affect and lower levels of negative affect). She suggests older adults are more effective at the self-regulation of emotions because their regulatory styles have become more inner-focused, directed toward reframing or reassessing negative events and feelings. In particular, she suggests older adults' greater experience may make them more facile at cognitively reappraising an event. If correct, older adults' negative mood states may be of shorter duration.

Those who have a tendency to evaluate age differences in regulation as indicative of a developmental process should remember Lazarus's (1996) contention that age differences in regulatory styles may reflect age-related changes in context and types of events that require some form of regulation. Quite simply, daily environmental contexts (and the problems/events that arise in those contexts) are likely to be very different for a 15-year-old girl living with parents as opposed to a 78-year-old widowed female struggling to maintain independent living. Put another way, different contexts may require different regulatory responses. Lawton et al. (1992) explored age differences in attempts to control or regulate the course of experienced emotions. Lawton and colleagues found older adults were more likely to be engaged in behavior focused on controlling the course of emotions (i.e., avoiding emotional situations, actively working to remain calm in an emotional situation), and that this control was related to a decrease in frequency of negative experiences. For example, an older adult residing in a nursing home may resist visits from children if those visits consistently produce high levels of emotion and consequent dysphoria.

Gross et al. (1997) assessed the subjective experience of emotions, emotion-expressive behavior, and self-reported control of emotional experiences. As a general trend, older adults reported a decline in the experience of negative mood states. Consistent with an emotional control model, older participants reported greater internal control of emotional experiences, especially negative emotional experiences (Gross et al., 1997). Instead of relying upon self-reported emotional control, Carstensen et al. (2000) operationalized control as the maximizing of positive affect and/or the minimizing of negative affect. If this is the goal of emotion regulation, effective use of an emotion regulation strategy should produce positive mood states that are maintained for a longer period of time and/or negative mood states of shorter duration. Carstensen found older adults were more likely to maintain positive affective states while being less likely to maintain negative affective states, suggesting older adults are more efficient at regulating their emotional lives than younger or middle-aged adults.

A well-formulated perspective on emotion regulation in adulthood is Socioemotional Selectivity Theory (SST; Carstensen, 1993; Carstensen, Gross, & Fung, 1998; Carstensen, Isaacowitz, & Charles, 1999; Fredrickson & Carstensen, 1990). Like Magai and Passman (1998), Carstensen suggests older adults regulate emotions by acknowledging the social nature of emotional experience. SST emerged as an explanation for the extremely well-replicated finding of age-related declines in social interaction (Carstensen, 1992; Lang & Carstensen, 1994). Critical analysis of the decline reflects an active selection process, SST proposes that over time the individual increasingly chooses to invest limited personal and psychic resources in close emotional relationships that maximize opportunities for the experience of positive affect and/or the avoidance of negative affect. In other words, older adults manage emotional experiences by selectively managing the social context. Choosing to spend time with a small number of intimate associates, engaging in activities known to be pleasant, is an incredibly effective strategy for maximizing positive outcomes.

Lawton (1989, 1996) has explored the association between self-regulation of affect, emotional well-being, and quality of life among older adults, both those in the community as well as those in some form of institutional context. Lawton's thesis is that the psychological well-being of older adults reflects their ability to adapt to life events while modifying their social and environmental context (Lawton, 1996). Defining self-regulation of affect as the individual's attempts to control not only the input of affect but also the response to affect, Lawton believes there is evidence older adults self-regulate affect experiences (i.e., the frequency of experiences, the duration and intensity of experiences, and expression of experiences). For example, older adults are more likely to indicate that although the types of problems they experience have not changed, the extent to which they are bothered by those problems has declined (Lawton et al., 1992). It appears that older adults are quicker to recognize that dwelling upon negative events frequently does little to modify or change the event.

Other than a desire to maintain a positive emotional profile, the emotion regulation efforts of older adults may also reflect awareness that intense affective experiences (positive or negative) sometimes bring psychic costs (Diener, Colvin, Pavot, & Allman, 1991). For example, events that are experienced as extremely positive can begin to serve as the context within which other positive events are judged, with moderately positive events increasingly evaluated as less positive. Further, it appears that intense events (either positive or negative) may set the stage for a rebound effect. A thought-provoking study by Charles, Carstensen, and McFall (2001) explored age differences in emotional responses and associated coping strategies. After presenting younger and older adults with vignettes depicting common problems that arise in a nursing home, respondents were asked to describe the emotional response of the person in the vignette as well as what action he/she should take. Interestingly, younger participants typically reported anger as the perceived emotional response and believed the actor should take a more action-oriented approach to solving the problem. Older participants, on the other hand, typically reported sadness as the perceived emotional response and believed the actor should take a nonaction approach to solving the problem. Charles et al. (2001) suggest differences in emotional response and consequent coping strategies represent the influence of age on emotion regulation, reflecting older adults' belief that intense emotions (like anger) should be avoided because of the physical, affective, and cognitive costs to the individual.

In summary, emotion regulation is suggested as the mechanism through which individuals achieve their emotional goals, specifically, the maximizing of positive affect and/or the minimizing of negative affect.

Definitions of emotion regulation generally emphasize the role of the individual in managing their own affective state through efforts to control or modify the environment (Campos et al., 1989; Gross & Munoz, 1995; Magai & Passman, 1998). A limited research base suggests there may be an influence of age on emotion regulation, with older adults reporting greater effort to control the experience of emotion in their daily lives (Gross et al., 1997; Lawton et al., 1992).

EMOTION MANAGEMENT IN THE NURSING HOME

Our discussion thus far has briefly focused on the broad domain of affect and emotion. We have attended to the concept of emotion regulation, highlighting evidence suggesting age differences in the management of emotion. For the most part, our focus has been community-dwelling older adults. Moving forward to consider the very limited research on older adults in institutional settings, we will propose that what constitutes a positive emotional profile in the community may not represent the desired affective profile of older adults in nursing homes. Our reasons for suggesting this as a hypothesis reflect what Magai and Passman (1998) point out is the very social contextual nature of emotional experience. If Magai and Passman (1998) are correct, and the majority of emotional experiences are influenced by others, imagine how the regulation of emotions changes when the individual, in declining health with diminishing physical and psychic resources, relocates to an institutional setting.

Baltes is one of the few theorists to consider issues of well-being in the nursing home (Baltes & Carstensen, 1996; Baltes et al., 1991). Baltes and her colleagues have stressed the potential for successful aging in the nursing home environment, paying particular attention to research identifying criteria associated with successful aging. Baltes has urged theorists to move away from the belief that successful aging in an institutional setting can be identified using normative criteria. Rather, any model that attempts to describe processes of successful aging among LTC residents must conceptualize successful aging as adaptive functioning irrespective of the environmental context (Baltes et al., 1991).

Positive Adaptation and Affect Management

A perspective on successful aging applicable across contextual settings is the metamodel of selection, optimization, and compensation (SOC; Baltes & Baltes, 1990; Freund & Baltes, 1998, 1999). SOC conceptualizes successful aging as the individual's ability to minimize the impact of age-related losses (for example, age-related declines in sensory functioning) while maximizing potential gains in development (Baltes & Carstensen, 1996). We believe there are similarities between the metamodel of SOC and Lawton's thesis of affective management, as both argue the adaptive task of the individual is to maximize positive outcomes while minimizing the impact of negative age-related changes. Selection, the initial step in the model, recognizes that aging (and related changes in physical/cognitive resources) frequently leads to restrictions in domains of functioning. The task of the individual is to adapt by selecting those areas of functioning of highest priority that "represent a convergence of environmental demands, individual motivations, skills, and biological capacity" (Baltes et al., 1991, p. 314). Through reducing the amount of attention and energy devoted to lower priority domains, and increasing the focus on selected high-priority domains, the individual modifies personal goals. Optimization refers to those behaviors the individual takes to amplify or extend existing resources with the goal of improving functioning in selected high priority domains (Baltes et al., 1991). Compensation refers to behavioral or psychological efforts to adapt to a loss while maintaining functioning. In many ways, compensation reflects the adjustment that must be made when there is a lack of fit between the individual's level of skill and the demands of the context (Carstensen, Hanson, & Freund, 1995). In other words, SOC represents a transactional model emphasizing the interplay between the individual's behavior and the environment's support or lack of support for that behavior.

Baltes suggests the nursing home is an institutional representation of SOC (Baltes et al., 1991). Selection is the furnishing of an environment with restricted domains of functioning. Services (medical, social, technological) available to assist the individual whose functional capacity has declined below the level of necessary behavioral competence is an example of compensation, while optimization refers to opportunities provided by the home to enhance functioning in desired areas. On the individual level, the choice (or forced choice) to relocate to a nursing home may be viewed as an example of SOC. A final well-cited example of SOC in the nursing home is Baltes' concept of a dependency-support script (Baltes, 1988; Baltes & Carstensen, 1999; Baltes et al., 1991). As described by Baltes, staff and residents in nursing homes operate according to a social script in which resident dependent behavior is followed by staff support for resident dependent behavior. Baltes suggests the consistency with which the script is acted out demonstrates that residents accept not only their dependent behavior but compensatory behavior by staff. Further, when residents violate the script by engaging in independent behavior, they and their efforts are typically ignored by staff

(Baltes, 1988). Instead of suggesting the support of dependency by staff is universally detrimental, Baltes highlights the potential optimization functions of dependent behavior. Specifically, by giving up some independence (e.g., dressing oneself in the morning), the resident is able to optimize another domain, the social domain, by increasing the amount of social contact they have with staff. In other words, the resident selects the behavior to be given up (i.e., dressing) as well as the behavior to be emphasized (i.e., social interaction). From this perspective, it is easy to see that both resident and nursing home staff are reinforced for their activity.

The concepts of SOC suggest a number of ways nursing home residents may approach the regulation of emotion and maintenance of psychological well-being. An example taken from Lawton (1983) describes well-being as the outcome of transactions between the person and their environment. Within this framework, subjective well-being includes perceived quality of life and psychological well-being (i.e., feelings of subjective distress/negative affect as well as feelings of positive affect). Lawton argues that feelings of subjective distress are typically influenced by inner biological factors while positive affect is influenced by external social factors. Objective well-being includes elements of the objective environment as well as observable aspects of behavioral competence within the domains of health, ADLs, cognition, and social behavior. From this perspective, the quality of individual outcomes is reflective of the adjustment(s) made to accommodate changes in both individual competence and environmental demands (or press) (Lawton, 1985; Lawton & Nahemow, 1973). Specific to psychological well-being in old age, Lawton (1989) argues that affective experiences serve to motivate behavior (both selective and compensatory) aimed at environmental modification (or environmental optimization).

Affective Self-Management as Compensatory Behavior

From an individual perspective, the influence of affect on environment may reflect efforts to achieve an adaptive balance between need for security versus need for autonomy (Baltes et al., 1991; Lawton, 1985, 1989). While acknowledging the continued importance of personal autonomy, age-related changes contribute to an increased need for security, with context and individual competence influencing which need predominates. Lawton describes the autonomy-support dynamic in old age in terms of "reactivity" and "proactivity." Reactivity refers to the individual's response to externally initiated intervention(s) while proactivity reflects individual attempts to change, themselves or the environment, to achieve a desired outcome. We would like to propose Lawton's concept of affective self-management as an example of compensatory behavior by the individual. If either the individual or context limits autonomy (selection), proactive behavior by the individual (optimization) will be limited and positive affect (compensation) should be lower. It may appear we are suggesting the individual compensates for environmental restrictions by lowering positive affect. What we are suggesting is that the individual's residence in an institution that limits available behavioral repertoires will have as an outcome a more restricted range of both positive and negative affects. Specifically, affective experience in the LTC setting is the outcome of a dialectic between biological and environmental factors (Lawton, 1989, 1996).

Research supports Lawton's belief that older adults demonstrate increasing affective proactivity (Lawton et al., 1992). Defining self-regulation as the ability to influence the occurrence and content of emotion, older adults report selecting activities on the basis of desired stimulation ("emotional control") and actively structuring their activities and context to avoid extremes of emotion ("emotional maturity through moderation"). Interpreted in this light, the previously discussed data on emotional experience among older adults (i.e., a capacity to experience emotions intensely but a corresponding decline in affect intensity) suggest older adults' self-regulation of affect is demonstrated via selection of contexts and activities that are controllable by the individual (i.e., television viewing) (Goodwin, Intrieri, & Papini, 2005).

Additional support for Lawton's thesis of person–environment transactions and affective self-regulation comes from personality research. Diener and colleagues (Diener, Larsen, & Emmons, 1984; Emmons, Diener, & Larsen, 1986) have examined the relationship between personality and choice of daily situations. Although few of us have complete freedom to choose situations, the authors' expectation was that in daily life individuals elect to spend time in personality-congruent contexts. In a context (like a nursing home) where individual situational choices are limited, the interplay between person and environment may be particularly important. More critical is the hypothesized link between person–situation fit and affective experience in which a closer fit between the person, their personality, and their context produces more favorable affective experiences. Diener et al. (1984) found some evidence that personality influences choice of situation (e.g., people high on extraversion spent more recreational time in social situations). Emmons et al. (1986) examined person–situation fit and affective outcomes with a design that included individual's degree of choice over the situation. Results indicated individuals typically chose to spend more time in situations that reflected underlying personality traits and needs. Further, positive affect was higher when individuals chose to be in situations that were personality congruent (Emmons et al., 1986).

Behavior, Mood, and the Nursing Home Context

Our basic premise is that the personal qualities of nursing home residents and the environmental context of the nursing home influence the person–environment transaction and its consequent affective outcomes. Like Baltes, we believe successful adaptation (seen as positive emotional profiles) is possible within the nursing home, though we argue that what constitutes "positive" may differ from the community setting. Also like Baltes, we believe these successful outcomes represent transactional processes, generally operationalized via the regulation of emotion.

Research with community-dwelling older adults consistently finds mood profiles to be positive (i.e., similar or better levels of positive affect and lower levels of negative affect) compared to younger and middle-aged adults. The question is whether this apparent advantage in emotional well-being carries over to the nursing home setting. An exploratory study of mood states in the nursing home found residents experienced lower levels of anger-hostility, vigor-activity, and tension-anxiety than samples from the general population, though differences were generally not significant (Gueldner, Butler, Ray, Ricketts, & Schlotzhauer, 1994). The only mood state residents reported in higher levels was depression-dejection, though the difference was insignificant. In a follow-up comparing mood states of community-dwelling older adults with nursing home residents, community-dwelling adults reported lower levels of tension-anxiety, depression-dejection, and confusion-bewilderment and higher levels of vigor-activity (Gueldner et al., 2001).

We hypothesize these findings represent the outcome of the transaction between the individual's ability to actively select, optimize, and develop adequate compensatory strategies in the nursing home context. Specifically, the lower levels of generally positive mood states for residents may reflect the increased need for security and consequent reduction in the ability to proactively shape their environment.

The small body of research examining mood states in the nursing home suggests depression as the most prominent mood or emotional disorder. Although prevalence estimates of major depression in the nursing home range from 12 to 16% (Parmelee, Katz, & Lawton, 1989, 1992; Teresi, Abrams, Holmes, Ramirez, & Eimicke, 2001), estimates of depressed mood and/or depressive symptoms can be as high as 45% (Parmelee et al., 1989; Teresi et al., 2001). More compelling is that studies examining mood disorders in the nursing home have identified an inability by staff to recognize depressed affect or mood (Goodwin & Smyer, 1999; Teresi et al., 2001).

Given our earlier discussion about the social nature of emotional experience, a reasonable hypothesis among nursing home researchers is that residents' risk of social isolation (due to their removal from existing social networks) and the resulting absence of meaningful social interaction facilitates the presence of depressed or dysphoric mood states. Further, the best response is intervention to improve the social context of residents. This line of thinking suggests that resident access to supportive relationships should be related to mood and affective well-being. An interesting study by Carpenter (2002) explored the association between types of social relationships and mood among nursing home residents. Using the Affect Balance Scale and the Geriatric Depression Scale, depressed mood was significantly negatively correlated with perceptions of peer support as well as satisfaction with support from family and peers. Satisfaction with family and peer support was also positively correlated with positive affect, consistent with the earlier work of Farber, Brod, and Feinbloom (1991) who found perceived quality of relationships was related to more positive emotional well-being. Negative affect was unrelated to any measure of social support or quality of social relationships, a result consistent with Lawton's belief that negative affect is not influenced by external social factors. Interestingly, a recent study by Fessman and Lester (2000) found that social relationships with other residents, specifically the number of residents considered to be close friends, was negatively correlated with loneliness and depressed mood. In other words, those residents who identified a greater number of close friendships within the nursing home reported less loneliness and depression.

These results are understandable within the context of emotion regulation (Carstensen, 1992). In theory, family/peer relationships characterized by greater emotional intimacy are more useful as a tool for managing positive affect. Nursing home residents reduced access to those relationships should be related to lower levels of positive affect. We believe it is important at this point to re-emphasize the goal of emotion regulation (i.e., the maximizing of positive affect and/or the minimizing of negative affect). Although it is true that residents could work to establish new intimate relationships (and thereby improve positive affect), such efforts could also increase the risk of exposure to possible negative affect. Perhaps very late in life, with increasingly diminished physical and psychic resources, the primary emotional goal of a nursing home resident is avoidance of negative above the maximizing of positive. From this perspective, the previously discussed high levels of dysphoria among nursing home residents may be the outcome of disruptions in emotion regulation. Specifically, Gross and Munoz (1995) argue that depression, or the "dysregulation of emotions in which the frequency, intensity, and duration of negative emotions, especially sadness, are increased, and those of positive emotions, such as interest and enjoyment, are decreased" (p. 157) may reflect changes in cognitive-affective schema, changes in activity patterns, or changes in self-reinforcement resulting from the changing context. In other words, nursing home residents experience dysphoria because efforts to avoid negative affect have failed, further impairing the ability to seek out and experience opportunities for pleasant activities.

Further emphasizing the link between social context, behavior, and mood, intervention aimed at increasing rates of social interaction in the nursing home often fail to be sustained across time. Carstensen, Fisher, and Malloy (1995) suggest this failure reflects a mistaken belief that all social interaction is beneficial and meaningful and should be encouraged, even among residents who clearly do not wish to engage in social behavior or who are limited in their ability to engage in social behavior. For example, Carstensen and Erickson (1986) raised rates of social interaction among residents through the provision of refreshments during a social hour. However, content analysis of the interactions indicated the majority of increase was in ineffective communication (i.e., vocal comments directed toward an individual but not responded to or incoherent vocal comments). If this finding is characteristic of most interventions, perhaps they fail to sustain because they do not provide opportunities for people to make meaningful social contact, a critical requirement of social contact if it is to be helpful in maintenance of mood.

A potentially more important barrier to social interaction among residents, and theoretically related to increases in dysphoric mood, is cognitive impairment. Despite an assumption that cognitive functioning should be positively associated with rates of social interaction, Carstensen et al. (1995) found limited negative relationships between cognition and quantity of social interaction. For example, poorer performance on the Boston Naming Test was significantly related to more interaction while spatial memory correlated negatively with rates of positive interactions and positively with rates of negative interaction. Although these relationships were not strong, they suggest a pattern of social interaction between residents and staff consistent with Baltes' concept of a dependency-support script. Specifically, residents with poorer spatial memory, whose functioning is more impaired, are more dependent and have more positive social contact with staff due to their dependence. On the other hand, residents with better spatial memory, whose functioning is less impaired, are less dependent and have more negative social contact with staff. Baltes would suggest the higher rates of negative resident–staff interaction reflect the violation of the dependency-support script. Finally, while loneliness was not related to rates of interaction, there was a significant negative correlation between social anxiety and rates of positive interaction. Many residents indicated an unwillingness to join groups, preferring to be alone in their room. These residents explained their preference in terms of the cognitive impairments of other residents. Quite simply, they reported avoiding social contact because they found potential social partners to be unattractive or unappealing and perceived that social interaction would add little to their lives. Not only are these potential partners unlikely to fulfill the role of close emotional partner necessary for maintaining positive affect or emotion, they represent an unwise use of limited psychic resources unlikely to assist in optimizing affective outcomes.

In theory, the influence of cognitive impairment on social and affective experience should be most pronounced among nursing home residents suffering from Alzheimer's disease (AD) or other dementias. Research suggests AD patients show deficits in the ability to encode and decode emotional information (Albert, Cohen, & Koff, 1991; Zandi, Cooper, & Garrison, 1992). Given that the pathophysiological nature of dementia frequently renders AD patients unable to find the words to verbally express emotional feelings, interaction with AD patients often depends upon nonverbal cues (like facial expression) for insight into emotional experience. In addition to the impact of neuroanatomical changes associated with disease processes, the emotional experiences of dementia patients may also be understood using Lawton's (1983) model of relationships between positive and negative affect, and external and internal influences. Specifically, positive affect is related to engagement in external activities or relationships while negative affect is related to inner phenomenon. Given the hypothesized relationships, AD patients may show lower levels of positive affect and higher levels of negative affect (due to their inability to externally engage). Lawton, Van Haitsma, and Klapper (1996) compared the frequency of six affect states between demented and nondemented nursing home residents. Based on observer ratings, significant differences were found between the two groups for pleasure, interest, contentment, and anxiety. Pleasure, interest, and contentment were significantly more frequent among nondemented residents (who were more likely to be externally engaged) while anxiety occurred more frequently among demented residents. Despite the differences, evidence suggests affect states are reliably observable in demented nursing home residents, a finding supported by Magai, Cohen, Gomberg, Malatesta, & Culver (1996).

SUMMARY AND CONCLUSIONS

In summary, literature on emotion suggests some terminological confusion. Despite this, the consensus among theorists is that emotion refers to the individual's biologically based multidimensional response to a stimulus, leading to changes in physiological functioning, behavior, and subjective experience. The dependence of the emotion system on the physiological structures of the brain suggests a number of influences of age on emotion functioning. However, research exploring age differences in the experience of emotion finds few, if any, substantial changes in functioning. Research examining age and somatic activity finds the link between facial expression and autonomic activity maintained in old age. Further, research exploring the influence of age on affect intensity finds older adults capable of intense emotions, although the frequency of experienced intense emotions declines with age. Finally, research examining age differences in mood states finds older adults enjoy a more positive mood profile with higher levels of positive emotion and lower levels of negative emotion. A popular explanation for the stability of emotional well-being into late life is emotion regulation. In a broad sense, emotion regulation refers to efforts by the individual to maximize the presence of positive emotions while minimizing the impact of negative emotions. A limited research base suggests that older adults engage in more active regulation of their internal and external environment with the goal of establishing a positive emotional outcome.

The majority of research examining emotion regulation and functioning in older adults has focused on those in the community. The research base devoted to emotional functioning among nursing home residents is scant, and generally focused on depression. Data that does exist generally examine affective well-being within the context of SOC or person–environment transactions. Both Baltes et al. (1991) and Lawton (1985, 1989) conceptualize the interaction between the individual and their environment in terms of a need to find an adaptive balance between security and autonomy. Both suggest such an adaptive balance will be related to positive affective outcomes. For example, data from Lawton find that older adults report actively structuring their social context to achieve a desired affective state (Lawton et al., 1992).

Emotional experience is understandably social. Given that the source of mood states of nursing home residents has generally been sought within the social context of the nursing home. Specifically, researchers have reasoned the low levels of positive moods and occasionally higher levels of negative moods result from low rates of social interaction. However, we agree with Carstensen et al. (1995) that this line of reasoning may reflect a misunderstanding about the nature of social interaction in the nursing home as well as the resident's desire to shape their social context. Specifically, social interaction is only meaningful to the extent that it assists the resident in achieving emotional goals (i.e., the maximizing of positive affect and/or the minimizing of negative affect). Interaction with other residents, who are largely unknown and unknowable due to cognitive or physical deficits, provides little opportunity to optimize emotional goals while presenting a level of risk for negative interactions and corresponding depletion of individual resources. We suggest that late in life, as personal resources decline, the individual may select a reorganization of emotional goals, emphasizing the construction of a personal environment that limits the risk of exposure to negative affective experiences.

REFERENCES

Albert, M. S., Cohen, C., & Koff, E. (1991). Perception of affect in patients with dementia of the Alzheimer type. *Archives of Neurology, 48*(8), 791–795.

Baltes, M. M. (1988). The etiology and maintenance of dependency in the elderly: Three phases of operant research. *Behavior Therapy, 19*(3), 301–319.

Baltes, P. B., & Baltes, M. M. (1990). Selective optimization with compensation. In P. B. Baltes, & M. M. Baltes (Eds.), *Successful aging: Perspectives from the behavioral sciences* (pp. 1–34). New York: Cambridge University Press.

Baltes, M. M., & Carstensen, L. L. (1996). The process of successful ageing. *Ageing & Society, 16*(4), 397–422.

Baltes, M. M., & Carstensen, L. L. (1999). Social-psychological theories and their applications to aging: From individual to collective. In V. L. Bengston, & K. W. Schaie (Eds.), *Handbook of theories of aging* (pp. 209–236). New York: Springer.

Baltes, M. M., Wahl, H.-W., & Reichert, M. (1991). Successful aging in long-term care institutions. *Annual Review of Gerontology & Geriatrics, 11*, 311–337.

Cacioppo, J. T., Berntson, G. G., Klein, D. J., & Poehlmann, K. M. (1998). Psychophysiology of emotion across the life span. *Annual Review of Gerontology & Geriatrics, 17*, 27–74.

Cameron, P. (1975). Mood as an indicant of happiness: Age, sex, social class and situational differences. *Journal of Gerontology, 30*(2), 216–224.

Campos, J. J., Campos, R. G., & Barrett, K. C. (1989). Emergent themes in the study of emotional development and emotion regulation. *Developmental Psychology, 25*(3), 394–402.

Carpenter, B. D. (2002). Family, peer, and staff social support in nursing home patients: Contributions to psychological well-being. *The Journal of Applied Gerontology, 21*(3), 275–293.

Carstensen, L. L. (1992). Social and emotional patterns in adulthood: Support for socioemotional selectivity theory. *Psychology & Aging, 7*(3), 331–338.

Carstensen, L. L. (1993). Motivation for social contact across the lifespan: A theory of socioemotional selectivity. In J. Jacobs (Ed.), *Nebraska symposium on motivation* (Vol. 39, pp. 209–254). Lincoln, NE: University of Nebraska Press.

Carstensen, L. L., Charles, S. T., Isaacowitz, D. M., & Kennedy, Q. (2003). Emotion and life-span personality development. In R. J. Davidson, K. R. Scherer, & H. H. Goldsmith (Eds.), *Handbook of affective sciences* (pp. 726–744). Oxford: Oxford University Press.

Carstensen, L. L., & Erickson, R. J. (1986). Enhancing the social environments of elderly nursing home residents: Are high rates of interaction enough? *Journal of Applied Behavior Analysis, 19*(4), 349–355.

Carstensen, L. L., Fisher, J. E., & Malloy, P. (1995). Cognitive and affective characteristics of socially withdrawn nursing home residents. *Journal of Clinical Geropsychology, 1*(3), 207–218.

Carstensen, L. L., Gross, J. J., & Fung, H. H. (1998). The social context of emotional experience. *Annual Review of Gerontology & Geriatrics, 17*, 325–352.

Carstensen, L. L., Hanson, K. A., & Freund, A. M. (1995). Selection and compensation in adulthood. In R. A. Dixon, & L. Backman (Eds.), *Compensating for psychological deficits and declines* (pp. 107–126). Mahwah, NJ: Lawrence Erlbaum Associates.

Carstensen, L. L., Isaacowitz, D. M., & Charles, S. T. (1999). Taking time seriously: A theory of socioemotional selectivity. *American Psychologist, 54*(3), 165–181.

Carstensen, L. L., Pasupathi, M., Mayr, U., & Nesselroade, J. R. (2000). Emotional experience in everyday life across the adult life span. *Journal of Personality & Social Psychology, 79*(4), 644–655.

Charles, S. T., Carstensen, L. L., & McFall, R. M. (2001). Problem-solving in the nursing home environment: Age and experience differences in emotional reactions and responses. *Journal of Clinical Geropsychology, 7*(4), 319–330.

Davidson, R. J. (1992). Emotion and affective style: Hemispheric substrates. *Psychological Science, 3*(1), 39–43.

Diener, E., Colvin, C. R., Pavot, W. G., & Allman, A. (1991). The psychic costs of intense positive affect. *Journal of Personality & Social Psychology, 61*(3), 492–503.

Diener, E., & Larsen, R. J. (1993). The experience of emotional well-being. In M. Lewis, & J. M. Haviland (Eds.), *Handbook of emotions* (pp. 405–415). New York: Guilford Press.

Diener, E., Larsen, R. J., & Emmons, R. A. (1984). Person X situation interactions: Choice of situations and congruence response models. *Journal of Personality & Social Psychology, 47*(3), 580–592.

Diener, E., Sandvik, E., & Larsen, R. J. (1985). Age and sex effects for emotional intensity. *Developmental Psychology, 21*(3), 542–546.

Ekman, P., Levenson, R. W., & Friesen, W. V. (1983). Autonomic nervous service activity distinguishes among emotions. *Science, 221*(4616), 1208–1210.

Emmons, R. A., Diener, E., & Larsen, R. J. (1986). Choice and avoidance of everyday situations and affect congruence: Two models of reciprocal interactionism. *Journal of Personality & Social Psychology, 51*(4), 815–826.

Farber, H. J., Brod, M., & Feinbloom, R. I. (1991). Primary family contacts and emotional health in the institutionalized elderly. *Family Practice Research Journal, 11*(3), 309–317.

Fessman, N., & Lester, D. (2000). Loneliness and depression among elderly nursing home patients. *International Journal of Aging & Human Development, 51*(2), 137–141.

Fredrickson, B. F., & Carstensen, L. L. (1990). Choosing social partners: How old age and anticipated endings make people more selective. *Psychology & Aging, 5*(3), 335–347.

Freund, A. M., & Baltes, P. B. (1998). Selection, optimization, and compensation as strategies of life management: Correlations with subjective indicators of successful aging. *Psychology & Aging, 13*(4), 531–543.

Freund, A. M., & Baltes, P. B. (1999). Selection, optimization, and compensation as strategies of life management: Correction to Freund and Baltes (1998). *Psychology & Aging, 14*(4), 700–702.

Goodwin, P. E., Intrieri, R. C., & Papini, D. R. (2005). Older adults affect while watching television. *Activities, Adaptation, & Aging, 29*(2), 55–74.

Goodwin, P. E., & Smyer, M. A. (1999). Accuracy of recognition and diagnosis of comorbid depression in the nursing home. *Aging and Mental Health, 3*(4), 340–350.

Gross, J. J. (1998). Antecedent- and response-focused emotion regulation: Divergent consequences for experience, expression, and physiology. *Journal of Personality & Social Psychology, 74*(1), 224–237.

Gross, J. J., Carstensen, L. L., Pasupathi, M., Tsai, J., Skorpen, C. G., & Hsu, A. Y. C. (1997). Emotion and aging: Experience, expression, and control. *Psychology & Aging, 12*(4), 590–599.

Gross, J. J., & Levenson, R. W. (1993). Emotional suppression: Physiology, self-report, and expressive behavior. *Journal of Personality and Social Psychology, 64*(6), 970–986.

Gross, J. J., & Munoz, R. F. (1995). Emotion regulation and mental health. *Clinical Psychology: Science & Practice, 2*(2), 151–164.

Gueldner, S. H., Butler, S., Ray, J. K., Ricketts, J. L., & Schlotzhauer, P. (1994). A profile of mood in ambulatory nursing home residents. *Archives of Psychiatric Nursing, 8*(5), 320–325.

Gueldner, S. H., Loeb, S., Morris, D., Penrod, J., Bramlett, M., Johnston, L., & Schlotzhauer, P. (2001). A comparison of life satisfaction and mood in nursing home residents and community-dwelling elders. *Archives of Psychiatric Nursing, 15*(5), 232–240.

Izard, C. E. (1977). *Human emotions.* New York: Plenum.

Izard, C. E., & Ackerman, B. P. (1998). Emotions and self-concepts across the life span. *Annual Review of Gerontology & Geriatrics, 17*, 1–26.

Labouvie-Vief, G., Hakim-Larson, J., DeVoe, M., & Schoeberlein, S. (1989). Emotions and self-regulation: A life-span view. *Human Development, 32*(5), 279–299.

Lang, F. R., & Carstensen, L. L. (1994). Close emotional relationships in late life: Further support for proactive aging in the social domain. *Psychology & Aging, 9*(2), 315–324.

Larsen, R. J., Diener, E., & Emmons, R. A. (1986). Affect intensity and reactions to daily life events. *Journal of Personality & Social Psychology, 51*(4), 803–814.

Lawton, M. P. (1983). The varieties of well-being. *Experimental Aging Research, 9*(2), 65–72.

Lawton, M. P. (1985). The elderly in context: Perspectives from environmental psychology and gerontology. *Environment & Behavior, 17*(4), 501–519.

Lawton, M. P. (1989). Environmental proactivity and affect in older people. In S. Spacapan, & S. Oskamp (Eds.), *The social psychology of aging* (pp. 135–163). Newbury Park: Sage Publications.

Lawton, M. P. (1996). Quality of life and affect in later life. In C. Magai, & S. H. McFadden (Eds.), *Handbook of emotion, adult development, and aging* (pp. 327–348). San Diego: Academic Press.

Lawton, M. P., Kleban, M. H., Rajagopal, D., & Dean, J. (1992). Dimensions of affective experience in three age groups. *Psychology & Aging, 7*(2), 171–184.

Lawton, M. P., & Nahemow, L. (1973). Ecology and the aging process. In C. Eisdorfer, & M. P. Lawton (Eds.), *Psychology of adult development* (pp. 619–674). Washington, DC: American Psychological Association.

Lawton, M. P., Van Haitsma, K., & Klapper, J. (1996). Observed affect in nursing home residents with Alzheimer's Disease. *Journal of Gerontology: Psychological Sciences, 51B*(1), P3–P14.

Lazarus, R. S. (1996). The role of coping in the emotions and how coping changes over the life course. In C. Magai, & S. H. McFadden (Eds.), *Handbook of emotion, adult development, and aging* (pp. 289–306). San Diego, CA: Academic Press.

Levenson, R. W., Carstensen, L. L., Friesen, W. V., & Ekman, P. (1991). Emotion, physiology, and expression in old age. *Psychology & Aging, 6*(1), 28–35.

Magai, C., Cohen, C., Gomberg, D., Malatesta, C., & Culver, C. (1996). Emotion expression in mid-to-late stage dementia patients. *International Journal of Psychogeriatrics, 8*(3), 383–395.

Magai, C., & Passman, V. (1998). The interpersonal basis of emotional behavior and emotion regulation in adulthood. *Annual Review of Gerontology & Geriatrics, 17*, 104–137.

Malatesta, C. Z, Fiore, M. J., & Messina, J. J. (1987). Affect, personality, and facial expressive characteristics of older people. *Psychology & Aging, 2*(1), 64–69.

Malatesta, C. Z., & Kalnok, M. (1984). Emotional experience in younger and older adults. *Journal of Gerontology, 39*(3), 301–308.

Mroczek, D. K., & Kolarz, C. M. (1998). The effect of age on positive and negative affect: A developmental perspective on happiness. *Journal of Personality & Social Psychology, 75*(5), 1333–1349.

Parmelee, P. A., Katz, I. R., & Lawton, M. P. (1989). Depression among institutionalized aged: Assessment and prevalence estimation. *Journal of Gerontology: Medical Sciences, 44*(1), M22–M29.

Parmelee, P. A., Katz, I. R., & Lawton, M. P. (1992). Incidence of depression in long-term care settings. *Journal of Gerontology: Medical Sciences, 47*(6), M189–M196.

Plutchik, R. (1984). Emotions: A general psychoevolutionary theory. In K. R. Scherer, & P. Ekman (Eds.), *Approaches to emotion* (pp. 197–219). Hillside, NJ: Erlbaum.

Russell, J. A., & Snodgrass, J. (1987). Emotion and the environment. In D. Stokols, & I. Altman (Eds.), *Handbook of environmental psychology* (pp. 245–280). New York: John Wiley and Sons.

Ryff, C. D. (1989). Happiness is everything, or is it? Explorations on the meaning of psychological well-being. *Journal of Personality & Social Psychology, 57*(6), 1069–1081.

Schachter, S., & Singer, J. E. (1962). Cognitive, social and physiological determinants of emotional state. *Psychological Review, 69*(5), 379–397.

Schulz, R. (1982). Emotionality and aging: A theoretical and empirical analysis. *Journal of Gerontology, 37*(1), 42–51.

Schulz, R. (1985). Emotion and affect. In J. E. Birren, & K. W. Schaie (Eds.), *Handbook of the Psychology of Aging* (pp. 531–543). New York: Van Nostrand Reinhold Company.

Smith, J., & Baltes, P. B. (1993). Differential psychological ageing: Profiles of the old and very old. *Ageing & Society, 13*, 551–587.

Teresi, J. A., Abrams, R., Holmes, D., Ramirez, M., & Eimicke, J. P. (2001). Prevalence of depression and depression recognition in nursing homes. *Social Psychiatry & Psychiatric Epidemiology, 36*(12), 613–620.

Tomkins, S. S. (1962). *Affect, imagery, consciousness: The positive affects* (Vol. 1). New York: Springer.

Zajonc, R. B. (1984). On the primacy of affect. *American Psychologist, 39*(2), 117–123.

Zandi, T., Cooper, M., & Garrison, L. (1992). Facial recognition: A cognitive study of elderly dementia patients and normal older adults. *International Psychogeriatrics, 4*(2), 215–221.

CHAPTER NINE

Application of SOC Model to Care for Residents with Advanced Dementia

Ladislav Volicer and Joyce Simard

Advanced dementia is a result of progression of several degenerative neurological diseases. The most prevalent of these conditions is Alzheimer's disease that usually starts by development of memory problems, personality changes, and other cognitive impairments. Alzheimer's disease is very often combined with two other diseases: vascular dementia and dementia with Lewy bodies that can also cause dementia by themselves. Vascular dementia may cause dementia by multiple small infarcts, by a single infarct in a sensitive area, or by changes of small blood vessels that result in impairment of subcortical white matter (Binswanger disease). Early symptoms of vascular dementia are quite variable and depend on the location of brain damage. Early symptoms of dementia with Lewy bodies are hallucinations, falls, and fluctuating course of cognitive impairment. Individuals having dementia with Lewy bodies also have commonly adverse effects from antipsychotic medications used to treat their hallucinations. Another cause of advanced dementia is frontotemporal dementia that usually starts by development of personality changes and problem behaviors.

Dementia that progresses beyond the mild stage can be considered advanced. In the mild stage of dementia, individuals are still independent in their activities of daily living, although they may have to stop working and have impairment in some instrumental activities of daily living such as driving or paying bills. Advanced dementia can be divided into moderate, severe, and terminal stages of dementia. In the moderate stage, individuals require cueing or help with activities of daily living and may require constant supervision to prevent unsafe behaviors, such as leaving a home or a facility and using tools or appliances that can harm them or others. Once the individuals with dementia become unable to walk and eat independently, they progress into the severe stage of dementia. And when individuals are unable to ambulate even with assistance and become unable to communicate with others, they can be considered in the terminal stage of dementia. Progression through these phases is quite variable and unpredictable and the order of functional losses may differ. Very often, individuals progress more rapidly at a time and then become quite stable with little or no progression over a period of several months or even years. Rapid progression is often initiated by a physical illness, such as an infection or seizure, and may be a result of stress-induced damage of already compromised brain.

Although symptoms of individuals in mild and early moderate stage of dementia may differ according to dementia etiology, the symptoms in more advanced stages are very similar regardless of dementia etiology. These symptoms include cognitive impairment, behavioral symptoms, and medical problems. Cognitive impairment invariably results in functional deficits making the individual dependent on others in meeting their physical and psychosocial needs. The care providers may be family members of individuals with dementia living at home, or professional staff for individuals living in institutions. Family members are deeply affected when one of their relatives develops dementia and they require attention of health care professionals to a similar degree as the individual with dementia, because they are at high risk for development of psychiatric or medical diseases.

Despite intensive research in the area of Alzheimer's disease and other progressive degenerative dementias, there is still no treatment that would prevent, stop, or cure these diseases. Currently available treatment includes inhibitors of cholinesterase (donepezil, galantamine, and rivastigmine) that partially reverse cholinergic deficit present in Alzheimer's disease, dementia with Lewy bodies, and vascular dementia. These drugs result in temporary improvement of cognitive, functional, and behavioral symptoms in mild and moderate dementia but do not stop progression of the disease. Similar effect has a partial glutamate receptor antagonist, memantine, which is indicated in moderate and severe Alzheimer's disease. It is very likely that future therapeutic strategies will result only in transient symptomatic improvement or delay of progression of dementia. Therefore, we can expect that a large number of individuals will continue to progress into the severe and terminal dementia stages.

Clinical issues faced in caring for individuals with severe and terminal dementia can be framed by the SOC (selection, optimization, and compensation) model. The SOC model is well suited for caregivers with a variety of backgrounds and that is important because care for individuals with dementia requires multidisciplinary approach. This chapter will attempt to describe how application of the SOC model may improve care for these individuals.

SELECTION

Optimal management of individuals with advanced dementia requires selection of appropriate strategies for treatment of medical issues. Management of chronic conditions and risk factors has to take into consideration that advanced dementia decreases lifespan. Therefore, strategies that have only a long-term effect on risk factors for disease development, for example, low fat diet, may not be appropriate. Similarly, the inability of individuals with advanced dementia to report adverse effects of treatments, e.g., dizziness and hypoglycemic reaction, has to be taken into consideration for treatment of chronic conditions such as hypertension and diabetes mellitus. These conditions should not be treated too aggressively because the immediate danger of adverse effects of treatment is more significant than the potential long-term effects of less than optimal blood pressure or glycemia control.

Treatment of medical issues should be guided by overall goals of care. In some cases, individuals with dementia developed well thought out living wills or statements that define their wishes regarding goals of care. However, in most cases these statements are not specific enough because the individuals could not predict their future conditions. Since individuals with advanced dementia may not be able to understand issues they face and make decisions, these decisions have to be made by an individual's proxy. Some individuals have named a health care proxy or have a court-appointed guardian, but in most cases a family member acts as a proxy.

The proxy needs to understand the nature of the dementing process and current condition of the individual to make informed decisions. These decisions are based either on previous wishes of the individual with dementia, if known, or on the best interest of the individual as perceived by the proxy. It is possible to define three main goals of medical care: life prolongation, maintenance of function, and comfort (Gillick, Berkman, & Cullen, 1999). However, these goals may not be possible to achieve simultaneously in many situations. Treatment in an intensive care unit may prolong life but may result in loss of function and severe discomfort to individuals who do not understand why aggressive medical interventions are necessary and may require physical or chemical restraints. Treating a medical condition in a nursing home may be more conducive to maintenance of function but may not treat the condition as effectively as is possible in an acute care setting. And aggressive medical interventions, e.g., resuscitation and intravenous therapy, increase discomfort even in a nursing home setting. Therefore, it is necessary to determine the priorities of goals of care and adjust treatment strategies accordingly.

The main decisions that have to be made include use of cardiopulmonary resuscitation (CPR), transfer to acute care setting, use of tube feeding for artificial nutrition, and hydration and use of antibiotics for treatment of intercurrent infections. The proxy has to understand that there is a very low likelihood of successful CPR after a cardiac arrest in a nursing home, and that even individuals who do survive to be discharged from an acute care setting back to a nursing home are much more severely impaired on return than they were before the arrest. In addition, partially successful CPR often results in injuries and use of life support that produce severe discomfort in an individual with dementia who does not understand the need for these interventions. Therefore, CPR is not indicated if the primary goal of care is maintenance of function or comfort.

Transfer to an acute care setting may also not be in the best interest of an individual with advanced dementia. Such a transfer is clearly indicated if a treatment can eliminate a source of discomfort, for example, in an acute abdomen condition or in surgically correctable fracture. However, the proxy has to be informed that the mortality of individuals treated aggressively for a hip fracture was more than 50% in 6 months and that hip fracture may be more appropriately treated conservatively in individuals who had limited ambulatory ability before the accident. Development of pneumonia may also not require transfer to an acute care setting because treatment in a nursing home results in lowering 2 month mortality than treatment in a hospital (Fried, Gillick, & Lipsitz, 1997).

Artificial nutrition and hydration have very few, if any, benefits in individuals with advanced dementia (Gillick, 2000; Finucane, Christmas, & Travis, 1999). Tube feeding does not prevent aspiration pneumonia, does not promote healing of pressure ulcers, and may not even maintain adequate nutrition. At the same time, tube feeding has many possible adverse effects that include discomfort, need for restraints to prevent tube removal, diarrhea, vomiting, abdominal distention, infections, and others. Tube feeding also deprives individuals with dementia from taste of food and contact with caregivers that occurs during oral feeding. Unfortunately, there is an institutional bias in favor of tube feeding because it is less expensive for the facilities, while it results in higher levels of reimbursement than hand feeding (Mitchell, 2003).

The most common intercurrent infections in advanced dementia are urinary tract infection and pneumonia, which is also the most common cause of death. Intercurrent infections may be treated with oral or intramuscular antibiotics avoiding the need for intravenous therapy that often requires physical or chemical restraints. In terminal dementia, however, antibiotic treatment is not effective in prolonging survival (Fabiszewski, Volicer, & Volicer, 1990). This lack of effect is caused by a recurrent nature of these infections that are often caused by recurrent aspiration. At the same time, antibiotic treatment may have significant adverse effects that include diarrhea, rash, and even agranulocytosis. If the goal of care is comfort and includes avoidance of antibiotic therapy for generalized infections, the management also eliminates diagnostic procedures that are necessary for rational antibiotic therapy. Avoidance of these procedures increases comfort of the patient and the staff can concentrate on providing "high touch" instead of "high tech" care. It is important to realize, that patient's comfort can be achieved without antibiotic therapy, using analgesics, antipyretics, and oxygen (Van der Steen, Ooms, Van der Wal, & Ribbe, 2002). Of course, antibiotic treatment should be provided for localized infections, such as cellulitis or conjunctivitis, where comfort can be achieved by this therapy.

Discussions establishing the goal of care should be conducted soon after admission of an individual to a long-term care setting, before any crisis arises. This discussion should be organized as a meeting of family member(s) or other proxy with the interdisciplinary treatment team. It is important to discuss patient's condition with staff prior to the meeting to achieve a staff consensus and a recommendation that can be presented at the meeting. The meeting may be moderated by a social worker and should start by answering any questions the family members might have and establishing if the patient expressed any wishes before becoming demented. Staff recommendation should be presented and rationale for that explained. This avoids unnecessary stress to the family members that would be caused by not giving them any guidance. The result of such a meeting is an advanced proxy plan that specifies the goals of care and may be changed by the proxy at any time (Volicer et al., 2002). Establishing the proxy plan early avoids the need for decisions at a time of crisis and improves the chances for optimal management of the individual with dementia during the dying process.

OPTIMIZATION

Overall goals of care in advanced dementia are maintenance of quality of life, dignity, and comfort. The care has to be optimized to achieve these goals. Three areas have to be addressed to maintain quality of life: medical issues, meaningful activities, and behavioral symptoms (Volicer & Bloom-Charette, 1999). Medical issues are addressed above and meaningful activities will be discussed below. However, it is important to realize that both of these areas are very important in prevention and treatment of behavioral symptoms. Aggressive medical interventions increase discomfort and may induce or aggravate behavioral symptoms of dementia, while meaningful activities may prevent or reduce these symptoms.

The two main behavioral symptoms of dementia are agitation and resistiveness to care. Agitation is often induced by a physical condition, such as hunger, thirst, feeling cold or hot, etc. Very often, agitation may be a result of untreated or undertreated pain. Optimal pain control is necessary to exclude pain as a cause of agitation. This pain control should be continuous avoiding administration of analgesics on "as needed" schedule and monitored by frequent pain assessments. Pain assessment in individuals with advanced dementia is difficult because of the comprehension and communication difficulties. Pain scales that are used for cognitively intact individuals may not be useful in individuals with advanced dementia. A simple pain scale relying on observation of the patient was recently developed (Warden, Hurley, & Volicer, 2003) and may be used also by front-line staff. It is also important to realize that advanced dementia rarely, if ever, progresses into the persistent vegetative state (Volicer, Berman, Cipolloni, & Mandell, 1997). Therefore, even individuals in very advanced terminal dementia may still perceive pain and should be assessed and treated.

Agitation may also occur because of the dementia process itself, without any external causes. The possibility that it is a symptom of boredom should be excluded by involving the individual in a meaningful activity. If agitation persists despite this intervention, a pharmacological approach may be necessary. Agitation could be a symptom of mood disorder, or it can be caused by a disturbing hallucination and delusion. Mood disorders include mania and depression that induce anxiety and restlessness. The possible cause(s) of the agitation should be determined and the treatment may sometimes require combination of antidepressants, antipsychotics, and mood stabilizers.

Resistiveness to care should be distinguished from agitation because it requires different therapeutic approaches. Resistiveness to care is caused by the lack of understanding of the caregiver activity by the individual with dementia. The individual with dementia does not understand the need for caregiving and resists it. If the caregiver insists in providing the care, the individual with dementia might defend himself/herself and even strike out. Such an individual is often labeled as "aggressive" or "assaultive." However, it is actually the caregiver who is the aggressor because he/she did not respond appropriately to the resistiveness. The caregiver has to prevent escalation of the resistive behavior into combative behavior. This can be accomplished by just delaying the care until the individual with dementia forgets that he/she did not want it, or by distracting the individual with dementia by reminiscence or interaction with another staff member. Another effective management strategy is modification of the care approach. For instance, substituting a bed bath for a shower or tube bath decreases or eliminates resistiveness during bathing (Sloane et al., 1995). In some cases, resistiveness could be due to delusions and, if behavioral approaches are not effective, its management may require administration of an antipsychotic medication.

Provision of care should be optimized according to the remaining abilities of the individual with dementia. Care providers should be considered "care partners" instead of just caregivers or carers, because they should involve individuals with dementia in their care instead of just providing the care for them. Self-esteem of the individual with dementia is increased if he/she is allowed to make choices of cloth items to wear and is given time to dress himself/herself instead of being dressed by the caregiver. Involvement of the individual with dementia in his/her care also provides a meaningful activity that improves quality of life and may prevent behavioral symptoms.

COMPENSATION

Individuals with advanced dementia require compensation in two areas. The first one is compensation for functional deficits and for executive dysfunction that results in inability to plan and initiate activities. Both of these are the result of cognitive impairment. Functional deficits in advanced dementia include inability to dress, groom, toilet, eat, and ambulate independently. These deficits may be ameliorated initially by cueing and by partial help. For instance, setting up the clothes in an order in which they are to be put on will allow individuals to dress themselves even when they would not be able to select appropriate clothing and may put it on in a wrong order or in multiple layers. Individuals who have difficulties eating independently may be helped by being served one item at a time instead of the whole menu. Urinary incontinence may be prevented by a prompted voiding program (Ouslander et al., 1995). Independent mobility may be promoted by using a Merry Walker device that allows residents to ambulate without the danger of falling.

Executive dysfunction is compensated by providing meaningful activities for individuals who cannot initiate for themselves. Engaging the resident in meaningful activities throughout the course of Alzheimer's disease or any other type of progressive dementia is challenging. When this task is assigned just to the activity staff, the resident with dementia is often overlooked. Residents with dementia do not ask for something to do as the more alert resident will. As their dementia progresses they are increasingly difficult to be kept engaged during activities because of diminished executive skills as well as a short attention span. However, meaningful activities are especially important for them because they allow residents to continue feeling like a loved and valued person. An activity program that provides continuous programming throughout the majority of the residents waking hours is not only an effective way to reduce psychotropic medication, reduce falls, and social isolation, but it also helps residents live with some purpose and meaning in spite of the disease. An activity program that brings humor and fun to resident's lives is difficult to evaluate unless you count the laughter and smiles. Until the resident is in the terminal stage, laughter continues to be "the best medicine"!

Developing an activity program that features continuous programming takes the effort and support of the entire team in a long-term care facility. The administration must provide dedicated staff 7 days a week. The beneficial effects mentioned above, family satisfaction, and marketing edge over the competitors justify the cost of dedicated staff. Nursing support is key to the program's success. The activity professional needs someone else to stay with the residents during breaks, assist with serving beverages, and help if a resident needs personal care. As soon as the residents are left alone, they begin to leave the activity area. The rule for continuous programming is never to leave the room and the residents unattended.

The continuous programming for moderate dementia should begin after breakfast is served and residents are toileted and groomed. The activity professional prepares the room for the beginning of the day. Music is played in the background and the newspaper, puzzles, and pictures for reminiscence are placed on tables. The nursing assistants, housekeeper, or whoever sees the residents wandering or isolated in their room bring residents to the programming area. Coffee or another beverage is served as a welcoming way to begin the day. When the majority of residents are in the room, the programming begins. Residents with dementia seem to function better when a familiar routine begins their day. The Pledge of

Allegiance, patriotic song, newspaper, weather report are some examples of a morning routine that has been shown to be effective for residents with moderate dementia. Exercise programs are then scheduled as they reduce depression, lower the risk of falls, and increase bone density. The day incorporates beverages as people with dementia often forget to drink enough liquid. Snacks are served to increase weight for residents who have difficulty consuming enough calories. When food and beverages are served in a social atmosphere, residents tend to eat and drink more than at planned meals.

The day continues with a variety of programs designed to meet the needs of the residents. Some programs require physical activity such as games and walking. Others help to stimulate their minds like word games and spelling bees. All are no fail opportunities to have fun. Many residents in the moderate stage feel important and their self-esteem is enhanced by their "role" in the various programs. One resident may hold the flag while another reads a thought for the day. Another "assistant" helps to pass out songbooks and several men help move tables. The women become "hostesses" and some help other more impaired residents. At the end of the day, active participants are tired and ready for a video or movie, snack, and a peaceful sleep.

As residents' dementia progresses into the severe stage, it becomes more challenging to engage them in meaningful activities. They tend to sleep during programs and may have difficulty in communicating. Another level of programming, one that has more individual attention and has less physical activities, helps to meet their needs at this stage. Activity staff provides more touch, respects when the resident needs short "naps," and uses more visual cues. For instance, in the moderate stage the resident may be able to look outside and tell what the weather is for the day. In the severe stage, an umbrella may jog the memory that it is raining. Physical exercise may require the activity staff standing in front of the resident and modeling the movement, or assisting the resident to move their arms or legs. Fewer programs are scheduled but the activity professional is in the room with the residents so that when they are awake, they can be engaged. Music, old musicals, sensory stimulation, showing items from the past are some ways to engage residents in the severe stage of dementia.

Activity professionals have largely ignored residents in the terminal stage of dementia. They may provide individual visits several times a week or place them in a room where activities are taking place, but continuous programming for residents with terminal dementia is rare. However, the activities should be available even for individuals in the terminal stage because even these individuals have some contact with the environment (Volicer et al., 1997). Activities that could be done even in that stage include massage, pet therapy, and Snoezelen (Brown, 1999). It has been the responsibility of nursing to provide the majority of care, and in some facilities residents in the terminal stage are left in bed for the majority of day.

A new program, Namaste, which has recently been implemented in a long-term care facility, increased involvement of staff with residents, and staff and family satisfaction (Simard, 2005). Continuous programming begins right after breakfast as in the other two stages of dementia. The difference is the component of "being present" for the resident. This is an approach distinct from "leading" programs. When the resident is taken to the Namaste room, music is played and residents are placed in a comfortable chair. It may be a lounge chair or lying on a couch. Rehabilitation therapists are asked to evaluate the type of chair and positioning of residents. Comfort of the resident is a major goal of Namaste. Residents are not ambulatory in the terminal stage, so warm slipper socks replace shoes. Clothing is soft and nonbinding. Bras are not usually necessary and if they are needed for large breasted women, a sports bra is more comfortable.

The day begins with men receiving a shave, complete with warm towels, and scented shaving lotion. Just entering the room while someone is being shaved brings back warm memories of the past. Women have their faces washed and hair combed while the activity professional talks to them in soothing tones. Each resident receives a foot and leg massage and a range of motion exercises unless they show distress, then they are spoken to but not touched. An awareness of the day is evoked by soft stuffed birds making real bird sounds and by scents such as the scent of freshly cut grass and flowers in the summer and fir tree branches and cinnamon in the winter.

Beverages are served several times a day as well as puddings and high calorie snacks as some residents in the terminal stage have lost a considerable amount of weight. Nursing assistants help with nourishments and are often assisting activity staff with massages. When 10 to 15 residents are in the Namaste room, the staff has the time to assist activity staff or give bed baths to residents uncomfortable in a tub or shower. Videos of nature scenes are played several times during the day, and depending on the alertness of the resident individual conversation takes place. An "over the bed" table may be placed in viewing distance of the resident with pictures and items that relate to their past. Wives are asked to bring a perfume their husbands would remember. Perfume is sprayed on material and placed around the resident's neck.

Namaste means "to honor the spirit within." This program provides the person with terminal dementia the continuing presence of another person. Dame Cicely Sanders said "You matter to the last moment of life." Namaste and the concept of continuous programming, or in the terminal stage continuous presence, makes it clear that in long-term care a resident does matter until death occurs.

CONCLUSIONS

The SOC model is well suited to dementia care. Selection of appropriate strategies for management of medical issues is necessary for maintaining the quality of life of individuals with dementia. This selection should be based on the knowledge of burden and benefit of different treatment strategies, and on previous wishes of the individual with dementia or his/her best interest. It is important to make selection of treatment strategies as early as possible, before any crisis situation. Such a selection can be formalized into an "Advance Proxy Plan" that clarifies goals of care.

Optimization of care strategies is necessary to prevent or minimize behavioral symptoms of dementia. The care should be optimized according to the remaining functional abilities of the individual with dementia. Caregivers should realize that individuals with dementia do not understand the need for care and may resist it. Preventing escalation of resistiveness into combative behavior requires gentle approach or modification of care procedures.

Compensation is required in two areas: functional deficit and executive dysfunction. Habilitation strategies may be used to maintain remaining functions for as long as possible. Executive dysfunction results in inability to initiate meaningful activities and in the need to provide these activities for the individuals with dementia. Meaningful activities should be provided as continuous activity programming and adopted to the stage of dementia. By paying attention on the SOC model, it is possible to improve dementia care and maintain quality of life throughout the course of the disease.

REFERENCES

Brown, E. J. (1999). Snoezelen. In L. Volicer, & L. Bloom-Charette (Eds.), *Enhancing quality of life in advanced dementia* (pp. 168–185). Philadelphia: Taylor & Francis.

Fabiszewski, K. J., Volicer, B., & Volicer, L. (1990). Effect of antibiotic treatment on outcome of fevers in institutionalized Alzheimer patients. *Journal of the American Medical Association*, *263*, 3168–3172.

Finucane, T. E., Christmas, C., & Travis, K. (1999). Tube feeding in patients with advanced dementia: A review of the evidence. *Journal of the American Medical Association*, *282*, 1365–1370.

Fried, T. R., Gillick, M. R., & Lipsitz, L. A. (1997). Short-term functional outcomes of long-term care residents with pneumonia treated with and without hospital transfer. *JAGS, 45*, 302–306.

Gillick, M. R. (2000). Sounding board—Rethinking the role of tube feeding in patients with advanced dementia. *New England Journal of Medicine, 342*, 206–210.

Gillick, M., Berkman, S., & Cullen, L. (1999). A patient-centered approach to advance medical planning in the nursing home. *JAGS, 47*, 227–230.

Mitchell, S. L. (2003). Financial incentives for placing feeding tubes in nursing home residents with advanced dementia. *Journal of the American Geriatrics Society, 51*, 129–131.

Ouslander, J. G., Schnelle, J. F., Uman, G., Fingold, S., Nigam, J. G., Tuico, E., & Bates-Jensen, B. (1995). Predictors of successful prompted voiding among incontinent nursing home residents. *Journal of the American Medical Association, 273*, 1366–1370.

Simard, J. (2005). Namaste, giving life to the end of life. *Alzheimer Care Quarterly, 6*, 14–19.

Sloane, P. D., Rader, J., Barrick, A.-L., Hoffer, B., Dwyer, S., McKenzie, D., Lavelle, M., Buckwalter, K., Arrington, L., & Pruitt, T. (1995). Bathing person with dementia. *Gerontologist, 35*, 672–678.

Van der Steen, J. T., Ooms, M. E., Van der Wal, G., & Ribbe, M. W. (2002). Pneumonia: The demented patient's best friend? Discomfort after starting or withholding antibiotic treatment. *Journal of the American Geriatrics Society, 50*, 1681–1688.

Volicer, L., Berman, S. A., Cipolloni, P. B., & Mandell, A. (1997). Persistent vegetative state in Alzheimer disease—Does it exist? *Archives of Neurology, 54*, 1382–1384.

Volicer, L., & Bloom-Charette, L. (1999). *Enhancing the quality of life in advanced dementia*. Philadelphia: Taylor & Francis.

Volicer, L., Cantor, M. D., Derse, A. R., Edwards, D. M., Prudhomme, A. M., Gregory, D. C. R., Reagan, J. E., Tulsky, J. A., Fox, E., & Natl Ethics Comm Veterans Hlth Adm (2002). Advance care planning by proxy for residents of long-term care facilities who lack decision-making capacity. *Journal of the American Geriatrics Society, 50*, 761–767.

Warden, V., Hurley, A. C., & Volicer, L. (2003). Development and psychometric evaluation of the PAINAD (Pain Assessment in Advanced Dementia) Scale. *JAMDA, 4*, 9–15.

PART IV

Training

CHAPTER TEN

A Paradigm for Qualitative Research in Long-Term Care

Shannon L. Gould and Lee A. Hyer

Approximately 70 million Americans, or 20% of the US population, will be 65 years of age or older by the year 2030. This represents more than a 60% increase in the number of older adults, an age group that currently represents 12.4% of the US population (Administration on Aging, 2002).

The percentage of older adults that currently reside in a nursing home is estimated at 4.5%; however, this varies considerably with age group: only 1.1% of individuals ranging in age from 65 to 74 live in a nursing home, while 4.7% between the ages of 75 and 84, and 18.2% aged 85 and over live in a nursing home. Laditka (1998) estimated lifetime nursing home use to be 30.5% across the elderly population. In other words, approximately 3 out of 10 older adults will spend at least some portion of their lives in a nursing home. With the rapid growth of the older adult population, the number of older Americans in nursing homes is expected to double by the year 2030 (Siegel, 1996).

These statistics underscore the pressing need for research in long-term care. To that end, this chapter will present a paradigm for conducting qualitative research in long-term care. This paradigm was developed as part of the first author's doctoral dissertation, titled "Management of Challenging Behaviors Among Dementia Residents: A Case Study in Needs Assessment and Program Design" (Gould, Fishman, & Hyer, 2004). Although the focus of the dissertation research was challenging behaviors, the qualitative paradigm developed may be used for studying a variety of phenomena in long-term care and other settings.

BACKGROUND/RELEVANT CONTEXT

Approximately 2 years ago, the research team, which consisted of S. Gould, D. Fishman, and L. Hyer, was invited to attend an administrative/planning meeting at a medium-sized NJ nursing home (henceforth referred to as "The Home"). During this meeting, the administration at The Home relayed their concern regarding a trend that they had noticed, namely that the number of residents referred to external psychiatric facilities due to consistently unmanageable challenging behaviors had steadily increased over the past several years. This was troublesome to the administration, who reported that when these residents returned to The Home they were often "like zombies" due to being "overmedicated." Attempts to adjust/reduce these residents' medications often resulted in a return of the problematic behaviors.

The Home was in the process of expanding and considering the development of a behavioral special care unit (SCU) to accommodate the needs of these residents. Before proceeding with the development of such a unit, however, the administration wanted to evaluate the current nonpharmacological practices and procedures used to manage residents with challenging behaviors. In other words, they wanted to ascertain the "current state of behavior management" at The Home. Many questions came to mind as the team considered potential contributing factors to this trend. Were there changes in policies or procedures? Could staff turnover be a factor? Were employees receiving adequate training and supervision in behavior management techniques? Or, was this a function of a different "breed" of residents that were more difficult to manage? Answers to these questions would provide the administration with information that would inform their decision to develop a behavioral SCU.

After deciding to proceed with the project, IRB approval was obtained from both Rutgers University and University of Medicine and Dentistry of NJ and the study was initiated. Rather than focusing on the specific results of this study per se, this chapter will offer an in-depth analysis of the predominantly qualitative *process* used for assessing the "state of behavior management" at The Home. Embedded in the description of the process will be selected results, the research team's insights, and the reactions of research participants. This process will be divided into four manageable steps: entry, data collection, data analysis, and feedback (see Figure 10.1).

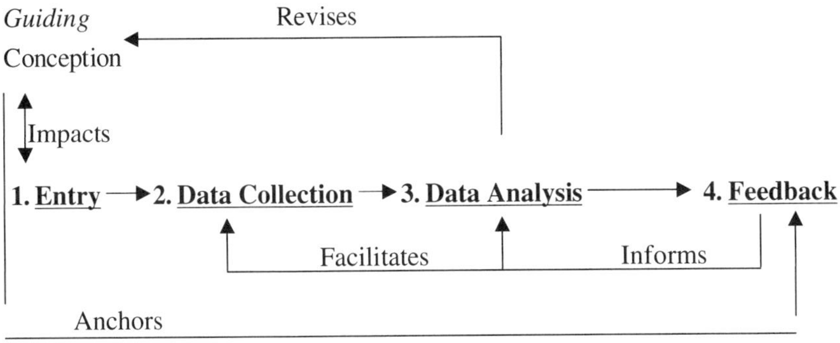

FIGURE 10.1 The four research phases with embedded feedback loops.

STEP ONE: ENTRY OR "LAYING THE FOUNDATION"

This phase of the research is without a doubt the *most* important. Without a solid foundation, the rest of the research project will be compromised. Therefore, this section will focus on the three key aspects of the *collaborative process* of "building" a solid foundation: development of an initial guiding conception, clarification of the research question(s), methods, and procedures, and adoption of the project by the administration.

Guiding Conception

After relevant research questions have been defined, the development of an initial guiding conception is the first step. Simply put, this is a framework that informs your entry and guides your research process. For example, in this study the research team took the broad approach that effective behavior management involves both individual and organizational factors, as well as their interaction. This conception (see Figure 10.2) was presented to the administration and they adopted, or believed in, this view. It is important to note that this conception is flexible and should be revised throughout the research process to accommodate new information. Therefore, your initial guiding conception may look quite different than your revised or expanded conception.

Clarification

Once a guiding conception has been developed and presented to the administration, the next step is clarification. This step allows for the

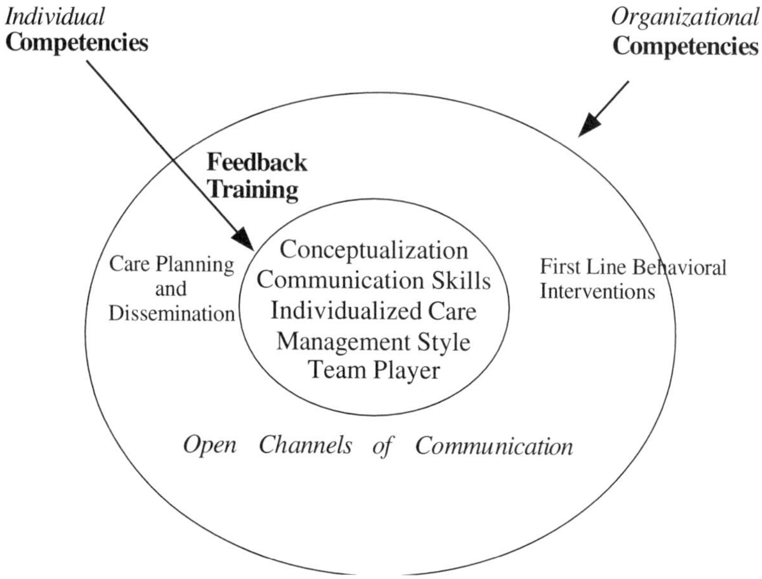

FIGURE 10.2 Guiding conception of the individual and organizational competencies of behavior management.

development of a shared understanding of the research process with the organization. Clear expectations are essential, regarding both what the administration expects of the research/consulting team and what the team expects of the research site. It is important for the administration to have a clear sense of what the final product will look like and what estimated steps are required to achieve this final product. Likewise, it is important to articulate to the administration the team's needs and the ways in which the administration can facilitate these needs.

The first level of clarification involves the research question(s). As seen in the case of our study, the initial question will often be quite broad, such as, "What is the current state of behavior management?" The clarification process allows an initial broad question to be transformed into several more targeted, mutually agreed-upon questions. This results in manageable research questions that can be answered within a specified period of time and which the administration views as reflective of their initial question.

The second level of clarification involves the methods and procedures utilized to answer the above, mutually agreed-upon research questions. Although at this point it is unnecessary to provide detailed specifics of how the data will be collected, a general overview of data collection methods and a timeline for their collection should be provided. Data collection should be broken down into phases, or distinct periods of time during which each data collection method will be utilized. In this study, individual interviews, focus groups, surveys, and observations were conducted, with each form of data collection conceptualized as a distinct phase of the study. The rationale for using these methods and the order of collection will be provided later in this chapter.

The third and final level of clarification involves the roles that the research team will play, in conjunction with the role that employees at the organization will play. This includes the logistical needs of the research, including procedures for recruiting and scheduling with research participants, the use of office space, recording equipment, etc. An important outcome of this step is a designated staff liaison, or an individual at the research site who is the direct contact. The staff liaison will play a critical role and it is important that he or she understands and accepts that role. For example, in this study the staff liaison was responsible for explaining the research project to participants, assisting in recruiting participants, insuring that adequate space was available, and troubleshooting if problems arose. In short, this individual plays a critical role in insuring the research runs smoothly.

Adoption

The result of a successful clarification process should be an organization that adopts the research project. This means, simply put, that they agree with the research team's view of the problem (guiding conception), believe in the methods that will be used to understand the problem, and are willing to make accommodations from a logistical standpoint to implement a successful study. If, on the other hand, any of these conditions are not met yet, it is imperative to continue "laying the foundation" until it is solid. Once a solid foundation has been established, data collection can be initiated.

STEP TWO: DATA COLLECTION

In this study, four phases of data collection were conducted over the course of 8 months: the first phase consisted of 21 semistructured individual interviews; the second phase consisted of five focus groups; the third phase consisted of surveys completed by 45 staff; and the fourth and final phase consisted of 20 hr of systematic observations of staff interactions with residents. Each phase of data collection will now be described in some detail.

Individual Interviews

During the first phase of this study, 21 semistructured individual interviews were conducted. Interviews were recorded and lasted for an average of 45 min. The primarily open-ended interview questions were developed in collaboration with the research team and The Home's administrative staff. In addition, the questions became more targeted after the first couple of interviews, when the most salient issues related to managing challenging behaviors became more relevant. Selected questions from the interview guide (see Table 10.1) are provided.

Recruitment for interviews was initiated by the staff liaison. Staff were approached by this individual, provided with a brief description of the research project, and asked if they would be interested in participating. They were informed that their participation was entirely optional and that their decision regarding participation would in no way impact their employment status. Interviews were scheduled by the staff liaison for times that were mutually convenient for the interviewee and interviewer. Every attempt was made to schedule interviews for times that were least disruptive to resident care and overall operations (e.g., no nurses were interviewed during care plan meetings and no CNAs were interviewed during AM or PM care). Individual interviews were conducted in private offices; participants provided informed consent. The investigator took detailed notes during each interview. After each interview, the audiotapes were reviewed to insure the accuracy of written information. Selected portions of the interviews were transcribed verbatim to highlight important themes.

An outcome of this phase of data collection was a compilation of staff-identified strengths and weaknesses in various domains. For example, in the domain of training, an identified strength was "many training programs are

TABLE 10.1 Sample Questions from the Interview Guide

1. What is your approach to working with challenging behaviors? How did you develop this approach (training, supervision, etc.)? If you were training someone, what would you emphasize?
2. Can you tell us about a success you had with the behavioral management of challenging behaviors?
3. Take a moment to remember the most behaviorally challenging resident you have worked with directly. Please describe the challenging behaviors you faced. What interventions did you try? What worked and what did not? In retrospect, would you have tried something different?
4. What else could be done at The Home to improve behavior management?
5. What is your assessment of The Home's strengths and weaknesses when it comes to behavior management?

offered on a variety of topics," while identified weaknesses were "poor attendance at trainings," "trainings may be too didactic," and "trainings not hands-on enough." In the domain of communication, identified strengths were "supervisors stay informed" and "interdisciplinary communication encouraged," although identified weaknesses were "important information may not trickle down to CNAs" and "CNAs not listened to." Other domains that were examined included staffing, resources, creativity, collaboration, atmosphere, and conceptualization of behaviors. By examining these various domains, an initial understanding of key organizational issues related to behavior management was developed. This understanding could then be applied to the next phase of data collection.

Focus Groups

During the second phase of the study, a total of 32 staff, representing all six departments at The Home, participated in one of five interdisciplinary focus groups. The focus groups lasted for an average of 75 min and each group followed the same format. Each group was presented with two fictional scenarios that described the challenging behaviors of two different residents, one of which had a dementia diagnosis and the other was cognitively intact. The groups were asked to discuss each scenario, answer a series of questions, and present their "care plans" to the facilitator. The scenarios and questions used in the focus groups were developed in a collaborative process between the dissertation committee and several employees at The Home.

Recruitment for the focus groups followed the same format as that of individual interviews. Three groups were conducted during the day shift and two groups during the evening shift to insure that a broad range of employees could participate. After participants consented, the first fictional scenario was presented and participants were informed that they could take notes if they desired.

The first scenario described a cognitively intact (alert, no dementia diagnosis) male resident. This resident had been at The Home for 6 months and had adjusted well during his first 4 months. During the past 2 months, however, the resident presented with several challenging behaviors that included refusal of both meals and groups, and verbal resistance to both AM and PM care. There was only one staff member for whom Mr Jones was cooperative, a CNA who would sing to him during AM and PM care. Although other staff members had tried singing to Mr Jones during care, he was not cooperative with them.

All groups were presented with the same scenario. After the scenario was presented, all groups were asked, "Is this a representative example

TABLE 10.2 Questions for Discussion (for Both Scenarios)

1. Is this a representative example of a scenario that could occur at The Home? If not, what elements could be altered to make it more realistic?
2. What are the target behaviors of concern?
3. Are there environmental factors that may be causing these behaviors?
4. Are there other factors that may be causing these behaviors?
5. What recommendations would you make for working with this resident? What questions might you ask him/her? What questions would you ask staff that have worked with this resident?
6. What would hinder your ability to provide care to this resident? What would enhance it?

of a scenario that could occur at The Home?" All groups agreed the scenario was realistic. Had any groups not agreed, the follow-up question would have been, "What elements could be altered to make it more realistic?" Groups were then provided with a list of questions to answer about the scenario (see Table 10.2). Larger groups (six or more) were divided into two smaller groups, while groups of five or less were not subdivided. Groups were instructed to work as a team to answer the questions and to act as if this were a "care plan meeting" and their job was to come up with a plan to work with the resident in the scenario. Groups were given approximately 15 min per scenario to work together to develop a care plan, during which time the facilitator observed the groups and took notes, both on ideas they were sharing and on the group members' behaviors. The groups then presented their ideas and the facilitator asked questions as needed to clarify group members' ideas. Group members frequently engaged in dialog about the scenarios.

After the participants presented their care plan for scenario 1, the second scenario was presented. The second scenario described Ms Smith, a female with Alzheimer's disease who resided at The Home for 4 years. Over the past 2 years, Ms Smith's ability to communicate had declined and she was no longer able to make requests for food or to be toileted. She becomes upset very easily and repeatedly asks for her husband, who passed away several years ago. She paces around The Home and often bangs her hand against the glass on the front door. As in scenario 1, group members agreed that scenario 2 represented a situation that could easily occur at The Home. Group members were then provided with a list of questions and instructed to work as a team to answer the questions. After about 15 min of discussion, participants shared their ideas and dialogued with each other and the facilitator.

After the second scenario was discussed, the group was asked several general questions about behavior management. These questions were intended to: (a) further assess what would enhance or hinder the implementation of the care plans developed by the groups; (b) obtain participants' reactions to participation in the group; and (c) provide participants with an opportunity to share additional thoughts, ideas, or concerns about behavior management. For example, participants were asked, "Given the plan of action that you described to me for managing the resident's behaviors, what would facilitate or hinder your ability to implement your plan?" A selected dialog between focus group participants, a recreation staff (REC) and a CNA, was as follows:

REC: You've got some people that think they know, excuse me, everything about the resident and they don't give you a chance to speak, and if you give them an idea or something to try they ignore you and sometimes you can walk up, you can explain to them something that you see, a change and everything, and if they didn't see it, am I right?

CNA: They ignore you.

REC: It's like—why do you bother?

CNA: We are the nurses aids—we have more contact with the patient—and if you tell a nurse about a behavior with a resident, most of the time she will ignore you, they don't want to listen; maybe it's because they have to write it down (referring to documentation in the resident's chart) that they don't want to do it.

REC: It's because they want to avoid the paperwork.

CNA: Somebody should listen to what we say because we know the patient.

REC: That's the point, I think again sometimes the administration, yeah actually, they do have a problem with that because if they say to nurses things like, punch out on time, they are going to be afraid of doing more paperwork. If you say, this nurse must punch out at 5 o'clock, it's like chasing the nurse, so the nurse can't be as flexible, she doesn't feel it's convenient to stay in the building after her stated time and that is another factor that, you know, that decreases the attention of the nurses to the behavior of the residents.

This section of the dialog reveals several themes. The participants in this focus group felt discouraged, ignored, and devalued. They wanted to share their knowledge about the residents but their attempts to do so were often ignored. This, in turn, decreased the likelihood that they would provide input in the future, as reflected in the statement, "It's like, why do you bother?" Simply stated, they were punished, rather than reinforced, for their attempts to provide input. These findings are consistent with studies that have found that at least one third of nursing assistants feel that their input is not valued and that they are not active participants in care planning (Curry, Porter, Michalski, & Gruman, 2000).

The focus groups served the role of expanding the research team's understanding of themes from the individual interviews. As seen above, highlighting selected portions of the dialog can be a powerful way of presenting relevant themes to the research site.

Surveys

Similar to the focus group scenarios, surveys were developed in a collaborative process with several staff at The Home, including two social workers, one recreation employee, and one administrator. The individual interviews and focus groups were reviewed and major themes were identified. These themes were then translated into survey questions. The survey consisted of a total of 36 questions, 25 of which were Likert-type responses, 4 that obtained background information, and 5 open-ended questions. The majority of Likert-type questions used the following scale: "never," "rarely," "sometimes," "often," or "always." The following dimensions were measured by the survey: demographic/employment information (five questions), frequency or exposure to challenging behaviors (two questions/one of which had multiple items), training in the management of challenging behaviors (six questions, two of which were open-ended), sense of belonging to a "team" (five questions), beliefs regarding challenging behaviors (three questions), confidence/skill in behavior management (three questions/one of which had multiple items), communication (six questions), recognition/feedback (four questions), ways to improve behavior management at The Home (one open-ended question), and obstacles to managing challenging behaviors (one open-ended question). In addition, the final question of the survey was open-ended and allowed for additional comments, recommendations, or questions.

A total of 47 surveys were completed, 45 of which were used in the final analysis (two surveys were discarded due to a significant number of omitted items). All participants provided informed consent. Surveys were completed in a conference room, with three to four staff seated around a large table. The researcher was present and answered participants' questions. Survey data was compiled and descriptive statistics were calculated. In addition, several one-way between-groups analyses of variance (ANOVAs) were calculated, using participants' department as the independent variable.

Rather than creating a "generic" behavior management survey that might have only provided general information, a customized survey was developed that targeted key areas of interest to this study. Alderfer and Brown (1972) found that a carefully designed questionnaire that relayed an understanding of several key organizational issues elicited more information that was threatening to the respondents than a questionnaire that was based on general topics. They found respondents were more likely to provide sensitive information with an "empathic" questionnaire compared to a more generic, theory-based one. At the time of survey distribution, the research team had been involved with The Home for nearly 6 months and had developed a sense of what some of the key issues were. This knowledge was reflected in both the content and context of the survey questions.

For example, one emergent theme was that direct care staff were not provided with feedback on their approach to working with challenging behaviors, nor were they recognized for their efforts. Two survey questions further explored these issues: "When I do a good job with a challenging resident, I receive recognition for my efforts," and "I have been provided with feedback regarding my ability to manage challenging behaviors." Each statement was rated using the Likert scale described above.

Overall, the survey information added to the findings of the individual interviews and focus groups, providing a quantitative perspective on several of the themes that emerged through these forms of data collection.

Observations

A total of 20 hr of observations were performed. Prior to the initiation of the observations, a total of 52 staff consented to being observed. These staff included CNAs, recreation employees, environmental services staff, nurses, administrators, and social workers. The majority of observations occurred on the Dementia Special Care Unit in the mid to late afternoon. This time was chosen due to the higher frequency of challenging behaviors reported at this point in the day. The unit was an ideal setting for the observations because of its relatively small size and the nature of its residents, all of which were diagnosed with a dementia and often had behavioral problems. The observation periods lasted for an average of 2 hr with a range of 1–3 hr. During most observation periods, there were one to two residents of focus. The researcher was positioned at a table in a common area with a clear view of the living room, kitchen, dining room, and outdoor patio. This way, multiple areas were scanned for instances of challenging behaviors.

During some observation periods, challenging behaviors were observed and the protocol was followed as planned. Immediately after the observation, the researcher approached the staff member who was most directly involved with the resident and followed the format described in the observation guide (see Table 10.3). At times, the participants were

TABLE 10.3 Guide for Observations

Procedures for observation
1. Identify staff to observe and obtain informed consent
2. Observe staff during their interactions with residents, particularly those residents who have a history of challenging behaviors
3. Record the following information: date, time, location, nature of the interaction (i.e., providing care, redirecting, engaging in activities), and length of interaction
4. Record the context and content of the interaction (i.e., describe what occurred, what was said, how it was said, etc.)
Postobservation questions (for staff)
5. During your interaction with the resident, what was (were) the behavior(s) of concern?
6. What were you attempting to do with the resident?
7. Is this the way that you would have typically handled this situation?
8. What about your approach increased your probability of success? Decreased it?
9. How would you rate the overall success of your approach, on a 1–10 scale, with 1 being completely unsuccessful and 10 being completely successful?

unable to speak immediately due to their responsibilities on the unit, in which case the interview was postponed until they were available. During a significant portion of the observation periods (approximately one-third) no challenging behaviors were observed. During these periods, the researcher made observations about what the residents and staff were doing that may have prevented challenging behaviors.

The observations added value to this study by "bringing to life" many of the themes that emerged from the interviews, focus groups, and surveys. For example, a common theme was that staff did not communicate with each other regarding optimal strategies for resident care. This theme was apparent in the following scenario: on a hot summer day, a resident was outside on the porch sitting quietly in her wheelchair. She appeared to be sweating. Without any notification, a staff member (staff A) came up behind the resident and began pushing her inside, which caused her to become quite irritated. She screamed out, "Leave me alone! I don't want to go inside!" Staff A encouraged her to "just come inside for a little while," explaining that it is very hot outside and that "you are sweating." The resident continued to resist going inside, both verbally (yelling) and physically (putting her feet down like brakes). Other residents who were outside took notice of this interaction and were distracted from the conversation that they had been having with another staff member, Staff B. The interaction between Staff A and this resident lasted for approximately 2 min before Staff B came over and intervened. Staff B approached the resident from the front and asked if she could take her for a walk, to which the resident responded favorably. She then took the resident and pushed her wheelchair around outside, talking with her in a calm voice. After about 2–3 min of walking with this resident, the resident agreed to come inside and cool off. Immediately after this interaction, the researcher was able to speak with Staff A. Staff A was visibly frustrated and explained that she was concerned that the resident was "overheating" outside and believed that she should come inside. She did not expect the resident to resist coming inside in the way that she did. She was surprised that the resident suddenly became cooperative after Staff B took her for a brief walk. When asked what she thought accounted for the resident's change, she replied, "I really don't know, sometimes that is just the way they are." When asked what she would do differently next time, she responded, "Take her for a walk. It would be much easier than pleading with her."

What was not observed after this interaction was any dialog between Staff A and Staff B about their different approaches to working with this resident. No one seemed to acknowledge Staff A's frustration or the difficulty that she had with the situation, and no one praised Staff B for the creativity in her approach. This example underscores the ability of observations to elucidate previous themes.

It is also important to note that by the time the observations were initiated, staff seemed to be comfortable with the primary researcher's presence and would go about their jobs without hesitation. On the other hand, if the primary researcher was a "stranger" from the outside, the staff who participated in the observations would have been less likely to work in their typical fashion. They may have adjusted their performance based on what they thought the research team was looking for. We believe that this relationship with The Home allowed for the minimization of the "Hawthorne Effect" (Roethlisberger & Dickson, 1939). In other words, staff were less likely to alter their typical behavior during the observation periods due to their familiarity and comfort with the research team.

STEP THREE: DATA ANALYSIS

This step can be the most exciting because it is an opportunity to make sense of the data. However, when faced with an abundance of qualitative data, data analysis can be an arduous and overwhelming task. Depending on the nature of the study, it may be necessary to transcribe all interviews and/or focus groups, which in and of itself is quite labor intensive.

Therefore, the following steps are proposed as a framework for data analysis: identification of cross-cutting themes, revision/expansion of the guiding conception, rating each domain of the guiding conception as a relative strength or weakness, and developing recommendations that target the key areas of weakness. In addition, to the greatest extent possible, data should be analyzed on an ongoing basis so that themes from each phase of data collection are elucidated and can be shared with the research site as applicable.

Identification of Cross-Cutting Themes

The identification of cross-cutting themes, or those that are consistent across multiple forms of data collection, is the first step in an integrated data analysis. This involves analyzing the themes identified from each phase of research for areas of convergence and divergence. This process may yield the following types of themes: (a) those that are cross-cutting, or consistent across two or more forms of data collection; (b) those that are supported by only one form of data collection; and, (c) those that are inconsistent. Cross-cutting themes can be presented with a reasonable degree of certainty, while themes that are supported by one type of data collection but not others should be presented as tentative. Themes that are inconsistent should be presented as inconclusive and areas for further research.

An example of a cross-cutting theme from this study was the existence of dysfunctional communication patterns between nurses and CNAs. After this theme was identified, a theory or theories was proposed to explain the etiology and maintenance of these communication patterns. This was achieved by using a psychological model or theory with adequate explanatory power as a framework for data analysis. For example, the cognitive model (Beck, 1995) was applied to this research to explain dysfunctional communication patterns between nurses and CNAs. The cognitive model states that distorted (or irrational) thinking is a common feature of all psychological disturbances. Although in this research the focus was not on psychological disturbances per se, the cognitive model remained applicable. Cognitive distortions such as minimizing, catastrophizing, overgeneralization, or emotional reasoning are common errors in thinking. These errors in thinking result in a less than accurate perception of the truth, yet the "thinkers" believe the thoughts are accurate ("If I think it, it must be true"). These irrational thought patterns negatively impact our relationships with others and the way we interact with our environment.

For example, the following findings were consistent across multiple forms of data collection: CNAs generally believed that their input was not valued, that no one wanted to hear what they had to say (especially not the nurses), and that they should serve a subordinate role. As a result, the CNAs often felt angry, frustrated, and/or discouraged, which influenced their interactions with nurses and other staff. CNAs typically kept to themselves and avoided opportunities for providing input, even though they frequently wanted to share their insights. At the same time, the nurses held an entirely different set of beliefs. They believed that the CNAs were disinterested in providing feedback and/or did not want to share what they knew. This resulted in frustration and anger on the part of the nurses, which in turn, made it less likely that they would solicit feedback from the CNAs. In both cases, the CNAs and nurses were overgeneralizing (cognitive distortion), or assuming that their beliefs were indicative of *all* nurses or *all* CNAs. Table 10.4 outlines a cognitive model for understanding these communication patterns between nurses and CNAs. This table shows how the thoughts/beliefs of the CNAs/nurses led to emotions, which then led to behaviors. It is important to note that these thoughts represented only perceptions of the truth, not the truth itself. In fact, most CNAs expressed a desire to provide input, although most nurses conveyed an openness and receptivity to hearing CNA input. Therefore, these thoughts were overgeneralizations that unnecessarily impaired communication between nurses and CNAs.

TABLE 10.4 A Cognitive Model for Understanding the Communication Patterns Between CNAs and Nurses

	Thoughts/beliefs	Emotions	Behaviors
CNAs	"My input is not valued"	Angry	Less likely to report behaviors
	"She won't believe what I have to say"		Avoid opportunities for providing input
	"I am not respected"	Sad	Detach from the "team"
	"What's the point in telling them what I see if they won't believe me"	Anxious	Avoid nurses Stay quiet
Nurses	"CNAs never speak their mind"	Frustrated	Less likely to solicit feedback from CNAs
	"They must not have anything to say"	Angry	Less likely to focus on CNAs during care plan meetings
	"They don't want to tell us what they see"		More likely to dominate
	"I feel like I'm pulling teeth"	Overwhelmed	meetings/discussions

As seen in Table 10.4, a psychological model was applied to the data to explain a cross-cutting theme. The model chosen should be accessible to the target audience, so that they can readily see the context in which the data is being interpreted. The cognitive model was chosen because it meets the above criteria and can be used to adequately explain a variety of phenomena.

Revision/Expansion of the Guiding Conception

Revision or expansion of the guiding conception is an ongoing process rather than a distinct step in data analysis. As previously discussed, the initial guiding conception should be viewed as a series of modifiable hypotheses about the research topic. The findings will serve the role of supporting, modifying, or disconfirming the initial hypotheses. In this study, the initial hypotheses involved the key individual and organizational elements of effective behavior management. These elements were developed through a review of the behavior management literature. The data then served the role of revising the guiding conception, i.e., customizing this conception for the research site.

Assessment of Strengths and Weaknesses

Each element of the revised, or customized, guiding conception can be examined and rated as a relative strength or relative weakness. This will provide the research site with a clear picture of areas that are in need of improvement, as well as areas that are generally sound. An example of a relative strength, conceptualization of challenging behaviors, and a relative weakness, teamwork, will be discussed.

Conceptualization

The vast majority of staff at The Home contextualized the residents' challenging behaviors. Rather than seeing residents as deliberately behaving in challenging ways, staff viewed their behaviors as part of a disease process. Behaviors that would typically be personalized in the "real world" were contextualized at The Home. This allowed staff to maintain a professional objectivity in their work with residents. For example, staff spoke about "being called names" or "derogatory comments" that the residents would make on occasion. Other staff spoke about certain residents' tendency to "play favorites," or be more cooperative with the requests of some staff over others. In these instances, staff described these behaviors as normative and attributed them to a disease process. Participants would say things such as, "It's the dementia," or "He has

Alzheimer's," clearly attributing the challenging behaviors to the resident's illness.

This ability to contextualize challenging behaviors is a crucial competency of behavior management. In general, studies have shown that staff who are able to do this on a consistent basis report more job satisfaction/enjoyment, increased confidence, and less frustration than staff who personalize challenging behaviors (Roper, Shapira, & Beck, 2001). The fact that the majority of staff contextualized resident behaviors was a clear strength at The Home.

Teamwork

A lack of teamwork was commonly cited as an obstacle to behavior management at The Home. For example, a CNA who was employed at The Home for more than 10 years shared her thoughts on the changing nature of "teamwork": "When I started as a CNA we would have 12–14 residents but it wasn't a problem because we worked as a team, three and three, we helped out each other—that's a problem even now, staff don't help each other." Another participant agreed, "They don't, that's a problem right there because teamwork, it has gone away because everyone feels they've got to do their own job and get it done." Many participants echoed this sentiment, noting that more of an emphasis should be placed on a team approach to care. At the same time, however, the vast majority of staff reported on the surveys a sense of "belonging" to a team and agreed that there was someone who they could turn to if they were in need. This begs the question: if most participants felt this way, then why was the need for more teamwork consistent across this study?

One possibility is that the communication barriers between departments (see Table 10.4) limit the ability of staff to feel unified with each other. Although staff may feel like they are part of a team, they may find it difficult to communicate their needs to other team members, particularly those who work in a different department. Furthermore, although they have someone they can turn to if they need help, this may be viewed as only appropriate in an emergency (for extreme behaviors). They may not utilize their team members in situations which are considered "less severe," but in which the help of another staff would make their job easier. Multiple staff at The Home, including social workers, recreation employees, and CNAs, expressed the belief that they were "underutilized" by other staff. In other words, these staff felt that there were situations in which they could have provided valuable assistance, but were not asked for their help or input. As communication is an essential element of teamwork, it stands to reason that enhancing communication may enhance teamwork. With improved teamwork at The Home, staff may feel that they are more adequately utilized in their work with challenging behaviors. This is an area that could be further explored at The Home in a follow-up study.

As seen above, each element of the revised guiding conception should be identified as a relative strength or weakness and discussed. If appropriate, direct quotes from participants that support your conclusions should be included. When presenting this analysis to the target audience, care should be taken to insure that they understand the concept of a *relative* strength or *relative* weakness. A simple way to frame this would be to say, "Relative to teamwork, conceptualization is a strength," or "Relative to conceptualization, teamwork is a weakness." The target audience should understand that if an area is a relative strength, it doesn't mean that the area is "perfect" or that nothing can be done to enhance that area. Likewise, a relative weakness does not confer that the area is awful or that drastic steps must be taken to improve the area. Often, simple changes will be highly effective at enhancing an area of relative weakness.

Development of Recommendations

The development of recommendations should serve the role of improving areas of relative weakness and maintaining or enhancing areas of relative strength. As seen in Figure 10.1, your recommendations should always be anchored to your revised guiding conception. Each recommendation should be presented in plain language and accompanied by a rationale for its implementation. For example, a sample recommendation for improving the areas of communication and care planning/dissemination, two areas of relative weakness, is presented below.

Adapt the Current Format of Care Plan Meetings So That More Staff Are Encouraged to Provide Input

In the first 5 min of a care plan meeting (or at some point beforehand), each participating staff should write down the key points that they would like to address in the meeting. All staff who cannot attend the meeting but who work in a meaningful way with the resident being discussed should be encouraged and provided with the opportunity to submit information/recommendations/suggestions regarding the resident of concern. In addition, the facilitator of each care plan meeting (Director of Nursing, Charge Nurse, or Social Worker) should elicit additional feedback from all staff before the end of each care plan meeting.

RATIONALE

In examining factors associated with staff turnover rates, Banaszak-Holl and Hines (1996) found that participation in care planning significantly lowered the turnover rates of CNAs. Their sample consisted of 250 nursing homes from 10 different states. Turnover rates were 30% lower in homes where nurses informally discussed the care plan with CNAs and were receptive to their advice or suggestions. Turnover rates were 50% lower in homes where CNAs were active participants in care plan meetings, which only occurred in 36% of the sample. The authors concluded that the added recognition associated with being an active participant in care plan meetings decreases that likelihood of CNA turnover.

Several staff at The Home, in particular the CNAs, reported the desire to provide input about a resident during care plan meeting but often felt unable to do so due to the current format of the meetings. Participants spoke about care plan meetings being "dominated by one discipline" and subsequently lacking collaboration between departments. Other CNAs spoke about a desire to attend care plan meetings but lacking the time to do so due to work demands. In addition, several participants felt as though nurses were not receptive to their input/suggestions.

This proposed adaptation provides CNAs and others with an alternative for providing input about the residents, regardless of whether they are present for the care plan meeting. However, it is ideal for these staff to be in attendance at the meeting whenever possible. These practices should promote increased interaction between the disciplines, an area for improvement identified by several staff at The Home.

In addition to individual recommendations such as the one above, "Principles of Behavior Management in Long-Term Care," were developed through the research The Home and a review of literature on behavior management in long-term care. These "principles" were conceptualized as elements of effective behavior management that, when combined, represented a comprehensive "package" of individual behavior management competencies. These principles are practical suggestions for enhancing or maintaining the individual competencies of behavioral management. Examples of principles included, "Know your residents," "Develop an understanding of challenging behaviors," "Use proper 'protocol' when interacting with residents," "Use a team approach to care," and "Be persistent and creative." Each of these principles was accompanied by adequate description and case examples, when applicable. In addition, a rationale that justified inclusion as a principle was provided, with references made to the literature when possible.

Recommendations and principles should be presented at the final feedback session (see below), but should be modifiable based on the feedback from the target audience. Any modifications should be submitted in a final report.

STEP FOUR: FEEDBACK AND RECOMMENDATIONS

Although this is labeled step four, the provision of feedback is a *two-way* continuous process that should occur throughout the research. As indicated in Figure 10.1, feedback facilitates data collection and informs data analysis. In this study, feedback from participants was essential in the modification of the individual interview guide, the creation of relevant scenarios for the focus groups, the development of an "empathic" survey, and determining the best way to perform the observations. Likewise, feedback was critical in "checking out" findings after each phase of data collection, understanding the broader context of cross-cutting themes, and the development of recommendations that were accepted by the target audience.

To insure that feedback can be provided at defined intervals throughout the research, data should be analyzed in a continuous fashion. It is important to keep in mind, however, that data from any one form of data collection is only part of the story. It is also important to relay this point when providing feedback and to frame your initial findings as tentative. Inform the target audience that the integrated feedback, to be provided after all data is collected and analyzed, will have conclusions that are grounded in more comprehensive data. Feedback sessions held after each phase of data collection should focus on the findings from that phase of data collection only; findings from any one phase of data collection should be framed as tentative, as they are only one part of the complete "picture."

The sequencing of the data collection, coupled with this continuous feedback process, allowed the primary research to gradually gain a "presence" within The Home. In this study, conducting the individual interviews was an opportunity to begin to build collaborative relationships with 21 of The Home's employees. By subsequently providing The Home with feedback regarding the preliminary findings from these interviews, the primary researcher was introduced to many other employees. Therefore, by the time the focus groups were initiated, most of the participants in these groups knew about the project and were comfortable with the primary researcher. A few participants relayed their trust and noted that this is the reason they were comfortable speaking candidly in the groups. If the primary researcher had attempted to conduct the focus groups without having been established as a "trustworthy" member of the organization, it is highly unlikely that the same degree of sensitive information would have been obtained.

In addition, the focus groups were a salient reminder that a needs assessment is often an organizational intervention, whether intentional or not. Specifically, we found that conducting the focus groups provided staff with an effective means for expressing themselves and sharing experiences. In fact, many participants approached the primary researcher after the groups, expressing their satisfaction and suggesting that these groups should be available to all staff on an ongoing basis. This led to the development of one of the recommendations—the implementation of a regular interdisciplinary behavior management group in which staff can discuss their ideas and experiences in working with challenging behaviors.

Again, providing The Home with feedback after the focus groups was another opportunity to reach out to staff members and reinforce our role in the organization. In addition, each feedback session served as a transition and set the stage for the next phase of data collection. By the time survey data was to be collected, the majority of participants knew the researcher. Many had participated in an individual interview or focus group, and some had participated in both. These individuals had a good understanding of the research and seemed to enjoy being part of it.

After collecting, compiling, and analyzing the survey data, feedback was provided via a power point presentation that represented data from all departments. Of the 20 or so attendees at the feedback, several asked questions about the results and expressed interest in knowing more about individual departments responses to the questions (at the time, the data was aggregated across all departments). It was clear that many staff were engaged in this research process and interested in understanding the findings and their implications for The Home. The goal from the beginning was to make this research as much of a two-way street as possible, and the collaborative tone of the feedback provided some clear evidence that this was the case.

The final feedback session was an integrated session that considered all forms of data collection, complete with overall conclusions and recommendations. The final session was attended by The Home's administration and lasted for approximately 2 hr. The overall consulting project was reviewed and cross-cutting themes were presented and discussed. In addition, "Principles of Behavior Management" that emerged from the data collection were reviewed. These "principles" represented what staff as a whole believed to be the key elements of behavior management. Finally, a series of recommendations were presented, both for improving current behavior management and for the development of a specialized unit, a project that The Home may undertake in the near future.

The continuous feedback provided to the research site kept the administration and other staff informed of emergent themes. It gave them a sense of where the research team was at with the research, what they could expect (logistically) with the next phase of data collection, and allowed them an opportunity to express questions or concerns. Equally important, it allowed the team to broaden their presence within the organization and reach out to staff who did not participate in the data collection. This process also seemed to sustain the administration's interest in the consultation and ultimately increased their ownership of the findings and recommendations.

This brings up a critical point: the research site's ownership (or valuing) of all aspects of the research is of critical importance. As discussed in step one (entry), the research site must value (or believe in) the guiding conception, the research questions, and the methods by which these questions will be explored. If this occurs, the likelihood that the administration will take ownership in the findings and any recommendations that emerge from these findings is significantly increased. Furthermore, recommendations that are valued are much more likely to be implemented than those that are not. Quite possibly, the best way to keep the ownership high is the implementation of a continuous feedback loop.

SUMMARY

This chapter outlined a four-step process for conducting qualitative research in long-term care (see Figure 10.1). The first step, entry, begins with the development of an initial guiding conception that reflects the research team's understanding of the phenomenon being studied. The next part of entry involves clarification of the research questions, methodology, and roles of the research team and the organization. This step is "complete" when the research site and the research team successfully negotiate these areas, resulting in adoption of the project. At the same time, however, entry is an ongoing process in that the research questions, methodology, and roles of participants may be modified over time.

The second step, data collection, should be conducted in distinct phases and special attention should be given to the sequencing of these phases. In this study, the data collection was deliberately conducted in the following order: individual interviews, focus groups, surveys, and observations. This sequencing, in conjunction with a feedback loop, allowed the research team to maximize the quality of the data collected.

Data analysis is the third step and consists of the following steps: identification of cross-cutting themes, revision/expansion of the guiding conception, assessment of the domains of the guiding conception as relative strengths or weaknesses, and the development of recommendations. Recommendations can serve the role of maintaining or enhancing areas of relative strength and improving areas of relative weakness. Each recommendation should be presented with a rationale for its implementation and should be modifiable based on feedback obtained in the integrated feedback session.

The fourth and final step, feedback, is a continuous process like entry rather than a distinct step. Feedback informs data analysis and facilitates data collection. Perhaps equally as important as entry, feedback keeps the target audience involved in the research and increases their ownership in all aspects of the project.

This four-step process represents what we believe to be an optimal approach for conducting qualitative research in long-term care. As the world's population continues to age, the demand for research in nursing homes will only increase. Qualitative research provides a unique perspective on the dynamics of behavior management in long-term care. As in this study, this perspective can be used to develop "road-tested" principles of behavior management that can be integrated in the future into an orientation package and/or an ongoing staff development curriculum. The rich descriptive data offered through qualitative research provides a window into the lives of nursing home employees and organizational currents in which these employees "swim." This perspective on the nursing home environment is valuable when considering ways for improving current practices or the development of specialized services (e.g., a behavioral unit). Qualitative research can be effectively used as a "stand alone" research paradigm in nursing homes, or it can be used in collaboration with quantitative research to enhance our understanding of statistical results. Finally, qualitative research makes it possible to study phenomena, such as staff interactions, communication and teamwork, that are not easily distilled into quantitative terms.

REFERENCES

Administration on Aging. (2002). *A profile of older Americans: 2002*. Washington, DC: Administration on Aging, United States Department of Health and Human Services.

Alderfer, C. P., & Brown, D. L. (1972). Designing an "empathic questionnaire" for organizational research. *Journal of Applied Psychology, 56*(6), 456–460.

Banaszak-Holl, J., & Hines, M. A. (1996). Factors associated with nursing home staff turnover. *The Gerontologist, 36*, 512–517.

Beck, J. S. (1995). *Cognitive therapy: Basics and beyond*. New York: Guilford Press.

Curry, L., Porter, M., Michalski, M., & Gruman, C. (2000). Individualized care: Perceptions of certified nurse's aides. *Journal of Gerontological Nursing, 26*(7), 45–51.

Gould, S. L., Fishman, D. B., & Hyer, L. A. (2004). Management of challenging behaviors among dementia residents: A case study in needs assessment and program design. Unpublished doctoral dissertation, Rutgers University, Piscataway, New Jersey.

Laditka, S. B. (1998). Modeling lifetime nursing home use under assumptions of better health. *Journal of Gerontology: Social Sciences, 53B*(4), S177–S187.

Roethlisberger, F. J., & Dickson, W. J. (1939). *Management and the worker.* Cambridge, MA: Harvard University Press.

Roper, J. M., Shapira, J., & Beck, A. (2001). Nurse caregiver feelings about agitation in Alzheimer's disease. *Journal of Gerontological Nursing, 27*(11), 32–29.

Siegel, J. (1996). *Aging into the 21st century* (HHS Publication No. 100-95-0017). Washington, DC: Administration on Aging, United States Department of Health and Human Services.

CHAPTER ELEVEN

Meeting the Needs of Nursing Home Residents and Staff

The Informed Teams Model of Staff Development

Alan B. Stevens and Angela K. Hochhalter

Staff training is one strategy for improving the care and quality of life of nursing home residents. Staff training provides staff members with knowledge and skills to identify and address the unmet needs of residents. Staff training interventions, however, seldom result in meaningful changes in staff behavior or skill use after the designated training period. Staff members can learn skills that will improve care, but they are not likely to continue to use those skills after training (Burgio & Stevens, 1998; Schnelle, Ouslander, Osterweil, & Blumenthol, 1993).

Characteristics of the nursing home work culture strongly contribute to staff performance and to the sustainability of new skills after initial training. Nursing home culture is affected by staffing levels and staff turnover, management and supervisory practices, opportunities for professional growth, incentives and recognition, regulatory demands, and the interprofessional and interpersonal relationships among staff members (Berlowitz et al., 2003; CMS, 2001; Shortell et al., 1995). Therefore, both the content of staff training and the culture into which new knowledge and skills are introduced are critical determinants of the impact that a staff development program has on staff behavior and resident care.

Staff training is an essential component in the development of a skilled and motivated nursing staff capable of identifying and meeting the needs of nursing home residents. The purpose of this chapter is to present a general model of staff development called *Informed Teams*. In the Informed Teams model, staff development supplements training with structured adoption of skills into routine use. According to the model, staff development programs should also address the unmet needs of staff members. Before introducing the model, we will briefly describe the need for staff development activities that address staff and resident needs in terms of Lawton's and Nahemow's (1973) theory of competence and environmental press. We will also touch on nursing home training research as a background for the Informed Teams model of staff development. The majority of our discussion is dedicated to a description of the Informed Teams model and to one example of its application in nursing homes.

COMPETENCE AND ENVIRONMENTAL PRESS IN NURSING HOMES

Lawton's and Nahemow's (1973; Lawton, 1982) theory of competence and environmental press is useful for understanding the characteristics of nursing home staff members and residents because the theory casts behavior and affective responses as dynamic functions of individuals' personal resources in the context of their environment. Changes in either competence or press produce changes in behavior and affect. Maladaptive behavior and negative affect result when either one's competence exceeds the demands of the environment or when the press of the environment exceeds one's competence. Although the theory describes older adults' adaptive behavior, it is also applicable to nursing home staff members in the context of the nursing home work environment.

Lawton (1982) defined environmental press as all stimuli associated with a behavior. A reasonable goal for nursing home staff development programs is to improve staff and resident outcomes by creating an environment that is manageably challenging for staff members and residents. For example, development of skills for delivering constructive feedback may ease the conflicts with supervisees that a licensed practical nurse (LPN) regularly encounters. Fewer conflicts may ease an LPN's stress and improve her ability to encourage and support the nursing assistants (CNAs) she supervises. Development of skills for time and stress management may improve a CNA's ability to complete her assigned tasks for the day and to accommodate residents' preferences and choices.

The Competence and Environment of Residents

Nursing home residents experience compromised competence. In addition to physical limitations, many experience psychiatric symptoms like depressed mood, agitation, and anxiety (Lopez et al., 2003). The 1999 National Center for Health Statistics National Nursing Home Survey (Jones 2002) found that nearly 75% of nursing home residents received help with three or more activities of daily living (ADLs). Over 26% of residents had a primary diagnosis classified as a mental disorder (including "senile dementia") or a disease of the nervous system and sense organs (including Alzheimer's disease). Still, all residents maintain some competencies, which include preserved health and abilities, preferences, and often the capacity for some degree of rehabilitation. Identification of those remaining competencies may require careful assessment. For example, communication problems like those associated with naming objects (i.e., anomia) sometimes make it appear that residents remember less than they actually know (Ford et al., 2001).

Residents' environments are complex. For example, their environments include the physical characteristics of the building, proximity of other residents (e.g., private or shared rooms), relative competencies of other residents, frequency and quality of involvement from family and friends, staffing ratios, nursing home policies and missions, nursing home work culture, and state and federal regulations that govern facility operations. There is quantitative and qualitative evidence that environment affects resident functioning and affect, including residents' quality of life (Kane et al., 2004). For example, residents spend more time in bed in facilities with low staffing than in those with high staffing. Residents who spend more time in bed also show lower social engagement and lower food/fluid intake, and spend more time asleep during the day than those who spend less time in bed (Bates-Jensen, Schnelle, Alessi, Al-Samarrai, & Levy-Storms, 2004).

Residents' needs can develop when the pressure induced by the nursing home environment far exceeds their competence. For people with dementia, pressure that exceeds competence can lead to what Algase et al. (1996) labeled *need-driven dementia compromised behaviors* (need-driven behaviors). Examples of need-driven behaviors include agitation, aggression, and repetitive questions. Lower cognitive and psychological (e.g., depression) competence are associated with the presence of need-driven behaviors (Beck et al., 1998). Need-driven behaviors can be adaptive for residents. For example, a resident confined to bed does not have the physical competence to navigate the environment well enough to engage in needed social interaction. Yelling repeatedly from the bed until a staff member comes to investigate can meet the resulting need for social interaction. In this example, yelling is adaptive in that it draws in another person and probably some conversation. The quality and quantity of interaction that results when a nursing home resident yells repeatedly for a staff member is probably not the ideal type of social interaction, but it is social interaction nonetheless.

Lawton and Nahemow (1973) argued that people who are less competent are vulnerable because their behavior is more heavily influenced by environmental forces than by personal forces like cognitive style. It follows that the nursing home environment is especially important for residents because of their reduced competence. Although this vulnerability can put residents at risk, it also means that small changes in the nursing home environment can have meaningful positive effects on residents. The nursing staff holds the most potential for bringing about important, small changes in residents' environments because they have regular direct contact with residents.

The Competence and Environment of the Nursing Staff

Staff members simultaneously contribute to and are influenced by the nursing home environment. The nursing staff in particular constitutes a large part of a resident's interpersonal environment and serves as a mediator between the resident and the physical environment. Staff members help residents navigate hallways, find recreational and private space, influence the level of noise and lighting, and insure that physical aids like wheelchairs are available in working order. Because CNAs usually have more contact with residents than other staff members, they will be the focus of our discussion on staff members.

CNAs possess an array of competencies. Most are young (<45 years). Nearly half are high school graduates, and an additional more than 25% have some college or a college degree (Yamada, 2002). We include their desire to help others, intimate knowledge of residents, skills for providing care, understanding of relevant regulations, and ability to plan a busy schedule of care routines among their cognitive competencies. Their expressed desire for additional training is also a competence (CMS, 2001; Scott-Caweizell et al., 2004; Walker, Porter, Gruman, & Michalski, 1999). However, even the most competent CNAs experience environmental press that may be overwhelming.

In general, the nursing home is a complex environment with few incentives to perform well. Between 1997 and 1999 nursing home aides earned a mean of $7.45 an hour (median = $7.00) and nearly 30% lived at or near the poverty level (Yamada, 2002). CNAs report feeling underappreciated and poorly supervised. Often the culture of their work environment is one in which too few people are available to provide the quality of care that they would like to provide (CMS, 2001; Deutschman, 2004). Very high turnover among staff members in all nursing home positions means that supervisors and coworkers come and go regularly (AHCA, 2002).

When CNA competences and environmental press are not well balanced in a nursing home, quality of care, staff performance, and workforce stability are threatened. For example, high work stress among CNAs is associated with reduced resident quality of life (Pekkarinen, Sinervo, Perala, & Elovainio, 2004). According to CNA reports, the most important influences on staff retention and satisfaction are the degree to which the nursing home values individuals, manages staff members as people with individual skills, and provides adequate supervision and a caring and supportive social system (Riggs & Rantz, 2001).

Research on Staff Development for Dementia Care

Resident and staff sensitivity to pressure from the nursing home environment requires a staff development program that acknowledges the complex interplay between the personal competencies of residents and staff and their environments. Staff training programs improve staff knowledge, skills, and behavior directly. They are one method of changing residents' environment to better match residents' competences. Although studies have tested the effects of staff training in a variety of care areas, we focus here on training to improve dementia care.

Research on training interventions to improve nursing home dementia care has usually focused on CNA training. Training traditionally includes basic information on dementia, communication skills, and recommended behavior management techniques for use with people who have cognitive impairment. Empirical findings show that skills are best learned when didactic sessions are followed by hands-on demonstration of the skills presented during those sessions (Beck et al., 1997; Burgio et al., 2001; McCallion, Toseland, Lacey, & Banks, 1999).

There is evidence that skills training can increase staff members' knowledge (Gilbert & McMahon, 2004; Martin, Rozon, McDowell, Cetinski, & Kemp, 2004), but changes in knowledge and skill use after staff training dissipate over time if steps are not taken to maintain and continue to develop new competencies (Burgio & Stevens, 1998). For example, McCallion, Toseland, Lacey, & Banks (1999) provided staff training on communication skills for use with residents who have dementia coupled with consultation-type monthly follow-ups. Resident depression and agitation improved after training. Staff members were more knowledgeable about strategies for managing problem behaviors 3 months after training, but the increase in knowledge did not persist 3 months after follow-up consultations ceased.

There are several reasons for the temporary effects of training in the typical nursing home work environment and culture. For example, if staff turnover remains high, new members of the care team may not have the skills learned in previous training. If supervisors do not encourage and expect continued skill use and do not provide the feedback necessary for skills to continue to develop, skill use will end. In some cases, the culture of the work environment discourages use of new skills by placing more emphasis on task completion than on quality of care.

Enduring improvements in skill use and in the quality of interactions with residents by CNAs are possible when skills training is accompanied by supervisory skills training for registered nurses (RNs) and LPNs who oversee care delivery (Boettcher, Kemeny, DeShon, & Stevens, 2004; Burgio et al., 2002; Hansebo & Kihlgren, 2001, 2004). Burgio et al. (2002) found that CNAs' knowledge of behavior management skills increased after 5 hr (three sessions) of training on the topic. In addition to paper-and-pencil knowledge, the same CNAs decreased their use of ineffective behavior management strategies and increased their use of several skills for communicating with residents with dementia. The improved knowledge and use of effective behavior management and communication skills were maintained for at least 3 months. When staff training was coupled with a management system that incorporated supervision and feedback about skill use into the routine of the nursing staff, the frequency of some skill use continued to increase over time (Burgio et al., 2002). Similarly, Boettcher et al. (2004) taught CNAs skills for delivering person-centered care and taught nurses to build mentoring relationships with CNAs through observation and feedback, and goal setting and problem solving. The combined training resulted in dramatic increases in skill use by CNAs. Increases in skill use were evident 2 months post-training.

Although evaluations of staff development interventions show promise for making lasting change in staff skill use and resident outcomes, we note that nursing home research takes place in facilities where leaders of the organization express support for quality improvement. By agreeing to take part in research on staff development, participating nursing homes show an interest in quality improvement on an organizational level. Even the best nursing home staff development efforts will not be put into practice if quality improvement is not a priority at the corporate or organizational level (Beaudin & Beaty, 2004;

Beck, Ortigara, Mercer, & Shue, 1999; Yeatts, Cready, Ray, DeWitt, & Queen, 2004).

The Informed Teams Model of Staff Development

We have developed a conceptual model of staff development entitled *Informed Teams* to aid in the design of successful staff development interventions. Informed Teams is a generic model that applies to a variety of health care settings. The model organizes principles that promote learning, use and continued development of new skills, and a supportive work environment into two core staff development components—skills training to improve the competence of people who deliver care and a system for structured adoption through initial implementation and long-term maintenance of skills. In nursing homes, the Informed Teams model calls skills training to improve staff competence and for culture-modifying supervisory support to balance staff competence and environmental press. Effective communication, incentives, and feedback systems enhance supervisory support, which makes up the structured adoption component of the Informed Teams model.

The Team Functioning model, developed by Strasser and Falconer (1997), influenced the Informed Teams model. The Team Functioning model describes variables that mediate outcomes for rehabilitation patients. Similar to nursing home staff members, rehabilitation health care professionals collaborate to provide in-patient therapeutic care. The Team Functioning model suggests that organization, treatment, and participant characteristics contribute significantly to the daily interactions and service delivered by team members (i.e., the team's functioning). According to Strasser and Falconer (1997), both relations and actions of the team influence the effectiveness of the team's functioning. Team relations include the social climate of the work environment and interprofessional interactions of team members. Team actions represent the mechanisms by which supervisors build relationships with and among staff members, and demonstrate consideration of staff accomplishments. Concrete team actions that facilitate the overall team process are effective communication, coordination, and group problem solving, which are all skills that have been successfully taught to nursing home staffs (Burgio & Stevens, 1998).

Similarities exist between care delivery in acute care rehabilitation settings and in nursing homes. In nursing homes, the staff plans, coordinates, and delivers daily resident care. Each resident's needs are unique, and quality care planning and actualization require input and actions by team members from several disciplines and in several positions.

The Informed Teams model relies on two major assumptions. First, similar to the Strasser and Falconer (1997) model of Team Functioning,

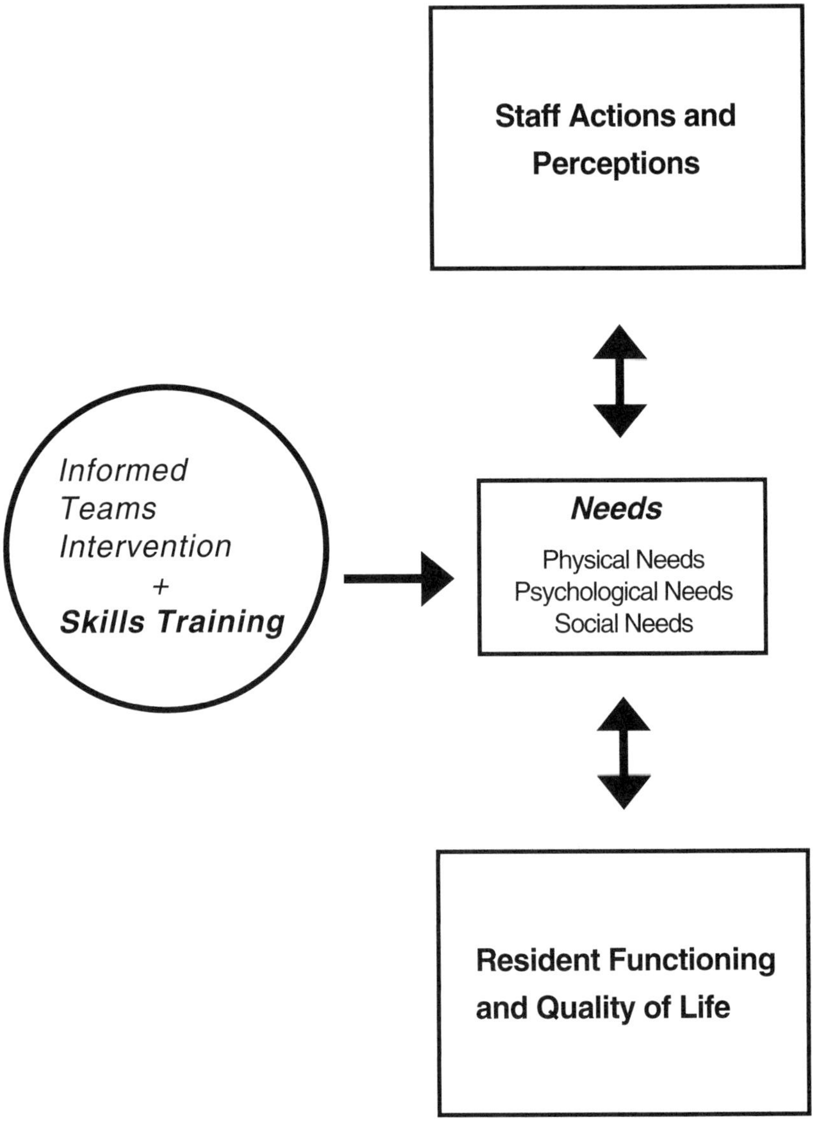

FIGURE 11.1 Role of Informed Teams interventions in changing the behavior and affect of staff members and residents.

the Informed Teams model assumes that the relations and actions of staff members as well as the overall organizational culture of the nursing home influence staff and resident outcomes. Figure 11.1 provides a schematic representation of how staff development interventions that follow the Informed Teams model of training and structured adoption bring about changes in the adaptive behavior and affective responses of health care providers and patients or residents. Two explanations are important for understanding this schematic. First, *needs* represent an imbalance between competence and environmental press, which results in behavior and affective responses that are not ideal (Lawton, 1982). We assume that staff members and residents make up an important part of the environment of everyone who works or lives at the nursing home. Needs of both staff members and residents must therefore be addressed by all nursing home interventions.

Second, the model does not account for the degree of organizational support for an intervention and does not include a component to convince the organization that staff development is important. Instead, active organizational support is a prerequisite. The Informed Teams model of staff development is not appropriate for application in an organization that does not value and actively support staff development or quality improvement.

We offer several specific suggestions for delivering interventions based on the Informed Teams model, which is based on our experiences and the experience of others conducting similar research (see Table 11.1; Boettcher et al., 2004; Burgio et al., 2002; Stevens et al., 1998).

1. Training is mandatory and time is allotted for new skill to develop. Enforcement of mandatory attendance policies is an indicator of an organization's commitment to a staff development program. If a nursing home administrator and director of nursing are not willing or able to require staff participation in training, then the organization is probably not ready for change.

TABLE 11.1 Informed Teams Staff Development Delivery Guidelines

Skills training	Structured adoption
• Mandatory training	• Supervisory and team-building skills training
• Multiple short interactive workshops	• One-on-one instruction and feedback for everyone
• Emphasis on respect and the importance of all roles and people	• Tools to guide skills use and active supervision
	• Incentives, praise, and encouragement for actions taken

2. Skill acquisition is not likely with didactic sessions alone. A combination of short interactive in-services, exercises, and on-the-job training is more likely to be effective than any of the three alone.
3. Effective teaching in a staff development program uses activities that demonstrate respect for staff members in all positions and for the designated duties of each position. Nursing home leaders and trainers must model respect for all staff members.
4. Supervisors in nursing homes require separate training on how to be a good supervisor. RNs and LPNs rarely have experience or training as a supervisor, and often feel unprepared to serve as a manager/supervisor (CMS, 2001). Although these skills come naturally to some, one should not assume that all supervisors have the skills needed to fill that role.
5. Incentives motivate staff members to try new skills initially. Continued motivation requires that staff members find new skills useful and that the culture of the work environment supports skill use with constructive feedback and recognition.

Working as Informed Teams: A Nursing Home Staff Development Project

Need-driven behaviors (Algase et al., 1996) are common among nursing home residents with dementia. Residents who have impairments in everyday functioning and communication behave in ways that may be adaptive in their environment, but their adaptive behaviors can create strain for the nursing staff. For example, CNAs are at risk if a resident physically resists care by hitting or pinching. In addition to pharmacological treatments, behavioral symptoms of dementia can and should be addressed with nonpharmacological interventions delivered in part by trained nursing home staff (Allen-Burge, Stevens, & Burgio, 1999; American Geriatric Society, 2003). The purpose of the WAIT Project (Working As Informed Teams) is to improve management of need-driven behaviors in nursing homes. The project applies the Informed Teams model of staff development to the issue of behavior management in nursing homes.

The goals of the WAIT Project are (a) to increase staff member use of care skills known to reduce need-driven behaviors, (b) to increase communication about the most effective care strategies for individual residents across shifts and levels of the nursing staff, and (c) to implement a system for continued skill use and development. If these goals are met, we hypothesize that resident need-driven behaviors will be reduced, that staff member variables like perceived effectiveness and job-related

TABLE 11.2 Components of the WAIT Project Classified in the Informed Teams Model

Behavioral skills training	Structured adoption
• In-services for RNs, LPNs, and RNs	**Initial implementation** • Key chain reminders and external reminders in rooms • Incentives for carrying key chains • One-on-one training for CNAs on behavioral care strategy use • Assistance from project consultant • Completion of Behavior Plans and introduction of plans on nursing units
• Workshops on writing Behavior Plans for the Care Plan Team and RNs	**Long-term maintenance** • Supervisory skills training for RNs and LPNs • One-on-one training for supervisors • Daily unit meetings • Skill-building sessions • Lottery drawings • Appointment of a facility coordinator to maintain the program

Jones, A. (2002). The National Nursing Home Survey: 1999 summary. In National Center for Health Statistics (Ed.), *Vital Health Statistics,* (Vol. 13(152)).

stress will improve, and that organizational factors like quality indicators and staff retention will improve.

Training for members of the direct care staff (CNAs, LPNs, and RNs) is the focus of the WAIT Project. As prescribed by the Informed Teams model, behavioral skills training is supplemented by a system for initial adoption and implementation of new skills and by a system for maintaining the use and continued development of those skills (see Table 11.2).

Behavioral Care Training

Eight behavioral care strategies form the foundation of the WAIT intervention. Every member of the nursing staff learns the eight strategies, which become the common "language" of behavior management at the facility. Examples of the strategies include giving instructions in small single steps and changing the level of stimulation in a room so that the environment is not too dull or busy for a resident. All CNAs, LPNs, and RNs attend two mandatory in-services on how to use the behavioral care strategies to reduce need-driven behaviors.

In addition to in-service training on the eight behavioral care strategies, the care plan team attends two 2-hr workshops on the construction of behavior plans. Behavior plans are documents that list appropriate behavioral care strategies and give specific ideas for customizing those strategies to meet the needs of each resident. Creation of each Behavior Plan requires input from the care plan team and from CNAs. The care plan team gathers CNA input through short structured interviews that the team learns to conduct during training. The behavior plans are dynamic documents that the care plan team updates as new ideas for successful behavior management emerge and as the need-driven behaviors change. Behavior plans are accessible to all CNAs, LPNs, and RNs.

Structured Adoption: Initial Implementation

Staff members who attend behavioral care training sessions will not necessarily use their new skills and knowledge. The WAIT Project therefore employs a structured system to insure adoption of the behavioral care strategies after training and timely completion and introduction of behavior plans to the nursing units. To generate a "buzz" about the new behavior management program, the nursing staff receives key chains with a short description and examples of each behavioral care strategy. Signs that are age appropriate and do not label residents are placed discretely in resident rooms to remind CNAs and LPNs of the behavioral care strategies that are most likely to be effective for each resident.

A project consultant (project staff member) is instrumental in the initial implementation portion of the WAIT Project. The consultant works closely with the care plan team, providing feedback and ideas for the behavior plans as needed. The project consultant, along with the care plan team, introduces the behavior plans to each RN, LPN, and CNA. In addition, all CNAs participate in two one-on-one training sessions with the project consultant on the nursing unit during usual resident care. One-on-one training includes review of the behavior plans and external cues, observation of a care routine, and feedback on the use of the behavioral care strategies listed in the behavior plans. The project consultant also periodically provides small rewards for the staff members who carry their reminder key chains on the unit.

Structured Adoption: Long-Term Maintenance

The key chains, small rewards, and regular presence of a project consultant generate excitement about the WAIT Project behavior plans and encourage initial use of the eight behavioral care strategies. Long-term use of the behavioral care strategies and behavior plans requires facility-wide changes, which are the focus of the structured maintenance portion of the intervention. The three major components of long-term maintenance are supervisory workshop and one-on-one training for LPNs, RNs, and the care plan team; three maintenance tools that are incorporated into the regular nursing unit routines; and a facility-maintained incentive system.

Supervision of the care provided by CNAs is necessary to promote the continued use of the behavioral care strategies by staff members who receive training and by new staff members. LPNs or RNs usually supervise the CNAs on each nursing home unit. All LPNs, RNs, and the care plan team attend two 2-hr workshops on supervisory skills training as part of the WAIT Project. The supervisors learn skills for effective communication, leadership, observation of supervisees, and the provision of constructive feedback. The workshops also introduce three tools for supervision of behavioral care strategy use. LPNs and RNs practice using the tools in one-on-one training with the project consultant.

One maintenance tool is a daily unit meeting about need-driven behaviors. Daily unit meetings are led by LPNs and are guided by a single-page agenda that calls for review of an existing Behavior Plan and group problem solving to address new or changing need-driven behaviors. Daily unit meetings last from 5 to 10 min. They are the primary source of suggested revisions to behavior plans or requests for new plans as new behaviors develop on the unit. Daily unit meetings are a formal opportunity for CNAs to provide input on resident care.

The other two maintenance tools are biweekly skill-building sessions for CNAs and for LPNs. The CNA sessions call for each CNA to meet with an LPN supervisor. The LPN observes delivery of care for a resident, provides feedback on care based on the resident's Behavior Plan, and works with the CNA to problem-solve as necessary and set goals for skill development. The LPN skill-building sessions call for each LPN to meet with an RN supervisor. The RN observes the leadership provided by the LPN during a daily unit meeting, provides feedback on the LPN's performance, and works with the LPN to coordinate needed changes in the behavior plans and to set goals for continued leadership skills development. Skill-building sessions last approximately 15 min each.

A lottery-style drawing run by the facility serves as the incentive system that promotes participation in daily unit meetings and skill-building sessions. CNAs and LPNs earn drawing entries by attending daily unit meetings and completing skill-building sessions. A facility-appointed coordinator maintains supplies of meeting agendas, drawing entries, and tracking sheets to mark completion of meetings and skill-building sessions. The coordinator also secures prizes, conducts the biweekly drawings, announces winners, and distributes prizes. With the appointment of a facility coordinator, the maintenance system for continued use of behavioral care strategies and behavior plans is handed over to the facility. The project consultant provides support initially to the facility coordinator, but the maintenance system is eventually run by the facility independent of project staff.

CONCLUDING REMARKS

Nursing home staff members are willing and able to demonstrate improved knowledge and skill use with training that may translate to improved quality of care for residents. However, the positive effects of training do not persist if the nursing home as an organization does not support improvements in quality of care and they do not persist without efforts to implement, maintain, and continue to develop new knowledge and skills. The Informed Teams model of staff development can guide the design of staff development interventions for nursing homes and other health care settings. The WAIT Project is an example of how the Informed Teams model can target a specific issue like need-driven behaviors in the nursing home.

REFERENCES

American Health Care Association. (2002). Results of the 2001 AHCA nursing position vacancy and turnover survey [Electronic Version]. Retrieved February 7, 2002 from www.ahca.org.

Algase, D. L., Beck, C., Kolanowski, A., Whall, A., Berent, S., Richards, K., & Beattie, E. (1996). Need driven dementia-compromised behavior: An alternative view of disruptive behavior. *American Journal of Alzheimer's Disease, 11*(6), 10–18.

Allen-Burge, R., Stevens, A. B., & Burgio, L. D. (1999). Effective behavioral interventions for decreasing dementia-related challenging behavior in nursing homes. *International Journal of Geriatric Psychiatry, 14*, 213–232.

American Geriatrics Society. (2003). Consensus Statement on Improving the Quality of Mental Health Care in U.S. Nursing Homes: Management of Depression and Behavioral Symptoms Associated with Dementia. *Journal of the American Geriatrics Society, 51*(9), 1287–1298.

Bates-Jensen, B. M., Schnelle, J. F., Alessi, C. A., Al-Samarrai, N. R., & Levy-Storms, L. L. (2004). The effects of staffing on in-bed times of nursing home residents. *Journal of the American Geriatrics Society, 52*, 931–938.

Beaudin, C. L., & Beaty, J. (2004). Strategies and innovations for successful quality improvement in behavioral health. *Nursing Care Quality, 19*(3), 197–208.

Beck, C., Frank, L., Chumbler, N. R., O'Sullivan, P., Vogelpohl, T. S., Rasin, J., Walls, R., & Baldwin, B. (1998). Correlates of disruptive behavior in severely cognitively impaired nursing home residents. *Gerontologist, 38*(2), 189–198.

Beck, C., Heacock, P., Mercer, S., Walls, R. C., Rapp, C. G., & Vogelpohl, T. S. (1997). Improving dressing behavior in cognitively impaired nursing home residents. *Nursing Research, 46*(3), 126–132.

Beck, C., Ortigara, A., Mercer, S., & Shue, V. (1999). Enabling and empowering certified nursing assistants for quality dementia care. *International Journal of Geriatric Psychiatry, 14*, 197–212.

Berlowitz, D. R., Young, G. J., Hickey, E. C., Saliba, D., Mittman, B. S., Czarnowski, E., Simon, B., Anderson, J. J., Ash, A. S., Rubenstein, L. V., & Moskowitz, M. A. (2003). Quality improvement implementation in the nursing home. *Health Services Research, 38*(1), 65–83.

Boettcher, I. F., Kemeny, B., DeShon, R. P., & Stevens, A. (2004). A system to develop staff behaviors for person-centered care. *Alzheimer's Care Quarterly, 5*(3), 188–196.

Burgio, L., Corcoran, M., Lichstein, K. L., Nichols, L., Czaja, S. J., Gallagher-Thompson, D., Bourgeois, M., Stevens, A., Ory, M., & Schulz, R. (2001). Judging outcomes in psychosocial interventions for dementia caregivers: The problem of treatment implementation. *The Gerontologist, 41*(4), 481–489.

Burgio, L. D., & Stevens, A. B. (1998). Behavioral interventions and motivational systems in the nursing home. In R. Schulz, G. Maddox & M. P. Lawton (Eds.), *Annual Review of Gerontology & Geriatrics* (Vol. 18, pp. 284–320). New York: Springer Publishing.

Burgio, L. D., Stevens, A. B., Burgio, K. L., Roth, D. L., Paul, P., & Gerstle, J. (2002). Teaching and maintaining behavior management skills in the nursing home. *Gerontologist, 42*, 487–496.

CMS. (2001). Report to Congress: Appropriateness of minimum nurse staffing ratios in nursing homes phase II final report. www.cms.hhs.gov/medicaid/reports/rp1201home.asp: Centers for Medicare & Medicaid Services.

Deutschman, M. (2004). What staff are saying: A firsthand report. *Nursing Homes: Long Term Care Management, 53*(10), 59–63.

Ford, J., Askari, N., Gabrieli, J., Mathalon, D., Tinklenberg, J., Menon, V., & Yesavage, J. (2001). Event-related brain potential evidence of spared knowledge in Alzheimer's disease. *Psychology & Aging, 16*(1), 161–176.

Gilbert, M. E., & McMahon, J. K. (2004). Nursing oriented in-services: Providing meaningful education to direct nursing care providers. *Journal of Gerontological Nursing, 30*(3), 54–56.

Hansebo, G., & Kihlgren, M. (2001). Carers' reflections about their video-recorded interactions with patients suffering from severe dementia. *Journal of Clinical Nursing, 10*, 737–747.

Hansebo, G., & Kihlgren, M. (2004). Nursing home care: Changes after supervision. *Journal of Advanced Nursing, 45*(3), 269–279.

Jones, A. (2002). The National Nursing Home Survey: 1999 summary. In National Center for Health Statistics (Ed.), *Vital Health Statistics,* (Vol. 13(152)).

Kane, R. L., Bershadsky, B., Kane, R. A., Degenholtz, H., Liu, J., Giles, K., & Kling, K. C. (2004). Using resident reports of quality of life to distinguish among nursing homes. *The Gerontologist, 44*(5), 624–632.

Lawton, M. (1982). Competence, environmental press, and the adaptation of older people. In P. G. Windley, & T. O. Byerts (Eds.), *Aging and the environment.* New York: Springer Publishing Co.

Lawton, M. P., & Nahemow, L. (1973). Ecology and the aging process. In C. Eisdorfer, & M. P. Lawton (Eds.), *Psychology of adult development and aging* (pp. 619–674). Washington: American Psychological Association.

Lopez, O. L., Becker, J. T., Sweet, R. A., Klunk, W., Kaufer, D. I., Saxton, J., Habeych, M., & DeKosky, S. T. (2003). Psychiatric symptoms vary with the severity of dementia in probable Alzheimer's disease. *Journal of Neuropsychiatry and Clinical Neuroscience, 15*(3), 346–353.

Martin, L. S., Rozon, L., McDowell, S., Cetinski, G., & Kemp, K. (2004). Evaluation of a training program for long-term care staff on bathing techniques for persons with dementia. *Alzheimer's Care Quarterly, 5*(3), 217–229.

McCallion, P., Toseland, R. W., Lacey, D., & Banks, S. (1999). Educating nursing assistants to communicate more effectively with nursing home residents with dementia. *Gerontologist, 39*, 546–558.

Pekkarinen, L., Sinervo, T., Perala, M., & Elovainio, M. (2004). Work stressors and the quality of life in long-term care units. *Gerontologist, 44*(5), 633–643.

Riggs, C. J., & Rantz, M. (2001). A model of staff support to improve retention in long-term care. *Nursing Administration Quarterly, 25*(2), 43–54.

Schnelle, J. F., Ouslander, J. G., Osterweil, D., & Blumenthol, S. (1993). Total quality management: Administrative and clinical applications in nursing homes. *Journal of American Geriatrics Society, 41*, 1259–1266.

Scott-Caweizell, J., Schenkman, M., Moore, L., Vojir, C., Connolly, R. P., Pratt, M., & Palmer, L. (2004). Exploring nursing home staff's perceptions of communication and leadership to facilitate quality improvement. *Journal of Nursing Care Quarterly, 19*(3), 242–252.

Shortell, S. M., O'Brien, J. L., Carman, J. M., Foster, R. W., Hughes, E. F. X., Boerstler, H., & O'Connor, E. J. (1995). Assessing the impact of continuous quality improvement/Total quality management: Concept versus implementation. *Health Services Research, 30*(2), 377–401.

Stevens, A., Burgio, L., Bailey, E. H., Burgio, K. L., Paul, P., Capilouto, E., Nicovich, P., & Hale, G. (1998). Teaching and maintaining behavior management skills with nursing assistants in a nursing home. *The Gerontologist, 38*(3), 379–384.

Strasser, D. C., & Falconer, J. A. (1997). Linking treatment to outcomes through teams: Building a conceptual model of rehabilitation effectiveness. *Topics in Stroke Rehabilitation, 4*(1), 15–27.

Walker, L., Porter, M., Gruman, C., & Michalski, M. (1999). Developing individualized care in nursing homes. *Journal of Gerontological Nursing, 25*(3), 30–35.

Yamada, Y. (2002). Profile of home care aides, nursing home aides, and hospital aides: Historical changes and data recommendations. *Gerontologist, 42*(2), 199–206.

Yeatts, D. E., Cready, C., Ray, B., DeWitt, A., & Queen, C. (2004). Self-managed work teams in nursing homes: Implementing and empowering nurse aide teams. *Gerontologist, 44*(2), 256–261.

PART V

Interventions

CHAPTER TWELVE

Cognitive-Behavioral Therapy for Long-Term Care Patients with Dementia

A. Lynn Snow, David Powers, and Debra Liles

The need for mental health services in nursing homes is enormous. About 80% of nursing home residents have diagnosable psychiatric disorders (Rovner, German, Broadhead, & Morriss, 1990). At least 19% suffer from mood and anxiety disorders (Sahyoun, Pratt, Lentzner, Dey, & Robinson, 2001). The next most prevalent disorders are psychosis, substance abuse, and behavioral disturbances (Reichman et al., 1998). Given that approximately 50% of nursing home residents suffer from dementia, the successful approach to mental health treatment in the nursing home environment must be adaptable to the unique needs of persons with dementia. In this chapter we will present cognitive-behavioral therapy (CBT) as such an approach. We will begin by presenting the basic tenets of CBT. We will then discuss the elements necessary for successful therapy with persons with dementia, as informed by review of the research evidence about different therapy approaches for persons with dementia. The bulk of this chapter will then be devoted to presenting an empirically informed SOC-based approach to modifying CBT for use with persons with dementia.

CBT BASIC TENETS

The CBT basic conceptual model is illustrated in Figure 12.1 (Thompson, Gallagher-Thompson, & Dick, 1995). Thoughts, behaviors, and emotions have strong reciprocal effects. Change in any one of these domains can result in change in the other domains. The target of therapy as conceptualized by the patient can be any of these domains, although generally patients tend to present their difficulties as problems within the emotional domain. Facilitating changes in behaviors and/or cognitions is posited to be the most effective way to bring about changes in emotions. The change targets in the cognition domain are unhelpful thoughts (sometimes referred to as dysfunctional or irrational thoughts), several major categories of which have been identified for ease in teaching the concept to patients. Many of these ideas are "automatic," occurring too quickly to notice. The goals in therapy would be to help the patient identify these thoughts, understand why they are unhelpful, learn how to be more aware of these thoughts, and learn how to modify these thoughts. The change targets in the behavior domain are maladaptive/dysfunctional behaviors. As with unhelpful thoughts, these behaviors

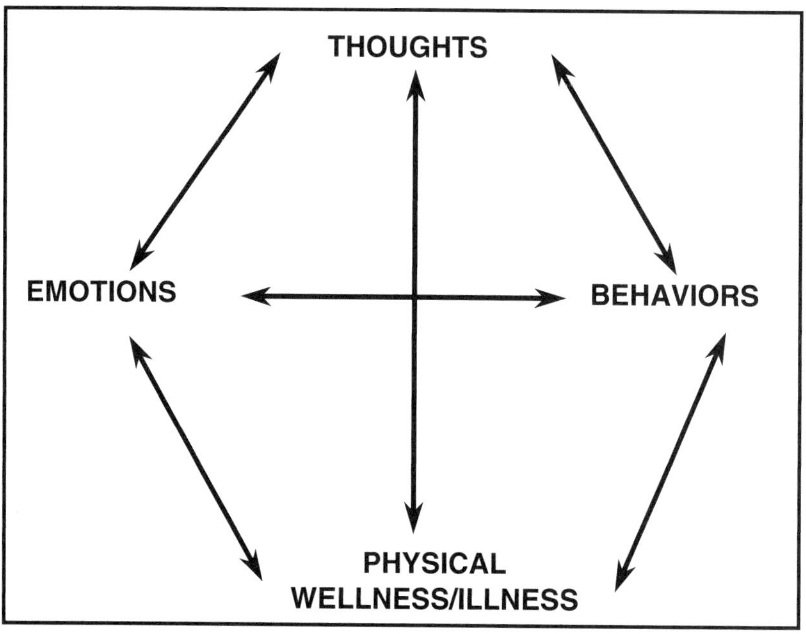

FIGURE 12.1 CBT basic conceptual model.

may not be fully in awareness. An action step in therapy would be to help the patient identify these behaviors and replace them with incompatible adaptive behaviors (e.g., planning pleasant events, introducing pleasant reinforcers, changing maladaptive interpersonal behavior). For example, a patient with depression may react to feelings of decreased energy by staying at home, refusing social invitations, and failing to exercise. An action step in therapy would be to help the patient understand how these behaviors contribute to and sustain depressed feelings, and develop a plan to become more active and seek social support. In sum, in CBT unhelpful thoughts and maladpative behaviors are conceptualized as responsible for causing and sustaining emotional disturbances, and thus changing thoughts and/or behaviors will lead to changes in emotions.

A second important tenet of the CBT approach is its foundation on empirical data. The severity and frequency of the presenting problems are quantified and recorded both at the beginning of therapy and throughout therapy. Hypotheses are developed about what cognitions and/or behaviors are causing/sustaining the problem, and a plan for changing those cognitions/behaviors is developed and implemented. Assessment data (which might include mood scales, thought logs, and activity logs) are examined to see if the expected effect is achieved; hypotheses and action plans will be modified as needed until the therapy goals are reached.

The third important tenet of the CBT approach is that work outside of the session is critical. The patient must take responsibility both for implementing action plans between sessions and for recording assessment data. The patient is in charge of his or her therapy and the therapist is the facilitator. Thus, the patient is taught the CBT conceptual model at the very first session, the patient sets the goals of therapy (with help from the therapist), and the therapist emphasizes the patient's responsibilities for accomplishing work outside the session.

WHAT IS DEMENTIA?

The Diagnostic and Statistical Manual of Psychiatric Disorders, fourth edition, defines dementia as a syndrome of acquired persistent compromise of mental function that includes: (a) memory impairment and at least one of the following cognitive disturbances: aphasia, apraxia, agnosia, disturbance of executive functioning (i.e., higher order cognitive processes such as abstract thinking and planning); (b) is sufficiently severe to interfere with social or occupational functioning; and (c) must not occur exclusively during delirium (American Psychiatric Association, 1994).

Alzheimer's disease is the most common type of dementia, followed by Lewy body dementia (26%), vascular dementia (18%), hippocampal sclerosis (13%), and frontotemporal dementia (5%) (Barker et al., 2002). Approximately 35% of persons with Parkinson's disease develop a dementia unique to that disease (MacKenzie, 2002). Rarer types of dementia include AIDS dementia, Huntington's disease, and Creutzfeldt–Jakob disease (MacKenzie, 2002). For the purposes of this chapter, we will discuss the presentation that is common for a person with Alzheimer's dementia. However, the approach discussed is applicable to other dementias as well; once a thorough assessment is completed so that the particular neuropsychological and functioning profile of the person is understood.

WHY CBT FOR PERSONS WITH DEMENTIA

A wide variety of psychosocial therapies have been investigated in persons with dementia, as detailed in several recent literature reviews (Cheston, 1998; Finnema, Droes, Ribbe, & van Tilburg, 2000; Gatz et al., 1998; Kasl-Godley & Gatz, 2000; Snowden, Sato, & Roy-Byrne, 2003). We recommend CBT over other therapy approaches for use with persons with dementia for a variety of theory-based and evidence-based reasons. First, the CBT conceptual model, based on the principles of learning, and its resulting combination of cognitive and behavioral techniques is particularly useful for persons with dementia because it easily accommodates cognitive disability and allows the therapist the flexibility to address the range of presenting problems common in dementia, from those that are more common in persons with mild dementia to those that tend to only affect persons with severe dementia. This is an advantage over other approaches, such as reminiscence therapy, support groups, and psychodynamic therapy whose strategies are dependent on at least partially intact language and executive function abilities.

The challenges faced by persons with mild dementia, as reported by persons with mild dementia in several qualitative studies, include working to accept the illness, grieving loss of abilities, adapting life to present abilities, loss of self-esteem, increased dependency on others, and increased tension in relationships due to strain of effects of the disease on caregivers and/or finances (Kasl-Godley & Gatz, 2000; Reichman et al., 1998). Such themes, which could not be adequately addressed by other approaches that are appropriate for more severely demented individuals (e.g., validation therapy, activities therapies, reality orientation, environmental manipulations) are well addressed in CBT by identifying unhelpful behavior or cognitive patterns that are contributing to the symptoms, and replacing them with incompatible helpful thoughts and behaviors. On the other end of the continuum, behavioral problems such as agitation and wandering are common in moderate-to-severe dementia (Teri et al., 1992). Other approaches that are appropriate for mildly demented individuals (e.g., reminiscence, support groups) require too much language and executive functioning ability for persons with moderate-to-severe dementia, yet behavioral approaches have been shown to be quite effective (Allen-Burge, Stevens, & Burgio, 1999; Fisher & Carstensen, 1990).

Further, there is a strong evidence base for CBT. One review using American Psychological Association criteria for empirically validated treatments concluded that CBT was a well-established treatment for depression in young and older adults, another review concluded it was probably efficacious for depression in older adults, and a third asserted that it was efficacious for depressive disorders in a wide variety of older adult patients (Chambless et al., 1996; Gatz et al., 1998; Laidlaw, Thompson, Dick-Siskin, & Gallagher-Thompson, 2003). Grant and Casey (1995) reviewed the literature on the use of CBT with older adults and concluded that CBT is an effective treatment for depression and other affective disorders of the frail elderly. More recently, there are randomized controlled trials in older adults showing positive effects of CBT for treating anxiety (Stanley et al., 2003; Wetherell, Gatz, & Craske, 2003), sleep disorders (Rybarczyk, Lopez, Benson, Alsten, & Stepanski, 2002), and promoting behavior change (Schneider, Mercer, Herning, Smith, & Prysak, 2004).

Unfortunately, there are no clinical trials of CBT in persons with dementia. However, there are four lines of evidence that converge to make a compelling case for the effectiveness of CBT in this population. First, there are positive case reports of success using CBT in persons with dementia (Koder, 1998; Teri & Gallagher-Thompson, 1991). Second, there is evidence that CBT is effective in other cognitively impaired populations. In addition to numerous case reports (e.g., Beail, 2003; Lindsay, Howells, & Pitcaithly, 1993; Romana, 2003), there have been two controlled trials of CBT for anger management in persons with mental retardation (both reported positive effects), two controlled trials of problem-solving therapy for problem behaviors in persons with mental retardation (one reported positive effects; (Beail, 2003)), and an uncontrolled trial of problem-solving therapy for sex offenders with mental retardation (positive effects were reported; (Nezu, Nezu, & Arean, 1991; Nezu, Nezu, & Dudek, 1998). Case reports have been published demonstrating positive effects of CBT in persons with traumatic brain injuries for insomnia (Ouellet & Morin, 2004) and problem-solving ability and social functioning (Suzman, Morris, Morris, & Milan, 1997), and a controlled study reported positive effects of a CBT intervention for acute stress disorder immediately following a mild traumatic brain injury (Bryant, Moulds, Guthrie, & Nixon, 2003). A randomized controlled trial of a CBT intervention in cognitively impaired patients with multiple sclerosis reported positive effects on social functioning (Benedict et al., 2000). Finally, a controlled study of problem-solving therapy for older persons with major depression and executive functioning difficulties found it to yield positive effects on depression and disability (Alexopoulos, Raue, & Arean, 2003).

Third, there is one randomized controlled trial that suggests CBT may not have the same cognitive requirements as other therapeutic approaches. The study of 32 older adults found that both a supportive treatment and a CBT treatment for anxiety produced positive effects. However, anxiety change scores were significantly and positively associated with fluid intelligence scores for those randomized to a supportive treatment for anxiety, whereas there was no association between fluid intelligence and treatment success in those randomized to a CBT treatment for anxiety (Doubleday, King, & Papageorgiou, 2002). The term fluid intelligence refers to those mental processes that are used to make sense of new information, such as problem-solving skills; such skills are impaired in persons with dementia.

Fourth, although there are no trials addressing the use of cognitive-therapy techniques in persons with dementia, there is a strong evidence base supporting the effectiveness of behavioral techniques in persons with dementia. The evidence for behavioral and environmental interventions for behavioral problems in persons with dementia was judged to be of the highest level using the American Psychological Association criteria ("well-established") in a review of therapies for older adults with dementia (Gatz et al., 1998). Evidence about the effectiveness of the involvement of collaterals in the therapy process is particularly important because, as will be discussed in detail later, the involvement of collaterals is a crucial element in the success of CBT in persons with dementia. Linda Teri and colleagues have completed several studies demonstrating the positive effects of behavior management when applied by caregivers on agitation (Teri et al., 2000) and depression in persons with dementia (Teri, Logsdon, Uomoto, & McCurry, 1997; Teri et al., 2003). Similarly, Louis Burgio and colleagues have demonstrated the positive effects of behavior management when applied by nursing home staff on behavioral problems in persons with dementia (Burgio et al., 2001, 2002). Finally, there is also a strong evidence base supporting the effectiveness of CBT in treating depression and increasing coping skills in caregivers (Akkerman & Ostwald, 2004; Gallagher-Thompson et al., 2003; Teri et al., 1997).

In sum, CBT offers an overarching conceptual model that informs therapeutic solutions for persons with dementia across the continuum of severity. Further, CBT is supported by an impressive research base that includes evidence for several of the significant elements of cognitive-behavioral therapy with persons with dementia (effectiveness with older people, persons with dementia, and caregivers and staff training), even though there have not yet been any clinical trials of cognitive-therapy approaches in persons with dementia.

SOC MODEL FOR MODIFYING CBT FOR USE WITH PERSONS WITH DEMENTIA

Therapy Needs of Persons with Dementia

To be successful with persons with dementia, CBT requires more modifications beyond those suggested for older persons. From an SOC perspective, to best understand what those modifications should be, one must have a firm understanding of the abilities and deficits of persons with dementia so that an approach that maximizes strengths and minimizes weaknesses can be devised. Short-term memory problems, such as forgetting what one had for breakfast, are the hallmark of Alzheimer's disease and usually the first symptom (Pitt, 2002). Language problems are also common in Alzheimer's disease and begin to present fairly early in the disease process. Expressive language difficulties include being unable to come up with a word (anomia), using the wrong word (paraphasia), and eventually language content with decreased meaning. Receptive language problems include decreased comprehension of spoken and written language. Visuospatial difficulties and calculation difficulties are common. Later in the disease process, the ability to intentionally control coordinated motor activities decreases (apraxia), as well as the ability to correctly recognize/perceive objects as what they really are (agnosia). Finally, throughout the disease process, executive functioning (higher order cognitive processes) progressively worsens. Examples of executive functions include: abstract thinking, logic, shifting mental set (ability to stop doing one activity and focus on something else—difficulty in this area leads to high distractibility and/or perseveration), initiation (ability to start an activity), sequencing (knowing the order of steps needed to do an activity, like making soup), choosing among options/decision making, planning/problem solving, judgment, quantity appreciation, and deficit awareness/insight.

Cognitive abilities that are preserved until late in the dementing process, and thus are strengths, include: repetition skills, procedural learning, ability to read aloud, social skills, memories of things that happened long ago, and matching/recognizing different shapes and sizes (Camp, Koss, & Judge, 1999). Successful modification of CBT for persons with dementia depends on exploitation of preserved abilities and use of compensatory strategies for impaired abilities.

One important approach to exploiting preserved abilities is teaching new information through spaced retrieval (SR). SR relies on procedural memory, which is relatively intact late into the progression of dementia. The technique consists of repeated trials of retrieving the target information at increasing intervals of time. When retrieval failure occurs, the participant is told the correct answer and is asked to repeat it immediately. The next retrieval interval is shortened to that of the last interval at which retrieval was successful. The interval continues to decrease until the participant provides the correct answer. At this point, intervals are once again expanded until an error occurs (Camp, 1989). Results from several studies indicate that persons with dementia can substantially benefit from interventions that incorporate SR training (Bourgeois et al., 2003; Cherry, Simmons, & Camp, 1999; Lekeu, Wojtasik, Van der, & Salmon, 2002; McKitrick, Camp, & Black, 1992; Schacter, Rich, & Stampp, 1985). Finally, SR has also been found to be effective with demented individuals when the technique is taught to and implemented by caregivers of persons with dementia (Arkin, 1991; McKitrick & Camp, 1993). Treatment manuals on the use of SR and on the use of an SR-based approach, Montessori-based activities, are commercially available (Brush & Camp, 1998; Camp, 1999).

Assessment

As discussed above, one of the tenets of CBT is that it is based on empirical data. When treating persons with dementia careful collection of baseline assessment data as well as outcome assessment data throughout the duration of treatment is even more imperative. The nature of the focal issues, therapeutic goals, patient functional abilities, and modifications to traditional CBT vary widely depending upon the profile of strengths and impairments in a particular individual. Thus, the first step is to conduct a multidimensional assessment of cognitive ability, functional ability, behavior problems, and emotional problems. In addition, a careful chart review should be undertaken and a medical evaluation should be requested if there is *any* possibility that the presenting problems might be due to drug side effects/interactions or physical problems (e.g., thyroid deficiency leading to depressed symptoms; undiagnosed urinary tract infection leading to aggression). The goal of the assessment is to understand what types of activities the patient will be able to engage in during therapy, and what modifications will be necessary to accommodate the patient's impairments. A secondary goal of assessment is to better understand the patient's environment, including those persons who provide care. Assessment should always include both direct observation and interview of the patient as well as interview of the primary caregiver(s) and, if possible, a visit to where the patient lives.

Regarding cognitive assessment, for the individual with mild-to-moderate dementia a cognitive screening instrument with subscales for individual cognitive abilities such as memory and language will often be sufficient; there are several such scales available that have been validated, including the Dementia Rating Scale-2 (Jurica , Leitten, & Mattie, 2001), the Cognistat (Kiernan, Mueller, Langston, & Van Dyke, 1987), and the Alzheimer's Disease Assessment Scale (Rosen, Mohs, & Davis, 1984). For a complete review of validated assessment instruments, we refer the reader to other sources (Lichtenberg, 1999; Teri et al., 1997), but we would like to mention a few instruments we have found particularly helpful.

One possible battery could include Physical Self-Maintenance and Instrumental Activities of Daily Living Scales or the Barthel Index to assess functional disability (Lawton & Brody, 1969; Mahoney & Barthel, 1965), the Behavioral Pathology in Alzheimer's Disease Rating Scale (Reisberg et al., 1987) or Cohen-Mansfield Agitation Inventory (Cohen-Mansfield, 1986) to assess behavior problems, and the Cornell Scale for Depression in Dementia (Alexopoulos, Abrams, Young, & Shamoian, 1988) or Neuropsychiatric Inventory (Cummings et al., 1994) to assess mood problems. Because executive functions are so integral to the patient's ability to engage in more complex psychotherapeutic activities, a screen of executive functioning such as the EXIT interview should be included if there is sufficient time (Royall, Mahurin, & Gray, 1992). Finally, we recommend that the assessor make the effort to characterize the severity of impairment by using a dementia staging scale, such as the Clinical Dementia Rating Scale (CDR) (Berg, 1984; Forsell, Fratiglioni, Grut, Viitanen, & Winblad, 1992; Hughes, Berg, Danziger, Coben, & Martin, 1982) or the Global Deterioration Scale (Reisberg, Ferris, de Leon, & Crook, 1982, 1988). Both of these scales rate severity by describing level of ability in several areas of functioning which are then aggregated into a severity category. For example, the CDR evaluates functioning in memory, orientation, judgment/problem solving, community affairs, and home/hobbies, resulting in classification as healthy (CDR = 0), questionable dementia (CDR = 0.5), mild dementia (CDR = 1), moderate dementia (CDR = 2), or severe dementia (CDR = 3). The Mini-Mental State Exam (MMSE) is often used as a cognitive screening, and its scores are often used as a common language among health care professionals, so it is also helpful to know the overlap off MMSE scores with CDR scores: MMSE score 18–27 ~ CDR 0.5–CDR 0.1; MMSE score 15–18 ~ CDR 1–CDR 2; MMSE score <15 ~ CDR 2–CDR 3. A dementia staging scale provides the clinician the opportunity to integrate assessment information with information from collateral interviews to better understand the relative strengths and impairments of the patient in a variety of dimensions.

Assessment of abilities and disabilities in persons with severe dementia presents a special challenge as many cognitive and functional instruments have little sensitivity at this end of the continuum. The test for severe impairment provides a good cognitive screen (Albert & Cohen, 1992), and the Minimum Data Set can provide helpful information about functioning for persons residing in nursing homes (Morris et al., 1990). The Myers Menorah Park/Montessori-based assessment system (MMP/MAS) is an innovative assessment system based on a set of Montessori activities that can be administered by activity professionals (as well as psychologists) to assess cognitive, motor, sensory, and social abilities in persons with severe dementia (Camp et al., 1997, 1999).

In closing, the therapist is reminded that the goal of the assessment is to identify abilities as well as disabilities. Although most assessment instruments, including the dementia staging instruments, focus on disabilities, the collateral interviews needed to complete the dementia staging provides a good opportunity to explore abilities. A discussion about what kinds of activities the collateral and patient engage in together, and how the patient fares with those activities, will also yield important information about abilities. Finally, assessment to identify ablities should be a continuous process that occurs throughout therapy. The therapist should carefully consider the tasks he or she is expecting the patient to engage in during and outside of session, and assure that the patient has the skills needed to complete those tasks, or assure that compensatory strategies are developed. Direct observation of the patient using the identified skills/engaging in the identified tasks during therapy, coupled with careful interview of the collateral regarding their observations of the patient engaging in those skills/tasks, will provide the information the therapist needs to develop a successful treatment plan. A comprehensive discussion of this task breakdown approach is provided by Weaverdyck (1990).

Next, we present an approach to modifying CBT for use with persons with dementia, stratified by CDR levels. However, we emphasize that there is wide individual variability within these categories, and the individual differences may necessitate flexibility in which recommendations work for particular patients. The goal of these recommendations is to help the therapist to "meet the patient where they are" in terms of their functional capacities, matching the therapeutic techniques as ideally as possible with the patient's abilities. Approaches that underestimate abilities may be as ineffective as those that overestimate a patient's abilities regardless of the patient's level of functioning. Meeting an older adult at the correct level can help keep them more engaged and invested. Therapists attempt to make such matches between patient and therapeutic technique across many patient populations, but this process requires more active consideration among older adults with dementia. Along these lines, the cognitive-behavioral approach becomes increasingly behavioral by necessity as memory impairment increases. Use of cognitive techniques with any severely demented patient, and with many moderately demented patients, is almost certainly an overestimation of the patient's abilities. The following discussion of modifications is informed by previous published case reports (Grant & Casey, 1995; Koder, 1998; Laidlaw et al., 2003; Teri & Gallagher-Thompson, 1991), as well as our own clinical experience, but some ethical and legal issues demand consideration prior to discussion of therapeutic technique.

Ethical/Legal Issues

Psychotherapists are appropriately trained to consider confidentiality to be critical to the therapeutic process, and nothing should be shared with anyone other than the patient without the patient's specific permission. However, it can be very helpful to have a trusted close associate of the patient (be that a friend, family member, or significant other) assist in some ways when working with an older adult with memory impairment. The level of involvement of the collateral support varies depending upon the nature of the problem and the severity of cognitive (as well as physical) impairment. In cases of very mild memory impairment, you may choose simply to interview the collateral support source at the beginning of treatment. In cases of mild impairment, that person may be enlisted in helping a patient remember when to do a particular homework assignment. It is important to note that older adults at this level of impairment are likely to have not yet set up legal protections such as guardianship or powers of attorney for health care or finances. An adjunct responsibility for the therapist may be to inform patients of these options and recommend their consideration.

Consent, Capacity, and Confidentiality

The issues of consent to treatment can become very complex when treating older adults with dementia. As a patient loses cognitive functioning he or she must increasingly rely on others for help with a variety of activities. Much of the work in meeting the patient where they are in this population involves balancing the autonomy of the patient with increased need for assistance from others. As dementia patients decline, they will eventually need legally to hand over decision-making authority in different domains to a collateral support person. A patient can designate power of attorney in different domains, including power of attorney for health care, legal, and financial decisions. These different responsibilities may be held by different people or may all be held by a single legal guardian. The therapist must be aware of whether someone else has power of attorney over health care decisions.

When someone else has legal decision-making authority for a patient, you must contact that person for legal consent to treatment and keep them appropriately updated as treatment progresses. It is also important that the dementia patient provides *assent* to treatment to the extent this is possible (it may not be possible in patients with severe dementia). When it is possible, the patient should be informed about treatment decisions in a manner commensurate with their capacity to understand them. Also, to the extent possible, their preferences and interests should be considered.

If the patient with dementia does not have someone with designated power of attorney for health care decisions, the situation may be more complex. In this situation, only the consent of the patient is technically required. However, it can be the case that patients have the legal right to consent for themselves, but their capacity to make health care decisions is in question.

Psychologists working with dementia patients are likely to encounter patients who retain their right to legally consent when they are in fact functionally unable to make such decisions for themselves. This is much more likely in outpatient settings than in residential care facilities, because such legal arrangements may be required prior to admission, and this situation may arise for a wide variety of reasons. For example, a patient may have an incredibly supportive family who make thoughtful decisions together and have not seen a need to change the patient's legal status. On the other hand, a patient may not have anyone close to them (a group now recognized as the unbefriended elderly), and therefore no one has adequately monitored their decline. Regardless of the reasons, this complicates the responsibilities of the psychologist in working with the patient and their family. For further information on assessment of capacity, the reader is referred to *Assessment of competency and capacity of the older adult: A practice guideline for psychologists* (Department of Veterans Affairs, 1997).

Psychologists should be aware of this issue, and discuss it with patients and their collateral supports when it arises. Patients and families may or may not be responsive to recommendations for capacity assessments, and such recommendations may not be acted upon immediately. In the meantime, the psychologist should strive to balance confidentiality and outside support in a manner that fits the best interest of the patient. We recommend that in such situations, a collateral support person be kept informed of the proceedings in therapy. However, the psychologist should clear all information to be shared with the client first. Agree with the client on what will be shared, and talk to the family member in the presence of the client whenever possible. Also, be aware of cultural differences in this process. It has been our experience that patients from some minority groups prefer that you speak with their family members outside of their presence, or that several family members be involved with the therapeutic process.

Goals

There are some goals in which a patient or caregiver may be interested that may not be appropriate with demented older adults. Patients and caregivers should understand that therapy will not cure their cognitive functioning difficulties, and it may be necessary to state this explicitly. Also, it is unwise in our opinion to attempt core personality change (deep schema work, in cognitive terms), because it requires concentration and sustained attention abilities that are very significantly impaired in demented patients. Finally, use caution when the therapeutic goals primarily benefit someone else besides the patient. This can be appropriate in particular cases, such as behavioral modification of yelling in severely demented patients. However, if a mildly demented patient is referred because of excessive complaining about institutional food quality, for example, the referral problem may quickly become secondary to other issues that are in the patient's best interest to address first.

Very mild and mild dementia

Basic insight work is possible with some patients in these categories, particularly in older adults with very mild dementia. These older adults often have an overall ability to connect thoughts and feelings with previous experiences, to see another person's perspective, and generally self-reflect. Older adults with very mild dementia can generally understand and discuss abstract concepts and complicated emotional difficulties. They may also be able to address interpersonal issues in a fairly complex way. Not everyone may be able to do it, but it is possible.

Along with the typical issues older adults address in therapy, these patients may have particular issues specifically related to the effects of dealing with dementia. For example, many older adults in the early stages of dementia are aware of some degree of loss of abilities, and some participate in support groups for early-stage dementia patients. They may want to discuss the impact of dementia as well as specific techniques for minimizing the impact of their memory problems. Increased difficulties with dementia result in increased responsibility for family members and friends who support them. It can be difficult for the demented older adult to discuss their problems with those closest to them because of the burden they already feel they are placing on their loved ones. Furthermore, increased levels of dependency can result in a host of conflicted feelings and relationship problems between the demented older adult and family members or friends who are serving more and more as caregivers. As memory problems increase, an older adult in the new role of care recipient may alternately (or simultaneously) feel guilty, frustrated, jealous, and/or more emotionally distant relative to their friends and family. Psychotherapy can serve an important role as a place to address such difficult and conflicted feelings.

Moderate dementia

With decline from mild-to-moderate dementia, therapy should generally include increased structure and a further shift from cognitive to behavioral techniques. Insight is more limited in this population. Patients can generally discuss present feelings, reminisce, and socialize, but may not be able to maintain attention for the length of a typical therapy session. Along with memory difficulties, patients at this stage of dementia also have difficulties with executive functioning. Therefore, issues addressed in therapy should be limited in scope and concrete.

General Features of Therapy

Very mild and mild dementia

Organizational skills, however, are more likely to decline earlier on, resulting in the need for the therapist to take more responsibility for directing how time is spent within (and outside) the session. However, as these skills vary among everyone else, so do they vary among people with very mild and mild dementia. If therapy is being provided in an outpatient setting, the therapist should consider at least one visit to the patient's residence in order to gain firsthand knowledge of their living arrangements.

Rapport remains critical with this population. A thoughtful, caring therapeutic relationship with the patient and anyone who may be a collateral support may be a bond that lasts and supports them well into the patient's cognitive decline. Your concern can help raise a family's spirits, and a strong relationship will be very important when discussing increasingly difficult issues such as cognitive decline, guardianship, and perhaps nursing home placement. This is a fundamental part of CBT, and is the topic of the first chapter of Beck, Rush, Shaw & Emery's (1973) original book on treatment of depression.

Several modifications to the session structure can be helpful in this population. In very mild dementia, it is possible to address multiple themes in therapy (e.g., issues of marital strain due to dementia and depressive symptoms), but it is difficult to imagine more than two in a particular session. Although structure within the session is typical in a CBT approach, it is even more critical to structure and organize the time available in this situation. Furthermore, key points should be repeated during the session more often than with a typical patient. Key points that are repeated are much likely to be remembered, so it is important to repeat key points (I have repeated this statement several times, in hopes that it will help the reader remember it). For example, the typical summary at the end of the session could be extended so that key points are more fully reiterated. It can enhance patient recall if they are asked to state the key points themselves.

Along those lines, a "session notebook" can be very helpful (some older adults we have worked with did not like the term "therapy notebook"). CBT therapists use these to varying degrees, but they are particularly helpful with patients with very mild or mild dementia. Session notebooks can help both with continuity within sessions and with continuity outside of therapy. Writing in the notebook is more organized and simpler than using multiple handouts.

Moderate dementia

Highly structured cognitive techniques can be effective in this population, but the general approach could be considered "behavioral cognitive therapy," where the emphasis is on behavioral techniques supplemented with cognitive methods as appropriate. There is increasing responsibility on the therapist for directing the therapy in terms of both individual sessions and overall goals. The therapist should also be increasingly sensitive to when therapy does not appear to be appropriate to initiate or not helpful once it has begun. Individual sessions should have a single theme choosing a limited number of appropriate interventions, but it is generally best to focus on one key issue in any particular session.

Therefore, it is recommended that session length be shortened, perhaps to 30 min or less (other health issues may also warrant decreasing session length in patients with very mild or mild dementia), and we recommend that you focus on a single theme in any particular session. It is critical to have a collateral support person involved when attempting therapy with moderately demented patients, as discussed earlier in this chapter. The scope of their role may vary from full participation in sessions and homework to involvement at the end of sessions and reminding patients about homework. Their level of involvement will depend on the functioning of the patient, the wishes of the patient and the support person, the availability of the person, and their relationship with the patient. Any use of homework with this population should only be attempted if there is a reliable collateral support person who can assist in implementation. It is rare to see moderately demented patients in outpatient settings, but if that is the case we very strongly recommend at least one home visit.

Cognitive Techniques

All patients with whom cognitive techniques will be used should be able to express a presenting problem in some way, or understand and agree to work on a presenting problem if someone else has referred them. Cognitive therapy typically involves explaining the purpose and reasoning behind each step of the process to the patient, but in demented patients such explanation can interfere with effectiveness rather than improve it. Therefore, such explanation of process is minimized with very mild and mild dementia patients, and essentially eliminated with moderately demented patients. Interventions are likewise more directive. For example, Laidlaw et al. (2003) describe different types of unhelpful thoughts common among older adults with depression. These types of unhelpful thoughts are discussed in therapy with the older adult, who will then begin to categorize their own unhelpful thoughts as part of the homework. If the older adult has very mild or mild dementia, the therapist could be more directive in pointing out which types of unhelpful thoughts are present.

Therapists should also consider restricting corrective methods to one or two that appear to be particularly helpful for the patient, rather than teaching many techniques. Dick, Gallagher-Thompson, Coon, Powers, & Thompson (1996) present a list of several techniques for changing unhelpful thoughts. Rather than presenting the patient with a list to choose from, the therapist can think about one or two that seem most likely to help, present them one at a time, and stop adding techniques when one or two are found to be helpful.

Rather than presenting the patient with the full list, the therapist can think about one or two that seem most likely to help, present them one at a time, and stop adding techniques when one or two are found to be helpful.

MODERATE DEMENTIA

If cognitive interventions are implemented, they should be very highly structured. It is best to avoid trying to categorize unhelpful thoughts in any way, instead providing a specific way to challenge unhelpful thoughts in a supportive manner (the last point is added as a reminder that rapport continues to be essential). Write down the alternative thought, and have the collateral support person involved in helping them remember the alternative between sessions.

Behavioral Techniques

Behavioral interventions should include simplified instructions relative to similar interventions with nondemented patients. For example, a relaxation technique may be simplified such that muscle relaxation strategies or visualizations are streamlined. Also, instructions for such strategies might be recorded from the session for use between sessions.

As mentioned earlier, behavioral techniques are likely to be emphasized over cognitive techniques, particularly in homework assignments. It is also important to work with a collateral support person to plan behavioral homework interventions that challenge the unhelpful thought. For example, a nursing home resident may state "Nobody wants to talk to me." Instead of discussing how to categorize that unhelpful thought and explaining that you would like to "test the evidence," you could simplify your response by empathizing, reframing, and setting up a behavioral intervention. Perhaps offer alternatives to the patient's unhelpful thoughts, then work with a collateral support person such as a nurse's aid to increase the patient's time in the day room with other residents they could talk to.

Homework

The therapist can expect more difficulties between sessions if any homework is assigned, and may want to have a collateral support person involved in completion of any homework. Homework should also be very clear, with instructions written down, and it is best if there is a concrete plan for homework completion that is regularized across sessions. For example, if a patient is feeling frustrated about their memory problems, you may ask the patient to write down their thoughts about this every morning after breakfast (patients are often most alert in the morning), and perhaps have them place a reminder sign on the kitchen cabinet.

Demented and nondemented patients (of all ages) fail to complete therapy homework from time to time. When there are problems with homework completion among this population, the therapist should ask themselves the following questions:

Is the patient remembering to do the homework? If the patient cannot remember to complete the homework with appropriate cues and support, it is best to avoid using homework, and assess whether the patient's memory problems are preventing therapy from having positive effects overall.

Is the homework clear, is it too complicated? Keeping with the theme of meeting the patient where they are, think of ways to perhaps simplify the homework such that the patient can do the homework and it still contributes to the therapy goals.

Is the homework "hitting the mark"? Patients who are not cognitively impaired do not comply with homework in some cases because it appears to them to be busy work and does not seem to address their presenting problem. It is always important to make sure that the homework fits with therapeutic issues, or patients at any level of cognitive functioning will see it as a waste of time. The therapist has increased responsibility with impaired patients to make sure any homework assigned fits the problem, because the patient may be less able to make that judgment.

Is the patient motivated? Motivation can be an issue among older adults with dementia just as with everyone else, but may best be considered after ruling out the issues listed above.

A therapist should monitor their own responses very carefully when homework is partially or fully incomplete, because these patients can be very sensitive about their ability to do what was asked. Be aware of your verbal and nonverbal reactions to what patients do or do not do, and in all cases be supportive.

Moderate dementia

The collateral support can be very helpful in designing activities that the person will engage in and that will be effective. Furthermore, consulting with them in the planning of activities can increase their commitment to assist. The questions about homework completion for patients with very mild or mild dementia also apply here. However, these questions should now also be considered in regard to the collateral support person. The collateral support should understand the reasoning for any homework assignments and be sufficiently motivated to reliably implement them; therefore, it will be important to check in with the support person (or people if there are more than one) in case they have questions or concerns.

Severe dementia

Only behavioral techniques are appropriate among patients with severe dementia. These patients have severe memory impairment, and capacity for insight is limited and fleeting if it is present. They also have limited verbal communication skills at best, and may be noncommunicative. Interventions with patients who are severely demented are typically focused on modifying behaviors that are harmful or significantly disruptive for the patient or others around them. For example, a patient may be referred for wandering, yelling, or aggressive behavior. Interventions typically involve monitoring the patient's behavior, introducing behavioral modifications, monitoring for improvement, and adapting the applied interventions as necessary. The psychologist will typically also train caregivers (whether they be family, friends or institutional staff) to monitor the patient's behavior and apply the intervention. Much of the interaction will be between therapist and caregiver, with the patient involved for demonstrations and training. Lundervold and Lewin (1992) provide a comprehensive discussion of the use of applied behavioral analysis techniques with nursing home residents. Treatment can also be directed towards caregivers of severely demented patients. Although we are not focusing on interventions directed towards caregivers in this chapter, we would refer the reader to cognitive-behavioral approaches that have been developed for caregivers of dementia patients (Akkerman & Ostwald, 2004; Gallagher-Thompson et al., 2003; Lundervold & Lewin, 1992).

PUTTING IT ALL TOGETHER

Case Study 1

Marianne was a 78-year-old nursing home resident with mild-to-moderate dementia. She had been confined to her bed for the past several weeks due to severely twisting her ankle and subsequently developing bronchitis while recovering from her ankle injury. Her physician determined that she was now healthy enough to walk out of her room with the assistance of a walker, but Marianne reported symptoms of a panic attack (although not enough to meet DSM-IV criteria) when nursing assistants attempted to help her out of bed. Her formal diagnosis was recurrent major depression with anxious symptoms, along with mild-to-moderate dementia. Her score on the MMSE was 19, in the mild-to-moderate range. In the first interview with the psychologist, she reported that she had two concerns related to getting out of bed: that she would fall again, and that her friends would be angry at her for not coming out to see them the past two weeks. She also discussed several other general concerns about being distant from her brother and his family, as well as longstanding regret that she never had a family of her own. Sessions were one half hour in length. The first several sessions with the psychologist involved practicing relaxation breathing exercises and examining her beliefs that her friends would be angry at her. Between the second and third session, one of her friends visited her in her room. This was somewhat helpful, but Marianne continued to think that her friend was "just being nice" and still believed her friend was upset about Marianne not coming out.

The therapist challenged her beliefs by asking for worst case scenarios and discussing the likelihood of those. The therapist also discussed the friend's visit as an empirical test of the patient's belief about her friend's anger. One difficulty was that Marianne frequently discounted any gains she made, and often perceived setbacks that she believed were her fault. Cognitive strategies were used to address these beliefs, but the explanatory component of cognitive therapy was omitted due to the patient's cognitive impairment. For example, the basic premises of the approach were not discussed with the patient, and the categorization of the patient's negative cognitions was not discussed. Rather, Marianne was told "maybe there's another way to look at this that will help you feel better." She would agree to do this if she was then asked "do you want to try this to feel better?" Typically no more than one or two specific beliefs were examined in a session, and the strategies used to refute the beliefs were repeated within the session. Simple and direct homework assignments were written down and given to Marianne to use between sessions. For example, the first few weeks the assignment was "Breathe slow and deep when you feel tight." A later assignment was to "think positively about your friends." The nursing home did not allow these notes to be posted in her room, so a staff member who served as a collateral source reminded her to look at them once daily on days the staff member worked.

Marianne eventually agreed to sit in a chair in her room, and then agreed to leave her room in a wheelchair during a session. Once Marianne's anxiety was reduced to the point that she was ready to try the walker, she did not remember that she had been cleared by physical therapy to walk. PT agreed to visit the room with the psychologist present to "re-evaluate" her, and told her (again) that she was cleared to walk. Two months after cognitive therapy began, Marianne agreed to leave the room with a walker, but at first only with her psychologist present. Collateral support then became critical in encouraging Marianne to leave her room at other times, and one member of the nursing staff was particularly helpful in walking with Marianne and reminding her to use the relaxation breathing exercises she learned in the early sessions of therapy. Marianne began to re-establish relationships with her friends and eat meals in the dining room. Her mood improved substantially and her anxious symptoms declined significantly, although her ruminative concerns about never having had a family of her own persisted.

Case Study 2

George was a 54-year-old man rehabilitating in the nursing home from a right-side stroke with left hemiplegia, left visual field cut, and inoperable arterial emboli in the right hand and forearm that were controlled with medication. He was referred to the psychologist for feelings of depression. George obviously had suffered real losses due to his stroke, and reacted to these losses with symptoms of depression. His interpretation of the meaning of these losses and his coping skills for dealing with these losses were the focus of treatment. The primary goal for therapy was to improve mood, particularly through increasing pleasant activities. He was seen for 12 sessions over 4 months.

Assessments of functional status and physical status revealed that George's difficulties due to his stroke included the loss of use of his left arm (he kept it immobile and close to his body with the use of a sling), a left visual field cut that made it tiring (though still possible) to read and do detail work, frequent wheelchair use due to an ability to walk only short distances with a cane, chronic pain in his back and left side, frequent grogginess and fatigue, and poor sleep. The difficulty with emboli in his right arm meant that there is always the possibility that future complications could lead to loss of functioning in his right arm. A neuropsychological evaluation was ordered to better understand George's particular cognitive strengths and deficits (this was particularly important because cognitive deficits due to a stroke can vary widely). Results indicated that he had suffered significant cognitive impairment affecting his general intellectual functioning level, visual memory, and ability to integrate large amounts of complex information especially visually, and executive functioning. George's Geriatric Depression Inventory (short form) score was 9 out of 15, indicating significant depressive symptomology. Diagnoses were major depression and dementia due to stroke.

Treatment initially focused on orientation to the CBT model and Unhelpful Thought Records. Each session the therapist and George completed one or two thought records in session to practice the skill. The therapist wrote a few words large on a dry erase board, which provided a memory cue to keep the conversation focused. George was also asked to complete thought records outside of therapy. The therapist provided large type worksheets for George, always wrote down homework assignments, and all materials were kept in a folder. George's wife was engaged as a "helper" for therapy; she did not sit in on the therapy, but at the end George and the therapist would discuss with George's wife a schedule for homework assignments (although not necessarily the content of the homework, unless George wanted to share this information), and then his wife could help remind him to complete the homework during the week.

The two most prevalent themes were identified for the focus of therapy. These were that his wife saw him as a burden and only stayed with him because she was Catholic and would not divorce, and that he did not want to make goals or try to improve his lot in life because he would just be disappointed. He said "I will continue to have strokes and die from them like my mother—that's a terrible way to live." He also said "whenever I get hope things will get better something else goes wrong (like with my arm because of the emboli) and the disappointment is too painful, so it's better not to hope." The most frequently used unhelpful thought patterns were mindreading, and filtering out the positive.

Once these patterns were identified, treatment focused on learning ways of challenging these unhelpful thought patterns and on learning about the link between engaging in these unhelpful thought patterns and mood level. With his wife's help, George kept daily mood ratings and ratings of engaging in the thought patterns. For example, George was encouraged to "collect evidence" rather than engaging in mindreading; one homework assignment was for him to ask his wife to write down the reasons she stayed with him. He then reviewed this list with the therapist who discussed this empirical evidence against his assumption that she really wanted to leave him. When he found himself engaging in mindreading, he would also look for connections between when he used mindreading and what his mood ratings were. Finally, treatment also focused on increasing activity level through generating a list of pleasant events and eventually tracking those events to encourage an increase in activity level.

At the end of therapy, a "survival manual" was developed for George, and after discussing the manual with him privately, and with his permission, the manual was discussed with both he and his wife. The manual included reminders about what was learned in therapy, what to do to keep his mood up, and signs to look for that would indicate that he should consider coming back to therapy or at least coming in for a booster session.

CONCLUSIONS

Cognitive-behavioral techniques can be used with older adults who are experiencing cognitive decline as a result of dementia. This chapter provides research-informed general guidelines for intervention that will hopefully be replaced as research in this area expands. It is critical in this (or any) therapeutic approach that the therapist "meet the patient where they are," working with them at a level of cognitive and emotional complexity that is commensurate with their level of functioning. As decline continues, emphasis is shifted increasingly from cognitive to behavioral techniques, and assistance from one or more collateral supports is necessary to insure that interventions are appropriate and effective. The involvement of collateral supports requires consideration of issues of confidentiality, patient capacity, and consent. When this approach is thoughtfully used in the best interest of the patient, it can enhance the well-being of this population. Their lives continue to be important and valuable both to them and to those who hold them dear.

ACKNOWLEDGMENT

This material is based upon work supported by the Veterans Affairs Health Services Research and Development Service Career Development Award to Dr. Snow (RCD 01-008-1).

REFERENCES

Akkerman, R. L., & Ostwald, S. K. (2004). Reducing anxiety in Alzheimer's disease family caregivers: The effectiveness of a nine-week cognitive-behavioral intervention. *American Journal of Alzheimer's Disease & Other Dementias, 19*, 117–123.

Albert, M., & Cohen, C. (1992). The test for severe impairment: An instrument for the assessment of patients with severe cognitive dysfunction. *Journal of the American Geriatrics Society, 40*, 449–453.

Alexopoulos, G. S., Abrams, R. C., Young, R. C., & Shamoian, C. A. (1988). Cornell scale for depression in dementia. *Biological Psychiatry, 23*, 271–284.

Alexopoulos, G. S., Raue, P., & Arean, P. (2003). Problem-solving therapy versus supportive therapy in geriatric major depression with executive dysfunction. *American Journal of Geriatric Psychiatry, 11*, 46–52.

Allen-Burge, R., Stevens, A. B., & Burgio, L. D. (1999). Effective behavioral interventions for decreasing dementia-related challenging behavior in nursing homes. *International Journal of Geriatric Psychiatry, 14*, 213–228.

American Psychiatric Association. (1994). *American Psychiatric Association: Diagnostic and statistical manual of mental disorders* (4th ed.). Washington, DC: American Psychiatric Association.

Arkin, S. M. (1991). Memory training in early Alzheimer's disease: An optimistic look at the field. *American Journal of Alzheimer's & Related Disorders Care & Research, 6*, 17–25.

Barker, W. W., Luis, C. A., Kashuba, A., Luis, M., Harwood, D. G., Loewenstein, D., Waters, C., Jimison, P., Shepherd, E., Sevush, S., Graff-Radford, N., Newland, D., Todd, M., Miller, B., Gold, M., Heilmann, K., Doty, L., Goodman, I., Robinson, B., Pearl, G., Dickson, D., & Duara, R. (2002). Relative frequencies of Alzheimer disease, Lewy body, vascular and frontotemporal dementia, and hippocampal sclerosis in the State of Florida Brain Bank. *Alzheimer Disease & Associated Disorders, 16*(4), 203–212.

Beail, N. (2003). What works for people with mental retardation? Critical commentary on cognitive-behavioral and psychodynamic psychotherapy research. *Mental Retardation, 41*, 468–472.

Beck, A. T., Rush, A. J., Shaw, B. F., & Emery, G. (1973). *Cognitive therapy of depression*. New York: Guilford Press.

Benedict, R. H. B., Shapiro, A., Priore, R., Miller, C., Munschauer, F., & Jacobs, L. (2000). Neuropsychological counseling improves social behvior in cognitively-impaired multiple sclerosis patients. *Multiple Sclerosis, 6*, 391–396.

Berg, L. (1984). Clinical dementia rating. *British Journal of Psychiatry, 145*, 339.

Bourgeois, M. S., Camp, C., Rose, M., White, B., Malone, M., Carr, J., & Rovine, M. (2003). A comparison of training strategies to enhance use of external aids by persons with dementia. *Journal of Communication Disorders, 36*(5), 361–378.

Brush, J. A., & Camp, C. J. (1998). *A therapy technique for improving memory: Spaced retrieval*. Beachwood, OH: Menorah Park Center for the Aging.

Bryant, R. A., Moulds, M., Guthrie, R., & Nixon, R. D. (2003). Treating acute stress disorder following mild traumatic brain injury. *American Journal of Psychiatry, 160*, 585–587.

Burgio, L. D., Allen-Burge, R., Roth, D. L., Bourgeois, M. S., Dijkstra, K., Gerstle, J., Jackson, E., & Bankester, L. (2001). Come talk with me: Improving communication between nursing assistants and nursing home residents during care routines. *Gerontologist, 41*(4), 449–460.

Burgio, L. D., Stevens, A., Burgio, K. L., Roth, D. L., Paul, P., & Gerstle, J. (2002). Teaching and maintaining behavior management skills in the nursing home. *Gerontologist, 42*, 487–496.

Camp, C. J. (1989). Facilitation of new learning in Alzheimer's disease. In G. Gilmore, P. Whitehouse, & M. Wykle (Eds.), *Memory and aging in dementia: Theory, assessment, and treatment* (pp. 212–225). New York, NY: Springer.

Camp, C. J. (1999). *Montessori-based activities for persons with dementia (Vol. 1)*. Beachwood, OH: Menorah Park Center for the Aging (available at http://www.myersresearch.org/home.html).

Camp, C. J., Judge, K. S., Bye, C. A., Fox, K. M., Bowden, J., Bell, M., Valencic, K., & Mattern, J. M. (1997). An intergenerational program for persons with dementia using Montessori methods. *Gerontologist, 37*(5), 688–692.

Camp, C. J., Koss, E., & Judge, K. S. (1999). Cognitive assessment in late-stage dementia. In P. A. Lichtenberg (Ed.), *Handbook of assessment in clinical gerontology,* (pp. 442–467). John Wiley & Sons.

Chambless, D. L., Sanderson, W. C., Shoham, V., Bennett Johnson, S., Pope, K. S., Crits-Christoph, P., Baker, M., Johnson, B., Woody, S. R., Sue, S., Beutler, L., Williams, D. A., & McCurry, S. (1996). An update on empirically validated therapies. *The Clinical Psychologist, 49*, 5–18.

Cherry, K. E., Simmons, S. S., & Camp, C. J. (1999). Spaced-retrieval enhances memory in older adults with probable Alzheimer's disease. *Journal of Clinical Geropsychology, 5*, 159.

Cheston, R. (1998). Psychotherapeutic work with people with dementia: A review of the literature. *British Journal of Medical Psychology, 71*(Pt 3), 211–231.

Cohen-Mansfield, J. (1986). Agitated behaviors in the elderly. II. Preliminary results in the cognitively deteriorated. *Journal of the American Geriatrics Society, 34*, 722–727.

Cummings, J. L., Mega, M., Gray, K., Rosenberg-Thompson, S., Carusi, D. A., & Gornbein, J. (1994). The neuropsychiatric inventory: Comprehensive assessment of psychopathology in dementia. *Neurology, 44*, 2308–2314.

Department of Veterans Affairs. (1997). *Assessment of competency and capacity of the older adult: A practice guideline for psychologists.* Milwaukee, WI: National Center for Cost Containment.

Dick, L., Gallagher-Thompson, D., Coon, D., Powers, D., & Thompson, L. W. (1996). *Cognitive-behavioral therapy for late-life depression: A patient's manual.* Stanford, CA: VA Palo Alto Health Care System and Stanford University.

Doubleday, E. K., King, P., & Papageorgiou, C. (2002). Relationship between fluid intelligence and ability to benefit from cognitive-behavioural therapy in older adults: A preliminary investigation. *British Journal of Clinical Psychology, 41*, 423–428.

Finnema, E., Droes, R. M., Ribbe, M., & van Tilburg, W. (2000). The effects of emotion-oriented approaches in the care for persons suffering from dementia: A review of the literature. *International Journal of Geriatric Psychiatry, 15*, 141–161.

Fisher, J. E., & Carstensen, L. L. (1990). Behavior management of the dementias. *Clinical Psychology Review, 10*, 611–629.

Forsell, Y., Fratiglioni, L., Grut, M., Viitanen, M., & Winblad, B. (1992). Clinical staging of dementia in a population survey: Comparison of DSM-III-R and the Washington University Clinical Dementia Rating Scale. *Acta Psychiatrica Scandinavica, 86*, 49–54.

Gallagher-Thompson, D., Coon, D. W., Solano, N., Ambler, C., Rabinowitz, Y., & Thompson, L. W. (2003). Change in indices of distress among Latino and Anglo female caregivers of elderly relatives with dementia: Site-specific results from the REACH national collaborative study. *Gerontologist, 43*, 580–591.

Gatz, M., Fiske, A., Fox, L. S., Kaskie, B., Kasl-Godley, J. E., McCallum, T. J., & Wetherell, J. L. (1998). Empirically validated psychological treatments for older adults. *Journal of Mental Health & Aging, 4*(1), 9–46.

Grant, R. W., & Casey, D. A. (1995). Adapting cognitive behavioral therapy for the frail elderly. *International Psychogeriatrics, 7*, 561–571.

Hughes, C. P., Berg, L., Danziger, W. L., Coben, L. A., & Martin, R. L. (1982). A new clinical scale for the staging of dementia. *British Journal of Psychiatry, 140*, 566–572.

Jurica, P. J., Leitten, C. L., & Mattie, S. (2001). *Demential rating scale-2: Professional manual.* Lutz, FL: Psychological Assessment Resources, Inc.

Kasl-Godley, J., & Gatz, M. (2000). Psychosocial interventions for individuals with dementia: An integration of theory, therapy, and a clinical understanding of dementia. *Clinical Psychology Review, 20*, 755–782.

Kiernan, R. J., Mueller, J., Langston, J. W., & Van Dyke, C. (1987). The neurobehavioral cognitive status examination: A brief but quantitative approach to cognitive assessment. *Annals of Internal Medicine, 107*, 481–485.

Koder, D. A. (1998). Treatment of anxiety in the cognitively impaired elderly: Can cognitive-behavior therapy help? *International Psychogeriatrics, 10*, 173–182.

Laidlaw, K., Thompson, L. W., Dick-Siskin, L., & Gallagher-Thompson, D. (2003). Psychotherapy with for older people. In K. Laidlaw, L. W. Thompson, L. Dick-Siskin, & D. Gallagher-Thompson (Eds.), *Cognitive behaviour therapy with older people* (pp. 15–25). West Sussex, England: John Wiley & Sons Ltd.

Lawton, M. P., & Brody, E. M. (1969). Assessment of older people: Self-maintaining and instrumental activities of daily living. *Gerontologist, 9*, 179–186.

Lekeu, F., Wojtasik, V., Van der, L. M., & Salmon, E. (2002). Training early Alzheimer patients to use a mobile phone. *Acta Neurological Belgica, 102*, 114–121.

Lichtenberg, P. A. (1999). *Handbook of assessment in clinical gerontology.* West Sussex, England: John Wiley & Sons, Inc.

Lindsay, W. R., Howells, L., & Pitcaithly, D. (1993). Cognitive therapy for depression with individuals with intellectual disabilities. *British Journal of Medical Psychology, 66*(Pt 2), 135–141.

Lundervold, D. A., & Lewin, L. M. (1992). *Behavior analysis and therapy in nursing homes.* Springfield, IL: Charles C. Thomas.

MacKenzie, J. M. (2002). Neuropathology: Other dementias. In J. R. M. Copeland, M. T. Abou-Saleh, & D. G. Blazer (Eds.), *Principles and practice of geriatric psychiatry* (2nd ed., pp. 259–263). West Sussex, England: John Wiley and Sons, Ltd.

Mahoney, F. I., & Barthel, D. W. (1965). Functional evaluation: The Barthel Index. *Maryland State Medical Journal, 14*, 61–65.

McKitrick, L. A., & Camp, C. J. (1993). Relearning the names of things: The spaced-retrieval intervention implementation by a caregiver. *Clinical Gerontologist, 14*, 60–62.

McKitrick, L. A., Camp, C. J., & Black, F. W. (1992). Prospective memory intervention in Alzheimer's disease. *Journal of Gerontology, 47*, 337–343.

Morris, J. N., Hawes, C., Fries, B. E., Phillips, C. D., Mor, V., Katz, S., Murphy, K., Drugovich, M. L., & Friedlob, A. S. (1990). Designing the national resident assessment instrument for nursing homes. *Gerontologist, 30*(3), 293–307.

Nezu, C. M., Nezu, A. M., & Arean, P. (1991). Assertiveness and problem-solving training for mildly mentally retarded persons with dual diagnoses. *Research in Developmental Disabilities, 12*, 371–386.

Nezu, C. M., Nezu, A. M., & Dudek, J. A. (1998). A cognitive-behavioral model of assessment and treatment for intellectually disabled sexual offenders. *Cognitive & Behavioral Practice, 5*, 25–64.

Ouellet, M. C., & Morin, C. M. (2004). Cognitive behavioral therapy for insomnia associated with traumatic brain injury: A single-case study. *Archives in Physical Medicine & Rehabilitation, 85*, 1298–1302.

Pitt, B. (2002). Clinical features of senile dementia and Alzheimer's disease. In J. R. M. Copeland, M. T. Abou-Saleh, & D. G. Blazer (Eds.), *Principles and practice of geriatric psychiatry* (2nd ed., pp. 237–240). West Sussex, England: John Wiley and Sons, Ltd.

Reichman, W. E., Coyne, A. C., Borson, S., Negr, A. E., Rovner, B. W., Pelchat, R. J., Sakauye, K. M., Katz, P., Cantillon, M., & Hamer, R. M. (1998). Psychiatric consultation in the nursing home: A survey of six states. *American Journal of Geriatric Psychiatry, 6*(4), 320–327.

Reisberg, B., Borenstein, J., Salob, S. P., Ferris, S. H., Franssen, E., & Georgotas, A. (1987). Behavioral symptoms in Alzheimer's disease: Phenomenology and treatment. *Journal of Clinical Psychiatry, 48*(Suppl), 9–15.

Reisberg, B., Ferris, S. H., de Leon, M. J., & Crook, T. (1982). The Global Deterioration Scale for assessment of primary degenerative dementia. *American Journal of Psychiatry, 139*, 1136–1139.

Reisberg, B., Ferris, S. H., de Leon, M. J., & Crook, T. (1988). Global Deterioration Scale (GDS). *Psychopharmacology Bulletin, 24*, 661–663.

Romana, M. S. (2003). Cognitive-behavioral therapy. Treating individuals with dual diagnoses. *Journal of Psychosocial and Nursing Mental Health Services, 41*, 30–35.

Rosen, W. G., Mohs, R. C., & Davis, K. L. (1984). A new rating scale for Alzheimer's disease. *American Journal of Psychiatry, 141*, 1356–1364.

Rovner, B. W., German, P. S., Broadhead, J., & Morriss, R. K. (1990). The prevalence and management of dementia and other psychiatric disorders in nursing homes. *International Psychogeriatrics, 2*(1), 13–24.

Royall, D. R., Mahurin, R. K., & Gray, K. F. (1992). Bedside assessment of executive cognitive impairment: The executive interview. *Journal of the American Geriatrics Society, 40*, 1221–1226.

Rybarczyk, B., Lopez, M., Benson, R., Alsten, C., & Stepanski, E. (2002). Efficacy of two behavioral treatment programs for comorbid geriatric insomnia. *Psychology & Aging, 17*, 288–298.

Sahyoun, N. R., Pratt, L. A., Lentzner, H., Dey, A., & Robinson, K. N. (2001). *The changing profile of nursing home residents: 1985–1997*. Hyattsville, MD: National Center for Health Statistics.

Schacter, D. L., Rich, S. A., & Stampp, M. S. (1985). Remediation of memory disorders: Experimental evaluation of the spaced-retrieval technique. *Journal of Clinical & Experimental Neuropsychology, 7*, 79–96.

Schneider, J. K., Mercer, G. T., Herning, M., Smith, C. A., & Prysak, M. D. (2004). Promoting exercise behavior in older adults: Using a cognitive behavioral intervention. *Journal of Gerontological Nursing, 30*, 45–53.

Snowden, M., Sato, K., & Roy Byrne, P. (2003). Assessment and treatment of nursing home residents with depression or behavioral symptoms associated with dementia: A review of the literature. *Journal of American Geriatrics Society, 51*, 1305–1317.

Stanley, M. A., Hopko, D. R., Diefenbach, G. J., Bourland, S. L., Rodriguez, H., & Wagener, P. (2003). Cognitive-behavior therapy for late-life generalized anxiety disorder in primary care: Preliminary findings. *American Journal of Geriatric Psychiatry, 11*, 92–96.

Suzman, K. B., Morris, R. D., Morris, M. K., & Milan, M. A. (1997). Cognitive-behavioral remediation of problem solving deficits in children with acquired brain injury. *Journal of Behavior Therapy & Experimental Psychiatry, 28*, 203–212.

Teri, L., & Gallagher-Thompson, D. (1991). Cognitive-behavioral interventions for treatment of depression in Alzheimer's patients. *Gerontologist, 31*, 413–416.

Teri, L., Gibbons, L. E., McCurry, S. M., Logsdon, R. G., Buchner, D. M., Barlow, W. E., Kukull, W. A., LaCroix, A. Z., McCormick, W., & Larson, E. B. (2003). Exercise Plus Behavioral Management in Patients with Alzheimer Disease: A Randomized Controlled Trial. *JAMA: Journal of the American Medical Association, 290*(15), 2015–2022.

Teri, L., Logsdon, R. G., Peskind, E., Raskind, M., Weiner, M. F., Tractenberg, R. E., Foster, N. L., Schneider, L. S., Sano, M., Whitehouse, P., Tariot, P., Mellow, A. M., Auchus, A. P., Grundman, M., Thomas, R. G., Schafer, K., & Thal, L. J. (2000). Treatment of agitation in AD: A randomized, placebo-controlled clinical trial. *Neurology, 55*(9), 1271–1278.

Teri, L., Logsdon, R. G., Uomoto, J., & McCurry, S. M. (1997). Behavioral treatment of depression in dementia patients: A controlled clinical trial. *Journals of Gerontology Series B, Psychological Sciences & Social Sciences, 52*, 159–166.

Teri, L., Truax, P., Logsdon, R., Uomoto, J., Zarit, S., & Vitaliano, P. P. (1992). Assessment of behavioral problems in dementia: The revised memory and behavior problems checklist. *Psychology & Aging, 7*, 622–631.

Thompson, L. W., Gallagher-Thompson, D., & Dick, L. P. (1995). *Cognitive-behavioral therapy for late-life depression: A therapist manual* (p. 3). Palo

Alto, CA: Older Adult and Family Center, Veterans Affairs Palo Alto Health Care System.

Weaverdyck, S. E. (1990). Dementia care: Patient, family, and community. Intervention-based neuropsychological assessment. In N. L. Mace (Ed.), *Dementia care* (pp. 32–73). Baltimore, MD: The Johns Hopkins Press.

Wetherell, J. L., Gatz, M., & Craske, M. G. (2003). Treatment of generalized anxiety disorder in older adults. *Journal of Consulting and Clinical Psychology, 71*, 31–40.

CHAPTER THIRTEEN

Montessori-Based Dementia Programming™ in Long-Term Care

A Case Study of Disseminating and Intervention for Persons with Dementia

Cameron J. Camp

> But if we observe them closely, we notice that they do not listen to the answers given them, but simply keep repeating the questions. What seems to be an eager curiosity is in reality a means of keeping a person they need near at hand. (Montessori, 1966, p. 162)

A long-term care resident living on a unit serving persons with advanced dementia was holding a full glass of water. She was repetitively saying, "Please get me something to drink. Please bring me some water." This had been going on for several minutes. If a staff member ignored the resident, her voice would rise and she would say, "Why won't you get me some water? You hate me—I can tell by looking in your eyes." Then, she would return to her original two repetitive statements.

What happened next was truly interesting. An activities therapist assigned to the unit asked the resident to come to "the meeting of the club." The resident put down her glass and followed the activities therapist, sat down with a small number of other residents from the unit, and a game of Memory Blackout Bingo™ was played (Camp, 1999a, b). This involved reading statements aloud, such as "Let me call you. . . . ," looking for the word that finished the phrase on cards placed in front of the players, and turning the matching card over if the match ("sweetheart") was found. The game continued for over an hour.

During the game, the resident who had previously been exhibiting repetitive vocalizations showed none of that behavior, took part in the activity appropriately, sang along with other residents when topics evoked songs and song lyrics, made appropriate comments, and displayed a calm demeanor throughout. This occurred in spite of the fact that strangers were present in the room with videocameras, lighting equipment, an overhead microphone, etc., recording the event. Returning later to a large room with nothing to occupy her attention, the resident reverted to her previous "problematic" behavior.

Psychologists and activities staff traditionally have had little contact with one another in long-term care settings. This should change. At least, that is the premise of this chapter. Physicians in general and psychiatrists in particular are the persons most often called upon to manage problematic behaviors in long-term care residents, and nursing staff generally provide and/or maintain medical interventions. Activities staff, on the other hand, focus on engaging long-term care residents (most of whom have dementia) in meaningful activities. When so engaged, persons with dementia do not exhibit problematic behaviors. This occurs as a by-product of engagement, for reduction of problematic behaviors is not the primary focus of activities. Activities staff are, in essence, at the front lines of dispensing psychosocial interventions in long-term care facilities. They are a mandated fixture of long-term care facilities, and as such represent an untapped source of allies for psychologists in these settings, as well as an important dissemination channel for psychosocial interventions (see Plautz & Camp, 2001).

The focus of this chapter is the dissemination of a cognitive intervention for persons with dementia initially researched and developed by psychologists—Montessori-Based Dementia Programming™. First, the intervention will be described. Research associated with this intervention, along with possible mechanisms responsible for effects produced by the intervention, will be reviewed. The dissemination of Montessori-Based Dementia Programming™ in long-term care environments will then be presented as a case study illustrating the process of adoption of psychosocial interventions for persons with dementia in the very real world of long-term care.

MANAGING PROBLEMATIC BEHAVIORS IN PERSONS WITH DEMENTIA

> "Meaning and meaningful activities, then, are our goals, our purpose, and our challenge. What we bring or do not bring is all these individuals we serve will or will not have." (Rancourt, 1991, p. 10)

If frailty brings a lessened prevalence of the types of high positive-affect experiences associated with a more vigorous early life, it may well be that one begins to savor smaller pleasures just as readily as the earlier ones. . . . It is possible that events of sufficiently positive impact occurring at a rate exceeding a particular individual's minimum requirement may reinforce the wish to live. . . . (Lawton, 1991, p. 20).

> "Their faces were expressionless, their eyes bewildered as if they had never seen anything before in their lives." (Montessori, 1966, p. 115)

As noted in this book, behavioral disturbances among persons with dementia are consistently reported to be among the most stressful aspects of providing care to these individuals. Research has shown that between 50 and 90% of persons with moderate to severe symptoms of dementia may display clinically significant behavioral problems at some point during the course of their illness (Davis, Buckwalter, & Burgio, 1997; Swearer, Drachman, O'Donnel, & Mitchell, 1990; Zimmer, Watson, & Treat, 1984). Behavioral disturbances among persons with dementia include agitation, verbally disruptive behavior, physically aggressive irritability, wandering, and mood lability (Burgio, 1996; Camp, Cohen-Mansfield, & Capezuti, 2002; Camp & Nasser, 2003; Cohen-Mansfield, 2001; Cole & Dastoor, 1987; Drevets & Rubin, 1989), as well as apathy (Mega, Cummings, Fiorello, & Gornbein, 1996). Of these, apathy, physical aggression, agitation and verbal disruption have been found to be the most common behavior problems (Holm et al., 1999; Mega et al., 1996). However, apathy may less likely be targeted for intervention as its expression does not result in as much stress or strain on caregivers as other behavioral disturbances.

Most services for persons with dementia have focused on the presumption that because they have a progressive disorder, maintaining adults with dementia at their current level of functioning and providing a nonchallenging, comfortable environment is the best approach. In long-term care, for example, this has led to the establishment of special care units (SCUs) in nursing homes. These usually focus on persons in early-stage dementia where ADLs and self-care are not problematic.

The idea is to create the atmosphere of a group or boarding home as much as possible. A similar philosophy is behind the rapid expansion of assisted living facilities for older adults. Under the best of circumstances, a medical model of care is replaced by a psychosocial support system.

An innovative approach to managing problems associated with dementia is based on the philosophy of reducing disability through reducing demands of the task environment. The emphasis is on recapturing lost or abandoned abilities, or restructuring activities so that they can be successfully accomplished in spite of deficits attributable to dementia. Interventions which could accommodate or compensate for losses in cognitive abilities should have a substantial impact on reducing problematic behaviors in persons with dementia (Camp et al., 2002). For example, researchers in cognition and aging report that normal older adults' most preserved abilities, on which interventions should be based, involve the use of environmental supports and cues found in familiar surroundings, along with the use of aspects of cognition that are relatively spared by aging, such as automatic skills and implicit memory (Hess & Pullen, 1996; Howard, 1996; Smith & Earles, 1996). Although this research has been conducted with normal populations, a similar approach and philosophy can be applied to persons with dementia (Camp, 1999b).

This approach can be viewed within The Disablement Model proposed by Verbrugge and Jette (1994). From this perspective, for persons with degenerative dementias, a reasonable approach to reducing their level of disability is to modify the demand level of the task environment. Verbrugge and Jette (1994) note: "Disability can be diminished swiftly and markedly if the physical or mental demands of a given task are reduced." (p. 9). This can be accomplished by presenting persons with dementia tasks not exceeding their capabilities and yet still providing challenge and stimulation.

The Disablement Model has similarities with Lawton's (1982; Lawton & Nahemow, 1973) Environmental Press Model. In that model, an individual's environment is also viewed as making demands (environmental press), and an individual's ability to meet those demands (person capacity) is viewed as his/her level of competence. When environmental press and competence are not in balance, negative affect and maladaptive behavior result. An important point in Lawton's model is that the gap between environmental demands and person capacity can be driven by stimulation levels. Within the Disablement Model, therefore, interventions in environments that provide appropriate levels of stimulation might prove effective in reducing Disability.

Williams, Wood, Moorleghen, and Chittuluru (1995) described a decision model to assist in the selection of interventions to reduce chemical and physical restraint of residents with dementia in long-term care settings. A major component of the model focuses on finding appropriate (i.e., optimal) levels of stimulation. They state, "In our experience, too little stimulation can result in disruptive, stimulus-seeking behavior, while too much stimulation yields behavioral excesses. . . . Optimal stimulation is considered a baseline condition for effective caregiving; . . . Prevention or reduction of catastrophic reactions and agitated behavior of whatever form, frequency or intensity, is the yardstick for success." (p. 23). This approach is quite similar to Lawton's call for a balance between environmental press and competence at the level of the individual.

Similarly, Cohen-Mansfield (2001; Camp et al., 2002) has written extensively about the need to determine the underlying cause of problematic behaviors associated with dementia. She ascribes such behaviors as generally associated with unmet basic human needs and states that the most common of these needs are for social and physical stimulation, which are often not available to persons with dementia because of a combination of the effects of dementia and the monotony of a typical nursing home environment.

Quality activities programming, therefore, is gaining increased attention as a much-needed intervention for persons with dementia. For many people, activities are synonymous with living (Fazio, Chavin, & Clair, 1999). Although activities are beneficial for everyone, they are especially important for those living with dementia (Fazio et al., 1999; Volicer, 1997; Volicer & Bloom-Charette, 1999; Zgola, 1987). A strong argument can be made that appropriate activities programming for persons with dementia is a necessary condition for their maintaining a good quality of life. Fazio et al. (1999) state, "Activities are a fundamental component of Alzheimer care. They provide structure, security, and a sense of belonging for the person with dementia. They allow individuals to feel useful and in control, while providing enjoyment. In addition, activities are often the vehicle or medium for interaction, maintaining relationships, and establishing connection with others." (p. 149) Volicer (1997; Volicer & Bloom-Charette, 1999) has suggested that the crucial intervention for persons with dementia is involvement in meaningful activities. Such involvement can reduce agitation, improve mood, and prevent apathy.

Finally, OBRA 1987 requires activities for persons in long-term care (the majority of whom have dementia) that provide opportunities for (a) promoting self-expression, personal responsibility, and choice (empowerment); (b) maintaining or improving physical, cognitive, emotional, and social functioning (maintenance); and (c) offering the appropriate level of stimulation to residents (support). The reason for including activities in OBRA '87's regulations is the belief that such programming is critical to insure that residents are able to meet their cognitive, physical, social, and emotional needs (Laurenhue, 2000). Meeting these needs would appear to be requisite to ensuring that persons with dementia in long-term care achieve a reasonably good quality of life.

Good activities programming, therefore, encompasses the concept of *enablement* (Dawson, Wells, & Kline, 1993). Enablement emphasizes a focus on abilities rather than on losses associated with dementia. An enabling approach focuses on "emphasizing the person's capacity to engage as fully as possible in day-to-day living" (Dawson et al., 1993, p. 2). Tappen (1997) notes that within an enabling framework for intervention, efforts are made to enhance any ability that remains, even if it is unused. If an ability is absent, compensatory interventions are used to circumvent disabilities related to the lost ability. Past research has shown that, through the use of external memory aids and prompts, persons with dementia display an increased level of engagement with their environment, spend less time sleeping, and use an enhanced level of communication with others (Bourgeois, 1990; Judge, Camp, & Orsulic-Jeras, 2000; Orsulic-Jeras, Judge, & Camp, 2000; Orsulic-Jeras, Schneider, & Camp, 2000; Orsulic-Jeras, Schneider, Camp, Nicholson, & Helbig, 2001). Persons with dementia have even shown the ability to serve as teachers/mentors for preschool children when provided appropriate training and support (Camp et al., 1997; Camp, Orsulic-Jeras, Lee, & Judge, 2005), and to successfully lead small group activities for persons with more advanced dementia (Camp & Skrajner, 2004; Camp, Skrajner, & Kelly, in press).

For example, a long-term care resident with dementia might not be able to recall names of objects. This leads to inability to name grandchildren when they visit. However, by having grandchildren wear name tags during visits, the resident can name grandchildren by utilizing an ability that still remains (ability to read and understand words). Thus, the resident can compensate for loss of word finding if the information sought is stored externally and can be accessed by an ability that is still present. Enabling the resident to name grandchildren can increase positive affect that can lead in turn to increased willingness to try other interventions. One such intervention might involve creating name tags for use when grandchildren visit. This, in turn, involves exercising fine and gross motor skills.

In summary, what are the characteristics of successful activities programming for dementia? Dreher (1997) suggests that activities developed for those with dementia should be purposeful and useful. Activities have also been found to be successful when they challenge a participant both physically and mentally, and are not made too easy or too difficult

(Bocksnick & Hall, 1994; Jackson, Dunne, Lanham, Heitkamp, & Dailey, 1993). The primary focus of activities programming should be on providing the individual with an opportunity to succeed and engage in meaningful interactions (Nissenboim & Vroman, 1998). It is critical that activities provide sufficient external structure to allow each participant to remain as engaged as possible, while at the same time, to benefit from social interaction and reminiscence. The key challenge for designing such programming, therefore, is to find a system for matching the individual who has dementia with an activity that is appropriate for that person at that time. For assistance in this, we have turned to developmental sequencing in general, and to the Montessori Method of education in particular.

DEVELOPMENTALLY BASED ACTIVITIES FOR PERSONS WITH DEMENTIA

> "To accommodate the regression of developmental stages, researchers are exploring interventions tailored to the neurodevelopmental level of the patient. This area holds promise for developing interventions that minimize patients' frustration." (Beck, 1998, p. S42)

Many researchers have claimed that during the progression of dementia, cognitive abilities may be lost in reverse developmental sequence; i.e., first-in/last-out—the reverse of the order in which they developed in childhood (Auer, Sclan, Yaffee, & Reisberg, 1994; Beck, 1998; Bickel, 1996; Biringer & Anderson, 1992; Camp et al., 1993; Lipinska, Bäckman, & Herlitz, 1992; Nolen, 1988; Reisberg, 1985, 1986; Reisberg et al., 2002; Sclan, Foster, Reisberg, Franssen, & Welkowitz, 1990; Thornbury, 1992). A common term for this concept is "retrogenesis" (c.f., Reisberg, et al., 2002). A somewhat parallel conceptualization has been forwarded by Emery (2003), known as "retrophylogenesis"—the idea that abilities in dementia are lost in reverse evolutionary sequence; i.e., in the reverse of the sequence in which they were acquired by our species over evolutionary time.

If this concept represents at least a useful heuristic, developmental sequencing of cognitive abilities may be a useful guide and basis for creating interventions and programming for persons with Alzheimer's disease and related dementias that will provide optimal levels of stimulation (Camp et al., 1993; Vance, Camp, Kabacoff, & Greenwalt, 1996). Also, "developmentally based" sequencing of activities represents the use of rehabilitation principles—e.g., breaking down tasks into their simplest components, then slowly increasing the complexity of a task; moving from concrete to abstract representations of constructs; extensive use of external cueing, etc. Therefore, such an approach incorporates rehabilitative principles for creating and implementing activities for persons with dementia, regardless of the ultimate veracity of first-in, last-out conceptualizations (Camp, 1999a,b, 2001, 2004; Camp & Mattern, 1999; Plautz & Camp, 2001). But the question then becomes one of selecting an approach on which to base a broad array of activity-based interventions that would be effective across a variety of individuals and levels of dementia.

We decided to begin with an approach widely and effectively used to teach children cognitive, motor, sensory, and social skills, in addition to providing them with meaningful social roles—the Montessori method developed by Maria Montessori. It is worth noting that this method was initially developed for children who were impoverished, understimulated, and destroying property. Their disruptive behaviors vanished when they were engaged in meaningful activity (Montessori, 1966).

MONTESSORI-BASED DEMENTIA PROGRAMMING™

> "Identifying the person with dementia's cognitive and physical strengths enables caregivers to incorporate these abilities within all aspects of daily life activity." (Hellen, 1998, p. 3)

Montessori-Based Dementia Programming™ is designed to reduce environmental demand, capitalize on preserved abilities, modify the social and physical environment, and provide external (social, cognitive, and physical) supports to enable older adults to successfully take part in and complete meaningful activities that they could not perform without the intervention. In other words, Montessori-based activities make use of the practices of enablement by both utilizing existing abilities and finding methods of circumventing impaired abilities to enable disability to be decreased. This, in turn, should lead to improvement in quality of life.

Similarly, Wilson (1997) notes that cognitive rehabilitation refers primarily to a process by which professionals work together with a client to reduce disability and optimize performance by alleviating, remediating, or circumventing deficits. She states "As far as cognitive rehabilitation is concerned, we should be attempting to remediate disability . . ." (p. 490). Thus, interventions designed within the *enablement approach* also correspond well to principles of cognitive rehabilitation. We have argued for the use of such a cognitive rehabilitation perspective when designing interventions for dementia (Camp, 2001, 2004; Camp & Mattern, 1999; Plautz & Camp, 2001; Sterns & Camp, 1998). Research examining effects produced by Montessori-Based Dementia Programming™ will be described next.

USE OF MONTESSORI-BASED ACTIVITIES FOR PERSONS WITH DEMENTIA

The Montessori teaching method is used to train children in the areas of practical life (activities of daily living), sensorial experiences, language, math, engaging and maintaining the environment, science, and social skills. Developmentally and programmatically based, Montessori techniques seem well suited for persons with dementia. Each lesson is first presented at its simplest level and each subsequent lesson, increasing in complexity, is a variation of previously mastered skills or concepts. For example, children learn first to distinguish a rough versus a smooth surface by touch, and then they learn to discriminate between different levels of roughness by manipulating various grades of sandpaper. Later, children are shown a globe on which the continents are represented by sandpaper and the oceans by a smooth blue surface. This is their introduction to land and water as geologic forms, and to geography. Learning to distinguish and name the continents by their shape and location will follow.

Materials are taken from the everyday environment and are designed not to be "toys" but tools to prepare the person for independent living. Persons with dementia need structure and order in their environment and activities; changes in routine or physical surroundings may be upsetting (Vance et al., 1996). Maria Montessori said the same of her young students, and thus all activities involve a structure and order that both comfort and allow attention to be focused. Activities involve immediate feedback, high probability of success, and repetition. Tasks are broken down into steps that can be mastered and then sequenced, an approach familiar to occupational therapists. Montessori-based programming makes use of a number of rehabilitation principles and techniques, including: task breakdown, guided repetition, task progressions from simple to complex and abstract to concrete, etc. Such programming also takes advantage of principles for dementia interventions including: extensive use of external cues, reliance on procedural/nondeclarative/implicit memory rather than declarative/explicit memory, etc. Persons with dementia demonstrate the ability to learn through procedural or nondeclarative memory (Squire, 1992, 1994), a phenomenon remarkably similar to what Montessori described as "unconscious learning" in children (Bäckman, 1992; Camp et al., 1993; Vance et al., 1996). When children are engaged and their attention focused during meaningful activities, Montessori referred to the process as "normalization." The term is especially appropriate when applied to this process involving persons with dementia.

At the Menorah Park Center for Senior Living, where the Myers Research Institute is housed, we have been working with a variety of Montessori-based activities for persons with dementia. These include both individual and group activities, which have been implemented in nursing home settings as well as in assisted living and adult day health care (Camp, 1999a,b, 2004; Camp & Mattern, 1999; Camp & Nasser, 2003; Camp et al., 2005; Camp et al., 1997; Judge et al., 2000; Malone, Skrajner, & Camp, 2004; Orsulic-Jeras, Judge, et al., 2000; Orsulic-Jeras, Schneider, et al., 2000; Rose, Camp, Skrajner, & Gorzelle, 2003; Schneider, Diggs, Orsulic, & Camp, 1999; Schneider & Camp, 2002).

In a 3-year study funded by the Alzheimer's Association, we observed clients from adult day care, and residents in long-term care from a dementia SCU and an advanced dementia unit, in Montessori-based individual and group activities as well as in regularly scheduled activities programming. Results from all three sites demonstrated significantly more positive engagement and virtually no nonengagement on the part of participants in Montessori-based programming compared to during regularly scheduled activities programming (Judge et al., 2000; Orsulic-Jeras, Judge, et al., 2000; Orsulic-Jeras, Schneider, et al., 2000). In addition, Montessori-based activities produced significantly more positive affect than regular programming activities.

At the end of the research project, we successfully trained adult day care staff, activity staff on our long-term care units, and nursing assistants on those units to conduct Montessori-based individual and group programming with their respective clients and residents (Schneider et al., 1999; Orsulic-Jeras et al., 2001). In addition, educational modules were developed to train all activities staff on the use of Montessori-Based Dementia Programming™ at Menorah Park. We are currently modifying these training modules in a project focusing on training home health workers to implement Montessori-based activities as part of their job routine when delivering services to persons with dementia. We have also developed training modules to enable activities staff at other facilities to implement Montessori-Based Dementia Programming™, and are continually refining our methods. An ongoing research project funded by the National Institute of Mental Health (R21 MH063395, Camp, PI) has as its focus the development of training materials and procedures to allow staff in long-term care, assisted living, and adult day health care facilities to implement such programming (Malone et al., 2004).

The director of activities at Menorah Park Center for Senior Living believes that Montessori-based programming has given her staff a wider variety of options when planning programming. In addition to the options Montessori methods have given to the staff, she states that the benefits for the residents have been even more remarkable. Montessori-based programming seems to have given the residents an opportunity to "maintain their current levels of physical, cognitive, and social functioning." In support of Montessori-based programming, she states, "Using

Montessori principles is a wonderful way to enhance the programming we already have."

In an ongoing demonstration project at a for-profit skilled nursing facility of HCR ManorCare, Inc., in rural Bellefountaine, Ohio, a full-day program of Montessori-based activities has been implemented. The executive director of the facility and her director of activities were trained in the application of Montessori-Based Dementia Programming™ by staff of the Myers Research Institute. Next, the executive director chose six of her residents exhibiting a high frequency of problematic behaviors (e.g., going into other residents' rooms and dragging their bedspreads and sheets into the hall), and created an 8-hr (10:00 am to 6 pm) program specifically for these persons.

The program consists of 30-min segments of individualized and small group activities. Meals, hydration (e.g., "tea time"), etc. are embedded within the program. It is administered by a nurse assistant who is supervised by the director of activities. After one year of such programming, these residents are now "model citizens," who have formed their own community (an outcome similar to what Montessori achieved with her impoverished children—the "normalization" process mentioned earlier). After their program ends they eat dinner together and then sit together on sofas outside of the nurses station (their "front porch time"). Problematic behaviors have been eliminated, and these residents are able to take part in restorative nursing activities embedded within the program. The administrator has since established a parallel program for residents in wheelchairs with limited mobility, and we are working with the director and executives within HCR ManorCare's corporate headquarters to develop this approach as a template for restorative nursing programs that has the potential to be implemented on a large scale. We are also refining a set of Montessori-based activities to be used as an assessment tool to create better plans of care and for the design of restorative nursing interventions for long-term care residents with dementia (Camp, Koss, & Judge, 1999; Grant R01 AG021508, National Institute on Aging; Camp, PI). This also will help facilitate usage and dissemination of Montessori-based programming within the development of restorative nursing programs for residents with dementia.

DISSEMINATION OF MONTESSORI-BASED DEMENTIA PROGRAMMING™

The program implemented at Bellefountaine is but one example of a cascade of events resulting from a deliberate effort on the part of HCR ManorCare, Inc. and the Myers Research Institute to disseminate Montessori-Based

Dementia Programming™ throughout their long-term care facilities on a national scale. This process was inspired, in part, by a project funded jointly by HCR ManorCare, Inc., HCR ManorCare Foundation, and the Retirement Research Foundation (Camp, PI). This project involved staff of the Myers Research Institute developing a "train-the-trainer" program such that activities staff of HCR ManorCare, Inc. could become agents of disseminating Montessori-Based Dementia Programming™ within facilities affiliated with the corporation.

In the past, we have discussed the acquisition of new skills for psychologists that are necessary to enable transitions from efficacy to effectiveness to diffusion in research focusing on interventions for persons with dementia (Camp, 2001). Our current efforts focus heavily on the process of dissemination of innovation in health care systems, using a model outlined by Berwick (2003). Previously, we have discussed components of that model involving three basic clusters of influence that relate to the rate of spread of change—perception of the innovation; characteristics of the people who adopt the innovation (or fail to do so); and contextual factors. This discussion used a cognitive intervention for persons with dementia (spaced retrieval) we have researched heavily at the Myers Research Institute to illustrate these clusters (Camp, in press).

In this chapter, we will discuss seven rules put forward by Berwick (2003) for dissemination of innovations within the context of health care delivery systems. We will illustrate these rules with examples from our efforts to disseminate Montessori-Based Dementia Programming™. These seven rules are as follows.

Find Sound Innovations

Care communities must find psychosocial interventions that they wish to apply. How will they find interventions developed by psychologists for implementation in long-term care settings? The answer is that they will not be combing scientific journals. This is not to say that research is not valued, or that care providers are not seeking evidence-based practice. However, their sources of information are usually trade journals, advice from colleagues, and/or viewing program abstracts and attending conferences where such interventions may be discovered. This also means that organizations delivering care to older adults with dementia must have and support persons actively seeking such innovations. In our case, staff from the Myers Research Institute presented results of our research on Montessori-Based Dementia Programming™ at an education conference on caregiving sponsored by the national Alzheimer's Association. Administrative staff from HCR ManorCare, Inc. were in attendance, and initial contact was made between the two agencies.

Find and Support Innovators

In addition to sending staff to conferences, HCR ManorCare, Inc., was interested in discovering and implementing innovative programming. This made sense on many levels. Given that all providers of long-term care claim to be providing a good quality of care, to stay competitive in the market place means being able to stay at the cutting edge of dementia care practices. Companies that understand this concept—high-quality care must be provided both for its own sake and because it is critical for a company's long-term survival—support innovators. As Berwick (2003) noted, novel ways to solve chronic problems tend to come from outside the current system. As a result, it is crucial to support the process of finding and testing innovations. After initial contact between our two agencies, staff from the Myers Research Institute were invited to give a presentation of our research at corporate headquarters. This led to our receiving initial funding from the corporation to examine the effects of Montessori-Based Dementia Programming™ within some of the company's facilities, and to examine effects produced by a train-the-trainer program for disseminating Montessori-Based Dementia Programming™ on a small scale.

Invest in Early Adopters

It is important to find individuals who have the curiosity and courage to test changes, as well as the pragmatic intelligence to recognize what is reasonable and what constitutes successful adoption. These are the translators who take ideas from innovators (generally originating from outside care systems, as described earlier) and test these ideas within local facilities or systems. By encouraging our meeting and interacting with the executive director of the Bellefountaine facility and her staff, HCR ManorCare, Inc. was directly supporting this step in innovation diffusion. Staff from the Myers Research Institute, in turn, emphasized the importance of this pilot program to corporate administrators and encouraged extending collaborations between the Institute and staff of this facility.

Make Early Adopter Activity Observable

As Berwick succinctly states, "Spread requires social interaction." (2003, p. 1974). Memoranda or policy statements do not produce lasting change.

Individuals within an organization who are not early adopters are interested in implementing improvements, but only if they are confident that innovations been tried and proven useful by persons they know and trust. The administrator at HCR ManorCare, Inc. who had originally invited a presentation of Montessori-Based Dementia Programming™ at corporate headquarters instituted a series of conference calls among facility staff who first attempted implementation of this innovation. These chats among colleagues allowed for frank discussion of barriers to implementation, sharing of success stories, and brainstorming the creation of new adaptations of the intervention. To further facilitate this process, staff of the Myers Research Institute created corporate training modules to enable staff from within the company to train their colleagues in the implementation of Montessori-Based Dementia Programming™. Now known as "Mature Montessori" and "Engagement Therapy" within this system, the innovation has since been implemented on a national scale.

Trust and Enable Reinvention

This maxim may be especially hard for psychologists to embrace. The concept of reinvention involves acknowledging that innovations will be adapted to fit the perceived needs of specific locations. Components of interventions that are deemed superfluous will be cast away by those who adopt them. In addition, innovations will be modified by persons who were not involved in their creation. To psychologists trained to implement manualized treatment regimens in all their pristine complexity, and to insure that only psychologists or those closely supervised by them apply interventions, this maxim may seem heretical. So be it. For interventions in long-term care to have widespread dissemination, reinvention must be not only tolerated but also embraced and encouraged.

To illustrate, activities therapists trained by staff of the Myers Research Institute found that they needed to supply activities to residents with dementia on an individual basis on second and third shifts. They developed "Activity Stations," where the materials were placed in conjunction with printed instructions for completing activities. A station, for example, might have a stack of facility newsletters that would have to be folded and placed into envelops. Residents learned to go to the Activity Stations when they were "looking for something to do." Activities therapists would then replace materials and instructions at the Activity Stations on a regular basis. Although the creation of such stations was not a part of their initial training, this example of reinvention worked so well that instructions for their creation are now part of the training provided by Institute staff.

Create Slack for Change

As Berwick states, "Leaders who want innovation to spread must make sure that they have invested people's time and energy in it." (2003, p. 1974). There must be a commitment of time and money to support the process of discovering innovations, testing them, reinventing them, and disseminating them. This may be especially challenging in long-term care facilities where management strategies are reactive rather proactive, and where declining revenues from Medicaid and other revenue sources are putting increasing pressure on health care costs. But a long-term survival strategy dictates that a continuing process of innovation adoption and reinvention is critical. We continue to work with HCR ManorCare staff and administrators to test and implement variations on our initial research with Montessori-Based Dementia Programming™. Our work with the Bellefountaine facility is an example of this approach. It has been our good fortune to work with a company that views dissemination of innovation as good business practice.

Lead by Example

We must be prepared to put our ideas into practice. In this case, we began this process by first implementing Montessori-Based Dementia Programming™ within our own facility—Menorah Park Center for Senior Living. Over time, our activities therapists have incorporated this approach into their standard job routines. They also train activities staff from other facilities, appear on radio, TV, and newspaper stories about the innovation, and have made the intervention part of our corporate culture. During initial negotiations with HCR ManorCare, Inc., the ability of our activities staff to discuss and support implementation of Montessori-Based Dementia Programming™ from a practitioner's point of view made a powerful statement to their colleagues from other facilities, and to their supervisors, in turn.

Although the speed of dissemination of innovation can appear to be glacial at times, and the path occasionally nonlinear, we are encouraged by what has been accomplished so far. In the year 2004, Menorah Park Center for Senior Living was presented an "Innovation of the Year" award by the American Association of Homes and Services for the Aging for its "Montessori-Based Programming for Long-Term Care Residents." In that same year, the American Society on Aging presented a

"Health Care and Aging Award" jointly to the Myers Research Institute of Menorah Park Center for Senior Living and to HCR ManorCare, Inc., for our collaboration on "Montessori-Based Dementia Programming in Long-Term Care Residents with Dementia."

> A social change of this type cannot come from the ideas or energies of individual reformers but from a slow and steady emergence of a new world in the midst of the old. (Montessori, 1966, p. 207)

ACKNOWLEDGMENTS

Preparation of this manuscript was supported by grant R01 AG021508-01A1 from the National Institute on Aging and by grant R21 MH063395-01A2 from the National Institute of Mental Health, C. Camp, PI. The author would like to express his thanks and appreciation to the staff of the Myers Research Institute of Menorah Park Center for Senior Living for their input and editorial comments. Thanks also to Mr Charles Batcher of HCR ManorCare, Inc., for his support of the dissemination process and for his friendship.

REFERENCES

Auer, S. R., Sclan, S. G., Yaffee, R. A., & Reisberg, B. (1994). The neglected half of Alzheimer's disease: Cognitive and functional concomitants of severe dementia. *Journal of the American Geriatrics Society, 42*, 1266–1272.

Bäckman, L. (1992). Memory training and memory improvement in Alzheimer's disease: Rules and exceptions. *Acta Neurologica Scandinavica, 84*, 84–89.

Beck, C. K. (1998). Psychosocial and behavioral interventions for Alzheimer's disease patients and their families. *American Journal of Geriatric Psychiatry, 6*(2, Suppl 1), S41–S48.

Berwick, D. M. (2003). Disseminating innovations in health care. *Journal of the American Medical Association, 289*(15), 1969–1975.

Bickel, H. (1996). The Hierarchic dementia scale: Usage. *International Psychogeriatrics, 8*, 213–224.

Biringer, F., & Anderson, J. R. (1992). Self-recognition in Alzheimer's disease: A mirror and video study. *Journal of Gerontology, 49*, 383–388.

Bocksnick, J. G., & Hall, B. L. (1994). Recreation activity programming for the institutionalized older adult. *Activities, Adaptation, & Aging, 19*(1), 1–25.

Bourgeois, M. (1990). Enhancing conversation skills in Alzheimer's disease using a prosthetic memory aid. *Journal of Applied Behavior Analysis, 23*, 29–42.

Burgio, L. D. (1996). Interventions for the behavioral complications of Alzheimer's disease: Behavioral approaches. *International Psychogeriatrics, 8*, 45–52.

Camp, C. J. (Ed.). (1999a). *Montessori-based activities for persons with dementia* (Vol. 1). Beachwood, OH: Menorah Park Center for Senior Living.

Camp, C. J. (1999b). Memory interventions for normal and pathological older adults. In R. Schulz, M. P. Lawton, & G. Maddox, (Eds.), *Annual review of gerontology and geriatrics* (Vol. 18, pp. 155–189). New York: Springer.

Camp, C. J. (2001). From efficacy to effectiveness to diffusion: Making the transitions in dementia intervention research. *Neuropsychological Rehabilitation, 11*, 495–517.

Camp, C. J. (2004). Valoración cognitive e intervención en el deterioro cognitivo grave: Apuntes de Maria Montessori. *Geriatría Y Gerontología, 39*, 10–14.

Camp, C. J., Cohen-Mansfield, J., & Capezuti, E. A. (2002). Use of nonpharmacologic interventions among nursing home residents with dementia. *Psychiatric Services, 53*, 1397–1401.

Camp, C. J., Foss, J. W., Stevens, A. B., Reichard, C. C., McKitrick, L. A., & O'Hanlon, A. M. (1993). Memory training in normal and demented populations: The E-I-E-I-O model. *Experimental Aging Research, 19*, 277–290.

Camp, C. J., Judge, K. S., Bye, C. A., Fox, K. M., Bowden, J., Bell, M., Valencic, K., & Mattern, J. M. (1997). An intergenerational program for persons with dementia using Montessori methods. *Gerontologist, 37*, 688–692.

Camp, C. J., Koss, E., & Judge, K. S. (1999). Cognitive assessment in late stage dementia. In P. A. Lichtenberg (Ed.), *Handbook of clinical gerontology assessment* (pp. 442–467). New York: John Wiley & Sons.

Camp, C. J., & Mattern, J. M. (1999). Innovations in managing Alzheimer's disease. In D. E. Biegel, & A. Blum (Eds.), *Innovations in practice and service delivery across the lifespan* (pp. 276–294). New York: Oxford University Press.

Camp, C. J., & Nasser, E. H. (2003). Nonpharmacological aspects of agitation and behavioral disorders in dementia: Assessment, intervention, and challenges to providing care. In P. A. Lichtenberg, D. L. Murman, & A. M. Mellow (Eds.), *Handbook of dementia: Psychological, neurological, and psychiatric perspectives* (pp. 359–401). New York: John Wiley & Sons.

Camp, C. J., Orsulic-Jeras, S., Lee, M. M., & Judge, K. S. (2005). Effects of a Montessori-based intergenerational program on engagement and affect for adult day health care clients with dementia. In M. L. Wykle, P. J. Whitehouse, & D. L. Morris (Eds.), *Successful aging through the life span: Intergenerational issues in health* (pp. 159–176) New York: Springer.

Camp, C. J., & Skrajner, M. J. (2004). Resident-assisted Montessori programming (RAMP): Training persons with dementia to serve as group activity leaders. *Gerontologist, 44*, 426–431.

Camp, C. J., Skrajner, M. J., & Kelly, M. (in press). Early stage dementia client as group leader. *Clinical Gerontologist.*

Cohen-Mansfield, J. (2001). Nonpharamcologic interventions for inappropriate behaviors in dementia: A review, summary, and critique. *American Journal of Geriatric Psychiatry, 9*, 361–381.

Cole, M. G., & Dastoor, D. P. (1987). A new hierarchic approach to the measurement of dementia. *Psychosomatics, 28*, 298–304.

Davis, L. L., Buckwalter, K., & Burgio, L. D. (1997). Measuring problem behaviors in dementia: Developing a methodological agenda. *Advances in Nursing Science, 20*, 40–55.

Dawson, P., Wells, D. L., & Kline, K. (1993). *Enhancing the abilities of persons with Alzheimer's and related dementias.* New York: Springer.

Dreher, B. (1997). Montessori and Alzheimer's: A partnership that works. *American Journal of Alzheimer's Disease, 12*, 138–140.

Drevets, W. C., & Rubin, E. H. (1989). Psychotic symptoms and the longitudinal course of senile dementia of the Alzheimer type. *Biological Psychiatry, 25*, 39–48.

Emery, V. O. B. (2003). "Retrophylogenesis" of memory in dementia of the Alzheimer's type: A new evolutionary memory framework. In V. O. B. Emery, & T. E. Oxman (Eds.), *Dementia: Presentations, differential diagnosis, and nosology* (2nd ed., pp. 177–236). Baltimore, MD: The Johns Hopkins University Press.

Fazio, S., Chavin, M., & Clair, A. A. (1999). Activity based Alzheimer care: A national training program. *American Journal of Alzheimer's Disease, 14*(3), 149–156.

Hellen, C. R. (1998). *Alzheimer's disease: Activity-focused care.* Boston: Butterworth-Heinemann.

Hess, T. M., & Pullen, S. M. (1996). Memory in context. In F. Blanchard-Fields, & T. M. Hess (Eds.), *Perspectives on cognitive change in adulthood and aging* (pp. 387–427). New York: McGraw-Hill.

Holm, A., Michel, M., Stern, G. A., Hung, T., Klein, T., Flaherty, L., Michel, S., & Maletta, G. (1999). The outcomes of an inpatient treatment program for geriatric patients with dementia and dysfunctional behaviors. *Gerontologist, 39*, 668–676.

Howard, D. V. (1996). The aging of implicit and explicit memory. In F. Blanchard-Fields, & T. M. Hess (Eds.), *Perspectives on cognitive change in adulthood and aging* (pp. 221–254). New York: McGraw-Hill.

Jackson, L. T., Dunne, J., Lanham, G., Heitkamp, K., Dailey, S. (1993). Age-appropriate activities: Establishing guidelines. *Activities, Adaptation, & Aging, 17*(4), 1–9.

Judge, K. S., Camp, C. J., & Orsulic-Jeras, S. (2000). Use of Montessori-based activities for clients with dementia in adult day health care: Effects on engagement. *American Journal of Alzheimer's Disease, 15*, 42–46.

Laurenhue, K. (2000). Broadening horizons: Activities with people with dementia. *Alzheimer's Care Quarterly, 1*(2), 38–45.

Lawton, M. P. (1982). Competence, environmental press, and the adaptation of old people. In M. P. Lawton, & T. O. Byerts (Eds.), *Aging and the environment: Theoretical approaches* (pp. 33–59). New York: Springer.

Lawton, M. P. (1991). A multidimensional view of quality of life in frail elders. In J. E. Birren, J. E. Lubben, J. C. Rowe, & D. E. Deutchman (Eds.), *The concept and measurement of quality of life in the frail elderly*. New York: Academic Press.

Lawton, M. P., & Nahemow, L. (1973). Ecology and the aging process. In C. Eisdorfer, & M. P. Lawton (Eds.), *The psychology of adult development and aging*. Washington, DC: American Psychological Association.

Lipinska, B., Bäckman, L., & Herlitz, A. (1992). When Greta Garbo is easier to remember than Stefan Edberg: Influences of prior knowledge on recent memory in Alzheimer's disease. *Psychology and Aging, 2*, 214–220.

Malone, M., Skrajner, M., & Camp, C. (2004, November). *Maximizing the abilities of the dementia population using Montessori-Based Dementia Programming*. Poster session presented at the 57th annual scientific meeting of the Gerontological Society of America, Washington, DC.

Mega, M. S., Cummings, J. L., Fiorello, T., & Gornbein, J. (1996). The spectrum of behavioral changes in Alzheimer's disease. *Neurology, 46*, 130–135.

Montessori, M. (1966). *The secret of childhood*. New York: Ballantine Books.

Nissenboim, S., & Vroman, C. (1998). *The positive interactions program of activities for people with Alzheimer's disease*. Baltimore, MD: Health Professionals Press.

Nolen, N. R. (1988). Functional skill regression in late-stage dementias. *American Journal of Occupational Therapy, 42*, 666–669.

Orsulic-Jeras, S., Judge, K. S., & Camp, C. J. (2000). Montessori-based activities for long-term care residents with advanced dementia: Effects on engagement and affect. *Gerontologist, 40*, 107–111.

Orsulic-Jeras, S., Schneider, N. M., & Camp, C. J. (2000). Montessori-based activities for long-term care residents with dementia: Outcomes and implications for geriatric rehabilitation. *Topics in Geriatric Rehabilitation, 16*, 78–91.

Orsulic-Jeras, S., Schneider, N. M., Camp, C. J., Nicholson, P., & Helbig, M. (2001). Montessori-based dementia activities in long-term care: Training and implementation. *Activities, Adaptation, and Aging, 25*, 107–120.

Plautz, R. E., & Camp, C. J. (2001). Activities as agents for intervention and rehabilitation in long-term care. In B. R. Bonder, & M. B. Wagner (Eds.), *Functional performance in older adults* (2nd ed., pp. 405–425). Philadelphia: F. A. Davis.

Rancourt, A. M. (1991). Programming quality services for older adults in long-term care facilities. *Activities, Adaptation, & Aging, 15*, 1–11.

Reisberg, B. (1985). Assessment tool for Alzheimer's type dementia. *Hospital and Community Psychiatry, 6*, 593–595.

Reisberg, B. (1986). Dementia: A systematic approach to identifying reversible cues. *Geriatrics, 4*, 30–46.

Reisberg, B., Franssen, E. H., Souren, L. E., Auer, S. R., Akram, I., & Kenowsky S. (2002). Evidence and mechanisms of retrogenesis in Alzheimer's and other dementias: Management and treatment import. *American Journal of Alzheimer's Disease and Other Dementias, 17*(4), 169–174.

Rose, M. S., Camp, C. J., Skrajner, M. J., & Gorzelle, G. J. (2003). Enhancing the quality of nursing home visits with Montessori-based activities. *Activities Directors' Quarterly, 3*, 4–10.

Schneider, N. M., & Camp, C. J. (2002). Use of Montessori-based activities by visitors of nursing home residents with dementia. *Clinical Gerontologist, 26*, 71–84.

Schneider, N. M., Diggs, S., Orsulic, S., & Camp, C. J. (1999). N.A.s teaching Montessori activities. *Journal of Nurse Assistants, 6*(2), 13–15.

Sclan, S. G., Foster, J. R., Reisberg, B., Franssen, E., & Welkowitz, J. (1990). Application of Piagetian measures of cognition in severe Alzheimer's disease. *Psychiatric Journal of the University of Ottawa, 15*(4), 221–226.

Smith, A. D., & Earles, J. L. K. (1996). Memory changes in normal aging. In F. Blanchard-Fields, & T. M. Hess (Eds.), *Perspectives on cognitive changes in adulthood and aging* (pp. 192–220). New York: McGraw-Hill.

Squire, L. R. (1992). Memory and the hippocampus: A synthesis from findings with rats, monkeys, and humans. *Psychological Review, 99*, 195–231.

Squire, L. R. (1994). Declarative and nondeclarative memory: Multiple brain systems supporting learning and memory. In D. L. Schacter, & E. Tulving (Eds.), *Memory systems* (pp. 203–232). Cambridge, MA: MIT Press.

Sterns, H. L., & Camp, C. J. (1998). Applied gerontology. *Applied Psychology: An International Review, 47*, 175–198.

Swearer, J. M., Drachman, D. A., O'Donell, B. F., Mitchell, A. L. (1990). Troublesome and disruptive behaviors in dementia: Relationship to diagnosis and disease severity. *Journal of the American Geriatrics Society, 36*, 784–790.

Tappen, R. M. (1997). *Interventions for Alzhiemer's disease*. Baltimore: Health Professions Press.

Thornbury, J. M. (1992). Cognitive performance on Piagetian tasks by Alzheimer's disease patients. *Research on Nursing and Health, 15*, 11–18.

Vance, D., Camp, C. J., Kabacoff, M., & Greenwalt, L. (1996). Montessori methods: Innovative interventions for adults with Alzheimer's disease. *Montessori Life, 8*, 10–12.

Verbrugge, L. M., & Jette, A. M. (1994). The disablement process. *Social Science and Medicine, 38*, 1–14.

Volicer, L. (1997). Goals of care in advanced dementia: Comfort, dignity, and psychological well-being. *American Journal of Alzheimer's Disease, 12*, 196–197.

Volicer, L., & Bloom-Charette, L. (1999). *Enhancing the quality of life in advanced dementia*. Boston: University School of Medicine.

Williams, D. P., Wood, E. C., Moorleghen, F., & Chittuluru, V. C. (1995). A decision model for guiding the management of disruptive behaviors in demented residents of institutional settings. *American Journal of Alzheimer's Disease, 10*, 22–29.

Wilson, B. A. (1997). Cognitive rehabilitation: How it is and how it might be. *Journal of the International Neuropsychological Society, 3*, 487–496.

Zgola, J. (1987). *Doing things: A guide to programming activities for persons with Alzheimer's disease and related disorders*. Baltimore, MD: Johns Hopkins University Press.

Zimmer, J. G., Watson, N., & Treat, A. (1984). Behavioral problems among patients in skilled nursing facilities. *American Journal of Public Health, 74*, 1118–11121.

Index

Page numbers followed by f or t indicate figures and tables, respectively.